Encyclopedia of Parkinson's Disease: Rehabilitation

Volume IV

Encyclopedia of Parkinson's Disease: Rehabilitation Volume IV

Edited by **Kate White**

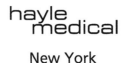

New York

Published by Hayle Medical,
30 West, 37th Street, Suite 612,
New York, NY 10018, USA
www.haylemedical.com

Encyclopedia of Parkinson's Disease: Rehabilitation
Volume IV
Edited by Kate White

© 2015 Hayle Medical

International Standard Book Number: 978-1-63241-192-1 (Hardback)

Contents

Preface

This book is a detailed, applicable and step-by-step medium helping students and researchers to understand Parkinson's disease. It provides the latest information pertaining to topics associated with this disease, including etiology, new methodologies to examine symptoms, multidisciplinary rehabilitation and invasive techniques to analyze Parkinson's disease. Researchers have currently started to focus on the non-motor symptoms of this disease, which are poorly identified and insufficiently treated by clinicians and have a considerable effect on the quality of life of the patient and mortality and include autonomic, sensory and gastrointestinal symptoms, and cognitive impairments. Detailed discussion of the use of imaging tools to analyze disease mechanisms is also given, with stress on the abnormal network organization in Parkinsonism. Novel approaches of early diagnostics, treatments and training programs have greatly enhanced the lives of people suffering from this disease in the latest years, significantly decreasing symptoms and delayed disability. This comprehensive book consists of information contributed by renowned veteran scientists from across the globe.

This book is a comprehensive compilation of works of different researchers from varied parts of the world. It includes valuable experiences of the researchers with the sole objective of providing the readers (learners) with a proper knowledge of the concerned field. This book will be beneficial in evoking inspiration and enhancing the knowledge of the interested readers.

In the end, I would like to extend my heartiest thanks to the authors who worked with great determination on their chapters. I also appreciate the publisher's support in the course of the book. I would also like to deeply acknowledge my family who stood by me as a source of inspiration during the project.

Editor

Part 1

Multidisciplinary Cognitive Rehabilitation in Parkinson's Disease

An Investigation into the Impact of Parkinson's Disease upon Decision Making Ability and Driving Performance

Jessica Davies[1], Hoe Lee[1] and Torbjorn Falkmer[1,2,3,4]
[1]School of Occupational Therapy and Social Work, Curtin Health Innovation Research Institute, Curtin University,
[2]School of Health Sciences, Jönköping University, Jönköping,
[3]Department of Rehabilitation Medicine, IKE, Faculty of Health Sciences Linköping University,
[4]School of Occupational Therapy, La Trobe University, Melbourne, VIC,
[2,3]Sweden
[1,4]Australia

1. Introduction

PD is a severe neurodegenerative disease that can impair functional driving performance and increase the risk of accidents and fatalities on Australian roads (Austroads, 2000). In particular, cognitive symptoms of PD can have a substantial influence on driving performance due to the complicated and demanding nature of the task (Uitti, 2009). PD can affect the neural pathways that facilitate essential cognitive processes; such as attention, information processing speed, memory and risk assessment. These processes are all integral to the decision making process (Cools, et at., 2001). Previous research has highlighted that the ability to make accurate and timely decisions is essential for safe driving performance. However, this has not yet been researched in relation to people with PD (Devos, et al., 2007).

1.1 Prevalence and aetiology of Parkinson's disease

PD is the second most common neurological disease in Australia; causing impairments in motor control, cognitive functioning and sensation (Access Economics, 2010). PD usually affects people over the age of 50 years. However, the rate of disease progression and severity of symptoms can vary greatly between individuals (Australian Bureau of Statistics, 2004). Australia's aging population is expected to increase the prevalence rate of PD by 40% by 2033 (refer to Figure 1) (Access Economics, 2010).

Recent improvements in the medical and psychosocial treatment of PD has dramatically increased life expectancy, as people with PD now live approximately 12 to 20 years past diagnosis (Access Economics, 2010). PD is currently the sixth highest cause of disease-related driving cessation in Australia (Access Economics, 2010). People with PD generally stop driving at the age of 68; eight years earlier than the general population (Access Economics, 2010). Research into the impact of symptoms upon functional ability will enable

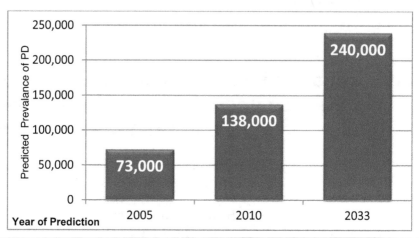

Adapted from: Access Economics, 2010

Fig. 1. Predicted prevalence of Parkinson's disease in Australia 2005-2033

the development of better screening tools and allow health professionals to differentiate between capable and unsafe drivers (Adler, et al., 2000). This may allow capable drivers with PD to retain their licences and current quality of life through active participation in occupations (Innes, et al., 2009). As the number of drivers with PD will rapidly increase due to the aging population, such an initiative will assist in improving road safety (Cordell, et al., 2008).

PD is caused by the progressive cellular death of dopaminergic neurons, predominantly in the basal ganglia in the brain (Arias-Carrión & Pöppel, 2007). Symptoms usually occur after the death of 70% of dopaminergic neurons; causing severe depletion of the neurotransmitter, dopamine (Jankovic, 2007). Dopamine has an extensive role in regulating movement, behaviour, mood and motivation; and may influence learning, time estimation, consequence prediction and awareness of the environment (Arias-Carrión & Pöppel, 2007). The cause of PD is unknown and as the disease cannot be detected prior to onset of symptoms, it is not currently possible to cure PD (Cools, et al., 2001). Severity of symptoms and rate of disease progression vary significantly between individuals. For example, some individuals may experience only minor symptoms 10 years after diagnosis, whilst other individuals may require full time high-support care within six months of being diagnosed with PD (Jankovic, 2007). It is not currently possible to predict how the disease will affect each individual's driving performance, and so assessment must be performed on a case-by-case basis (Jankovic, 2007).

1.2 Physical and cognitive symptoms of Parkinson's disease that affect driving

PD can cause a wide range of physical symptoms, which are known to affect driving ability. Common symptoms include motor tremors, bradykinesia, postural instability, rigidity, involuntary movements, generalised slowness and impaired balance (Adler, et al., 2000). People with PD can also experience alterations in sensation; including pain, burning, paresthesia and vestibular dysfunction (Jankovic, 2007). Driving is the most complicated activity of daily living, and even small mistakes can cause severe and potentially fatal crashes (Molnar, Marshall, & Man-Son-Hing, 2006). Driving requires numerous skills and behaviours to be learnt, coordinated and continuously adapted in a constantly changing environment with time-based pressures (Elvik & Vaa, 2004). Driving therefore places extensive demands upon cognitive abilities, requiring high levels of vigilance, concentration, multitasking, complex reasoning and decision making even when driving over short and/or familiar distances (Devos, et al., 2007).

Physical symptoms of PD have been systematically researched in relation to driving performance. This has contributed to a comprehensive evidence base on the physical effects of PD symptoms upon driving performance (Cordell, et al., 2008; Jankovic, 2007). Drivers with PD have reduced strength and speed of movement, slower reaction times and a diminished ability to turn their head to check mirrors (Adler, et al., 2000; Heikkila, et al., 1997). Drivers with PD also have difficulty in negotiating roundabouts, turning across traffic, driving at high speeds and driving in urban environments (Cordell, et al., 2008; Radford, et al., 2004; Uc, et al., 2009). Drivers with PD are often aware of how their physical limitations influence their driving performance (Kulisevsky & Pagonabarraga, 2009). Consequently, many drivers with PD self-regulate their driving habits by avoiding potentially difficult or risky situations, such as not driving on the freeway, avoiding peak hour or having a co-pilot (Amick, et al., 2007). Factor and Weiner (2002) claimed that the main contributing factors to poor driving performance are PD-related deficits in cognition and visual processing as self-regulating behaviours are very effective in compensating for physical deficits. Uitti (2009) claimed that decline of visual sensitivity, motion perception and cognition are the largest contributing factors to unsafe driving. Further research is required to confirm these claims.

Research into the impact of cognitive symptoms upon driving ability is limited and contradictory. It is difficult to detect the presence of cognitive impairment in PD and to determine the relationship and severity of cognitive impairment on driving performance. The exact prevalence of cognitive impairment amongst drivers with PD is unknown. People with mild to moderate PD have scored significantly lower upon psychomotor and cognitive assessments, showing that PD affects cognition and psychomotor ability at all stages of the disease (Heikkila et al., 1997). However, routine cognitive assessments, such as the Mini Mental Status Examination have low sensitivity, preventing the accurate detection of cognitive deficits in people with PD (Kulisevsky & Pagonabarraga, 2009). Adler and colleagues (2000) stated that 25 to 40% of people in the later stage of PD experience cognitive impairment whilst Factor and Weiner (2002) recorded a lower prevalence rate of 20% amongst another cohort in a similar stage of the disease. Tröster and Woods (2007), however, claimed that cognitive impairment is more common with an earlier onset, occurring in one third of people with only mild to moderate PD.

It is known that the prevalence of cognitive impairment significantly increases with disease progression. However, the number of drivers with PD in Australia who have cognitive impairment is unknown (Amick, et al., 2007). Inability to accurately screen for cognitive impairment is of concern to road safety, since people who are affected may not be aware of it. If drivers with PD are not aware of the need to self regulate driving behaviour and/or compensate for performance alterations, the risk to road safety is increased (Amick, et al., 2007). Drivers may not seek medical advice and/or driving assessments may not be sought as needed, as the potential impacts upon driving performance are poorly understood (Betz & Fisher, 2009). Jones (2009) found that the most frequently self-identified cognitive areas affecting driving amongst people with PD were decision making, complex attention, visual search, impulse control, planning and divided attention. They also conducted a meta-analysis, and found that these six areas have been associated with previous incidents of unsafe driving and traffic errors (Amick, et al., 2007; Innes, et al., 2009).

In a study of 150 people with PD, it was found that cognitive impairment had a significant impact upon the crash rate per miles driven, irrespective of the actual disease severity (Devos, et al., 2007). Other studies have found that drivers with PD have increased indecision at T-junctions and when changing lanes, as well as a slower information processing speed, reaction time and decision making speed (Heikkila, et al., 1997; Stolwyk, et al., 2006). The current study focuses primarily upon decision making ability, which has been identified as one of the most important contributing factors to safe driving.

1.3 Drivers with Parkinson's disease and road safety

In 2008, traffic collisions caused 1,402 preventable deaths in Australia (Australian Bureau of Statistics, 2008). Deaths and disabilities caused by traffic collisions result in extensive, long term, social and emotional costs to families, friends and communities (Elvik & Vaa, 2004). Traffic collisions have vast financial implications; including healthcare services, insurance premiums, property damage and clean up services (Australian Bureau of Statistics, 2008). Therefore, improving road safety through research is of high importance to save lives and prevent disabilities. Although the majority of traffic collisions are preventable, the number of collisions is actually predicted to increase substantially in the future. Escalating population density in cities, increased usage of vehicles and number of cars per household are resulting in Australian road networks becoming more complicated and demanding (Australian Bureau of Statistics, 2009). The fastest growing population of Australian drivers are aged over 70 years, as improvements in healthcare have enabled drivers, including those with PD, to retain their licences for longer (Australian Bureau of Statistics, 2004). The ageing population demographics, in combination with the increased complexity of road systems, mean that the risk of collision for drivers over 65 years is predicted to triple by 2030 (Australian Bureau of Statistics, 2004). This older population are also more likely to sustain serious injuries or death during collisions due to age-related deterioration of musculoskeletal and cardiovascular systems (Adler, et al., 2000).

Longer licence retention can be very beneficial in improving the quality of life of older Australians, since they are able to maintain independence, access to the community and preserve their self-efficacy (Radford, et al., 2004). However, older drivers must be able to compensate for their age-related deficits, since the increasing complexity of road systems place additional demands on cognitive, physical and sensory systems (Elvik & Vaa, 2004). Drivers with PD face further challenges as the PD symptoms as well as side effects of medication can interfere with driving performance. Research, both on-road and using driving simulators, has shown that drivers with PD commit more risky faults and driving offences, and have a significantly increased number of collisions per kilometre driven when compared to the average population (Devos, et al., 2007; Radford, et al., 2004). Despite the challenges faced by drivers with PD in continuing to drive, it is unethical to cancel their licences based upon diagnosis of the disease alone (Tröster & Woods, 2007). Many drivers with PD are able to overcome barriers using their extensive driving experience and knowledge of road systems or they can compensate for the declining ability through self-monitoring and self-regulation (Stolwyk, et al., 2006). For example, a person who becomes overwhelmed when driving at high speeds may change their route to avoid freeway driving (Tröster & Woods, 2007).

In Australia, like most of the developed countries, the guidelines regulating licence retainment and cancellation are based upon a system of subjective medical expert opinion (Adler, et al., 2000). There are no current national standards or requirements for how clinical driving assessments should be conducted (Innes, et al., 2009). Medical experts are often required to determine driving performance, even though the majority have not been trained in driving assessment, or actually observed their patient driving a car (Adler, et al., 2000). Specific clinical assessment batteries and criteria to renew or cancel driving licences have not been clearly defined in the Australian Assessing Fitness to Drive handbook; the combination of symptoms and/or the severity that could compromise driving ability are not defined (Cordell, et al., 2008). Therefore, the medical practitioner must make a subjective decision on the fitness to drive of their patients, even though they may not have been trained to do so (Cordell, et al., 2008). Most current methods of determining licence retainment or cancellation is through on-road driving tests and/or clinical psychometric assessments (National Road Transport Commission, 2003). On-road assessment is the gold standard. However, the process is costly and time consuming (Bedard, et al., 2010; Bryer, et al., 2006). A person who is unable to undergo a driving assessment as recommended by their medical professional is unlikely to be able to retain their licence (Anceaux, et al., 2008). The high assessment cost and need for drivers with PD to undergo annual driving reviews may contribute to the early cessation of driving (Access Economics, 2010).

The cheapest, most accessible and commonly used method for determining driving ability is through clinical assessment. Tools, such as the Timed Up and Go (measures ability to stand up, walk for 3 metres and return to the chair), Unified Parkinson's Scale and Mini Mental Status Examination (MMSE) are commonly used (Cordell, et al., 2008). However, the predictive validity of using these tools in driving assessment is frequently questioned in the literature (Anceaux, et al., 2008; Betz & Fisher, 2009; Cordell, et al., 2008; Stolwyk, et al., 2006). Radford, Lincoln and Lennox (2004) stated that an objective and reliable assessment tool to measure driving ability do not currently exist. Based upon an extensive literature review, Molnar, Marshall and Man-Son-Hing (2006) concluded that no office-based test had validated cut-off scores that correlated to on-road driving performance amongst people with dementia. Ernst and Paulus (2005) noted that it is difficult to assess risk-taking behaviours in an indoor, clinical setting without actually watching the person drive. In a double blind study using 20 people with PD and 20 age-matched controls; it was found that there was a 35% inconsistency in clinical assessment results conducted by a neurologist, compared to on-road driving assessment results provided by a driving instructor and occupational therapist (Heikkila, et al., 1997). Although these results need to be interpreted with caution due to the small sample size; it does highlight that assessment processes need to be improved. Moreover, the Heikkila el al study (1997) did suggest that visual memory, choice reaction time and information processing speed tests could potentially be used to assess fitness to drive; once more research is conducted to establish validity and reliability. Betz and Fisher (2009) suggested that further research into the detection of cognitive impairment and its potential implications for road safety is becoming more crucial in preventing fatal collisions as the population ages.

1.4 Impact of poor decision making ability of PD drivers on driving performance
PD-related cognitive deficits are believed to occur due the inefficient neurotransmission of dopamine-dependent neural connections between the basal ganglia and other areas of the brain (Tröster & Woods, 2007). The deprivation of dopamine, caused by the damage to the

basal ganglia, can directly affect the cognitive functions that are essential to decision making ability. These include; time estimation, working memory, executive function, compulsion, perseveration, attention, motivation and information processing speed (Cools, et al., 2001). Additionally, priority given to stimuli, error prediction, action planning, learning and interest in the environment are also affected (Ernst & Paulus, 2005). Furthermore, Nieoullon (2002) stated that the reduced amount of dopamine may interfere with a person's ability to perform an activity or behaviour, as well as alter a person's ability to adapt to environmental changes. Making decisions is a high-level cognitive function that involves the caudate nucleus and ventral striatum of the basal ganglia, as well as parts of the prefrontal cortex of the brain (Ernst & Paulus, 2005). The decision making process is reliant upon the neurotransmitter dopamine to transmit information via the mesocortical and mesolimbic pathways to the involved areas of the brain (Cools, et al., 2001). Due to the complexity of the decision making process, multiple high-level cerebral functions contribute to the ability to make a decision within a set period. These include attention, information processing speed and capacity, working memory, concentration, recall memory, planning, complex reasoning and risk assessment (Busemeyer & Stout, 2002; Kalis, et al., 2008). Fatigue, stress, emotions and medication can cause the speed and accuracy of decision making ability to fluctuate (Ernst & Paulus, 2005).

The Decision Making Process Model (see Figure 2) defines three important stages to making a decision: Option Generation, Option Selection and Action Initiation (Kalis, et al., 2008). PD can affect all of the components of decision making, although the severity of deficits vary from person to person (Stolwyk, et al., 2006; Tröster & Woods, 2007). This model has been employed in research to study PD in numerous activities other than driving (Levy & Dubois, 2006). Firstly, in Option Generation the person considers the requirements of the situation and thinks of possible courses of action. Then during the Option Selection stage, the person analyses each potential course of action for probable outcomes. Factors that can influence the selection of one course of action over the alternatives include: probability of the benefits and/or risks, the person's previous experiences, emotional state, values and preferences for one course of action (Ernst & Paulus, 2005). Finally, in Action Initiation, the decision is implemented through physical actions (Kalis, et al., 2008). The person then evaluates the results of the decision to promote learning for future situations. According to Busemeyer and Stout (2002), poor decisions can be due to a failure to anticipate consequences, poor perceptual sensitivity, problems in memory storage or retrieval, inability to determine possible courses of action, fatigue, poor concentration, difficulty in learning from mistakes, and/or impulsivity.

Decision making deficits have been recognised as a key area that could influence driving competence and safety amongst people with PD (Cools, et al., 2001). Dopamine has an important role in facilitating the cognitive processes that enable a person to make a decision. However, what this functionally entails for driving is poorly understood (Arias-Carrión & Pöppel, 2007; Cools, et al., 2001). Deficits in decision making are most apparent during activities, such as driving, that require spontaneous, complex information processing and reasoning within time constraints (Tröster & Woods, 2007). The driver may have to make multiple decisions in quick succession, which place extensive demands upon cognitive processes. The driver must quickly consider all components of the situation, generate and consider options, implement the choice, evaluate the result and then start the decision making process again (Busemeyer & Stout, 2002). The driver may also have to ignore multiple distracting auditory, visual and tactile stimuli from the car's radio, air conditioning, passengers and the visual environment (Ernst & Paulus, 2005). Medication, fatigue, other PD symptoms, co-morbid conditions and environmental distractions can also intensify the deficits experienced by drivers with PD (Tröster & Woods, 2007).

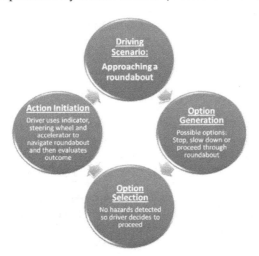

(Adapted from: Kalis, et al., 2008; Lefy & Dubois, 2006)

Fig. 2. Summary of the decision making process in driving

Decisions can be made either through conscious deliberation, for example, deciding if a parking space is large enough for the car, or through an unconscious process using previously learned behavioural patterns; for instance, automatically using the indicator when leaving a roundabout (Ernst & Paulus, 2005). PD can cause deficits in decision making ability at any of the decision making stages, and the resultant hesitancy, ambivalence or apathy may significantly impact upon road safety for the driver and other road users (Kalis, et al., 2008). As shown in Figure 2, if a driver is indecisive about whether to stop, slow down or to proceed through a roundabout, they could increase the risk of collision due to either incorrect use of signals, inappropriate speed or lane placement, sudden braking without checking review mirrors and/or impulsively increasing speed. All of these actions can directly result in a collision, especially as the other drivers may not be able to anticipate the indecisive driver's actions and react in time.

Numerous studies have identified that hesitancy and indecision contribute to a higher risk of crashing. However, the extent of the contribution is unknown (Bryer, Rapport, & Hanks, 2006; Stolwyk, et al., 2006). Drivers with PD frequently have a lack of cognitive flexibility and difficulty in shifting attention and multi-tasking, particularly when in stressful situations (Arias-Carrión & Pöppel, 2007). Drivers with PD often drive at slower speeds, have reduced reaction times and can fail to notice specific landmarks and traffic signs (Stolwyk, et al., 2006; Uc, et al., 2009). A study that surveyed 5,210 drivers with PD found that cognitive deficits are strongly associated with dangerous driving, with the most common causes of collision being indeciveness at T junctions and reduced usage of mirrors (Meindorfner, et al., 2005). A review of 42 driving studies concluded that the effect of a disease upon driving performance is difficult to determine due to numerous confounding factors. It is not currently possible to conduct an extensive randomised controlled trial into this area, since there is not yet enough information available to control all confounding variables (Elvik & Vaa, 2004). Therefore, the study reported in this chapter was valuable in trialling alternative assessment methodologies and making recommendations for future research projects. Information from the study may also contribute to the development of a successful assessment protocol for drivers with PD to improve road safety.

2. Methodology

2.1 Purpose of study

The aim of the research was to explore the impact of impaired decision making ability upon the driving performance of people with PD. To address the aim, a quantitative, pre-post case-control study design was employed to assess participants the decision making ability of drivers with PD and healthy controls, as well as their driving performance under time pressure, were examined. The objectives of the study are: **Objective 1:** To assess the decision making ability of drivers with PD using standardised psychometric assessment tools and the E-prime computer based assessment; **Objective 2:** To investigate the relationship between the decision making ability and driving performance of people with PD; and **Objective 3:** To compare the driving performance of people with PD to the healthy control group whilst driving under a time pressure in the driving simulator.

The first objective was addressed by administering an assessment battery of clinical psychometric tests to assess the main cognitive processes that contribute to decision making ability. The assumption was that drivers with PD would have lower scores on the psychometric assessments, due to PD-related cognitive impairments, when compared with the healthy control group. The second objective was addressed by assessing the driving performance of the groups on the driving simulator. The assumption was that drivers with PD would have poorer driving performance at baseline driving (Trial One) as well as driving under time pressure (Trial Two) when compared to the healthy control group. The third objective was addressed by analysing the results from stage one and two to determine if there is a correlation between driving performance and decision making ability. The assumption was that the ability of people with PD to make correct decisions whilst driving under time pressure would be significantly lower than the control group. Ethical approval was granted by the Curtin University Human Research Ethics. Data was collected from Sept 2009 until March 2010 at the Curtin University Driving Rehabilitation Clinic.

2.2 Participants

Convenience sampling was used to recruit participants by displaying advertisement posters at community centres, retirement villages, shopping centres and neurologists' offices. Advertisements were also placed in community newsletters, as well as the Western Australia Parkinson's Association newsletter. Study participants were required to be community living adults, aged 50 to 80 years old with a valid driving licence. They had to be current drivers, driving at least half an hour each week. To ensure adequate binocular acuity, a score of at least 6/12 corrected vision on the Snellen Acuity Chart was required. In the experimental group, each participant's diagnosis of PD had to have been confirmed by a general practitioner or neurologist. Participants were excluded from the study if they had severe hearing impairments or inadequate comprehension of written or verbal English as judged by the researcher, or any co-morbid diagnosis that may interfere with driving ability. Participants with the following conditions were excluded from the study: dementia, severe cognitive or physical impairment, depression and/or psychiatric conditions. Participants were withdrawn from the study immediately if they requested to do so. A reason for withdrawal was not required. Fifteen drivers with PD and 17 control group participants were recruited were contacted by phone to establish suitability to participate in the study.

To address Study Objectives 2 and 3, baseline-driving performance was established in Trial 1 and then a time constraint was imposed to create pressure upon the participants. In Trial 2, all participants were told to complete the same driving scenario 20% faster than in Trial 1. The percentage of reduction in time was based upon pilot study data. A 20% reduction represented a time that was perceived by the participants as being challenging, yet achievable within the driving assessment parameters. This time pressure forced the participants to make quicker decisions in response to the traffic conditions, without compromising on safety or breaking the road rules. Drivers with PD are more likely to experience decision making deficits whilst making complex decisions under pressure (Amick, et al., 2007). The study assumption is that drivers with PD are capable of making correct decisions; however, they require more time to do so. Important driving behaviours, such as appropriate signalling, use of mirrors and obeying the speed limit potentially could have been affected and/or forgotten as the participants concentrated upon negotiating the scenario faster. The driving performance of participants was measured using Driving Performance Score. A battery of psychometric assessment tools were administered to the participants to assess the cognitive processes that are essential to decision making ability. The cognitive processes included executive function, task switching, sustained, selected and divided attention, attention set shifting, memory, efficiency and accuracy of information processing systems, visual attention and decision making speed and accuracy. All psychometric assessment tools were time based, standardised instruments that measured speed and accuracy of response. The study assumption was that drivers with PD are capable of completing the assessments; however, they will require more time to do so. The confounding variables in the study are presented in Table 1 in next page. Measures have been taken to ensure that the data collected was valid.

2.3 Equipment used in the study
The following section describes the tools used for initial screening of participants, and psychometric assessments for measuring the main components of decision making in driving.

2.3.1 Initial screening of participant medical and driving history
Standardised clinical assessment tools and a Medical History and Driving History Checklist were used to screen for potentially confounding factors (refer to Table 2 and Table 3 for details of assessments). All assessments were administered in a quiet, distraction free room as per the instruction manuals to ensure the reliability of data. The research assistant was trained in administering these assessments prior to commencement of the data collection.

2.3.2 Psychometric assessment
Decision making ability cannot be directly measured. Instead, the main contributing components were all assessed using a battery of psychometric assessments. These components were attention set shifting, visual attention, memory, information processing speed and decision-making speed and accuracy (refer to Table 3). The psychometric

Variable	Potential Impact	Measures taken to improve validity
Medication	- Side effects of medication could affect functional performance. (Radford, et al., 2004).	- Drivers with PD were assessed during periods of optimal function, to ensure that motor and non-motor fluctuations in performance did not affect results (Radford, et al., 2004).
Co Morbid Conditions	- Symptoms and medications for co-morbid conditions could alter functional performance (Radford et al., 2004).	- People with co morbid medical conditions that could affect driving performance were excluded from the study. Refer to Exclusion Criteria and the Screening procedure.
Fatigue	- Fatigue may affect driving performance especially as participants are older (Radford, et al., 2004).	- Assessment periods were held during mid morning and early afternoon and frequent rest breaks with refreshments were offered.
Driving Experience	- People who have been driving either longer or more frequently are likely to be better drivers (Bedard, et al., 2010).	- The Driving History Checklist was used to seek a fair distribution of driving experience across groups. All drivers must have driven at least one half hour a week to ensure the maintenance of skills.
Gender	- Men have a greater risk of having a fatal crash (Adler, et al., 2005).	- A fair distribution of gender between groups was sought. Statistical analysis identified the gender-related difference in performance.
Age	Driving performance usually decreases after the age of 60 years (Adler, et al., 2000)	- A fair distribution of ages between groups was sought. Statistical analysis identified the age-related difference in performance.

Table 1. Confounding variables of the study

assessment battery comprised of the Symbol Digit Modalities Test (Smith, 2007), Digit Vigilance Test (Kelland & Lewis, 1996), Purdue Pegboard (Lafayette Instrument Company, 1985) and Trail Making Test – B (Corrigan & Hinkeldey, 1987).

The assessments were chosen based upon recommendations from literature to ensure high reliability, sensitivity, and/or validity of each test in assessing driving performance. For example, the Trail Making Test-B, Symbol Digit Modalities Test and Digit Vigilance are highly sensitive to detecting differences in cognitive performance (Smith, 2007). The Trail Making Test-B is one of the most frequently used tests in driving research and clinical settings, due to its high reliability and sensitivity to mild cognitive impairment (Arbuthnott & Frank, 2000; Ashendorf et al., 2008). The Symbol Digit Modalities Test was found in a study of 150 people to be the most reliable of 12 assessment tools in detecting mild cognitive impairment (Ashendorf, et al., 2008).

Screening Tool	Purpose of Assessment Tool	Administration and justification for Use
Medical Checklist	- To gather demographic medical information and screen for excluding factors.	- Based on medical screening assessments according to Australian Driving regulations (National Road Transport Commission, 2003).
Driving History Checklist	- To gather demographic driving information and screen for excluding factors.	- Based on current Driving History assessments at the Independent Living Centre and Australian driving regulations (NRTC, 2003).
Snellen Acuity Chart	- A standardised measure frequently used in driving assessment to screen for binocular acuity deficits (Lotfipour, et al., 2010)	- Adequate binocular vision was assumed based upon the ability to read a series of letters on a chart placed 6 metres away. Minimum standard for on road driving is 6/12 corrected vision (NR TC, 2003).
Cognistat (Kiernan, Mueller, Langston, & Van Dyke, 1987)	- Brief screening tool to detect cognitive impairment Subtests of attention, constructional ability, memory, calculations, reasoning and judgement were administered.	- Economical and efficient clinical screening tool that has high sensitivity to cognitive impairment (Adler, et al., 2000)

Table 2. Outline of Screening Tools

2.3.3 E-Prime computer based tool

The E-Prime software has been used in 104 research studies since 2001; including research projects into simulated situations, older adults and neurological conditions (Psychology Software Tools, 2010). The E-Prime software is capable of millisecond precision and is frequently used in research to increase the accuracy and reliability of data (Ranzini, et al., 2009). In the present study, the E-Prime computer program was set up to measure the speed and accuracy of the participants' decision making ability by administering a series of multiple choice questions (refer to Figure 3). The questions were based upon traffic situations in which drivers with PD are known to experience difficulty; such as roundabouts, traffic lights, freeway driving, city driving, over taking and right hand turns (Allen, et al., 2003; Anceaux, et al., 2008; Lee, et al., 2003). It took approximately 10 minutes to complete.

The "red", "yellow" and "green" button system (refer to Figure 3) had buttons that were large, visually distinguishable, and highly sensitive to touch, to enable people, who experienced PD-related physical symptoms to enter their decision as quickly as possible. The computer was placed in front of a blank, white wall and the researcher sat behind the participant, out of sight to prevent potential distractions. The questions were displayed in large, white writing on a black backdrop to improve readability. A black instruction screen was displayed to inform participants about how to answer the following question (refer to Figure 4).

Psychometric Tool	Purpose and Administration	Literature support for tool validity
Trail Making Test B (TMT-B) (Corrigan & Hinkeldey, 1987)	- To assess executive function, visual attention and task switching (Corrigan & Hinkeldey, 1987). Participants join alternating dots of letters and numbers (1, A, 2, B etc.).	- TMT-B is suggested for older driver assessment as a score of over 180 seconds could indicate increased driving risk (Betz & Fisher, 2009). Moderate predictive ability for increased crash risk (Bedard, et al., 2010).
Purdue Peg Board (Lafayette Instrument Company, 1985)	- To assess bilateral gross motor movements and dexterity of the fingers, hands and arms to distinguish between the influence of physical and cognitive PD-symptoms on results.	- Range of norms for people over 65 years available. High test-retest reliability (0.82 to 0.91), moderate sensitivity and moderate predictive ability for driving (Wood, et al., 2005). Suggested for assessing impact of neurological disease upon motor function (Wood, et al., 2005).
Digit Vigilance Test (Kelland & Lewis, 1996)	- To assess sustained, selected and divided attention, and information processing speed and accuracy. Participants scan rows of single digit numbers and circle all of the number sixes.	- High test-retest reliability and has been validated as a measure of sustained attention (Kelland & Lewis, 1996). Determines if participants were able to remember and attend to important information whilst disregarding excess stimuli (Radford, et al., 2004).
Symbol Digit Modalities Test (Smith, 2007)	- To measure the efficiency and accuracy of information processing systems. Participants had to convert geometric shapes into numbers as quickly as possible.	- Substitution tasks are highly sensitive to detecting cerebral dysfunction (Wood, et al., 2005). Norms provided for age and education levels. High test-retest reliability (0.80). Moderate predictive ability for driving ability (Wood, et al., 2005)
E-Prime Computer Based Assessment (Psychology Software Tools, 2010)	To assess decision making accuracy and response time - Multiple-choice questions based upon photographs of different driving scenarios.	- Software is capable of capturing the responses of participants with millisecond precision (Ranzini, et al., 2009). Standardised video instructions used for to improve inter-rater and intra-rater reliability.

Table 3. Outline of the Psychometric Assessment Tools

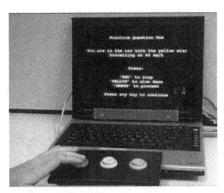

Fig. 3. The setup of the E-Prime Assessment tool

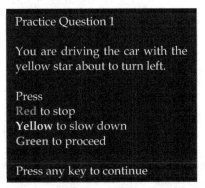

Practice Question 1

You are driving the car with the yellow star about to turn left.

Press
Red to stop
Yellow to slow down
Green to proceed

Press any key to continue

Fig. 4. E-Prime Instruction Screen

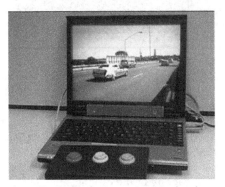

Fig. 5. The E-Prime Assessment Tool; displaying an example of a question

In each photograph there was a car labelled with a bright yellow star (refer to Figure 5). Participants were instructed to assume that he or she was the driver of the car with the yellow star and give the most appropriate response for each scenario. The participant had to decide whether they would 'stop', 'slow down' or 'proceed' based upon their interpretation of the hazards as shown in the photograph. Participants responded using one of the three buttons. The accuracy of answers and response time was automatically recorded by the E-Prime software to determine decision making ability.

2.3.4 Driving simulator in curtin driving rehabilitation clinic

A fixed-base, Systems Technology Incorporated (STI) driving simulator was used to assess driving performance in this study (Lee, et al., 2003). Driving simulators are frequently used in research and clinical practice to assess driving ability, since risk of injury and property damage is eliminated (Bedard, et al., 2010). The STISIM driving simulator enables the development of highly controlled and regulated traffic scenarios (Allen, et al., 2003). The STISIM simulator technology has been used in 61 different studies, whilst the STISIM simulator driving technology in particular has been used in at least 24 studies in the past eight years (Systems Techonology Inc, 2010). Low cost, fixed base driving simulators have been used in research on older drivers and on the effect of fatigue, drugs, cognitive impairment, Alzheimer's disease, PD, traumatic brain injury and numerous other conditions upon driving performance (Bedard, et al., 2010; Lee, et al., 2003). Driving simulators are becoming more affordable options; especially as on-road assessment costs are becoming more prohibitive due to the increasing fuel, car purchase and maintenance costs and higher insurance premiums (Bedard, et al., 2010).

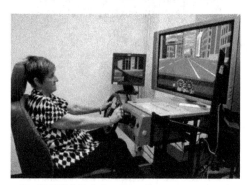

Fig. 6. The Curtin University STISIM Driving Simulator

Simulators are capable of distinguishing between safe and unsafe drivers (De Winter, et al., 2008; Lee, et al., 2003). Numerous studies have found high transferability of simulator-based behaviours to on-road driving behaviours (De Winter, et al., 2008; Lee, et al., 2003). Factor and Weiner (2002) found that driving simulators have a greater accuracy in predicting driving ability than the clinical psychometric assessments currently used by medical practitioners. High inter-rater and intra-rater reliability (correlation coefficients were 0.87 and 0.83 respectively) were recently established by Bedard and colleagues (2010). They used the simulator-recorded data and data manually recorded by a laboratory assistant in a similar STISIM simulator. The validity of the driving simulator used in this study has been established for assessing older adults (Lee, et al., 2003). A photograph of a participant being assessed on the Curtin University STISIM Driving Simulator is shown in Fig. 6.

2.3.5 Development of the STISIM driving scenario

Two driving scenarios were specially designed for the present study. They were based upon the Western Australian licensing standards, in combination with recommendations from driving simulator literature (Allen, et al., 2003; Factor & Weiner, 2002; Lee, et al., 2003; National Road Transport Commission, 2003). In the present study, the roadway geometry and intersections, position of traffic signals and markings, weather conditions, the responsiveness of vehicle controls, location of other vehicles and road users were all programmed to target decision making ability. The scenarios included small town, city and country driving, simple and complex intersections, curved roads, simulated emergency braking, varied speed control and visually obscured intersections. Auditory instructions were included in the simulator programming to ensure that all of the information and instructions were consistent throughout data collection.

To investigate the impact of PD-related decision making deficits upon driving performance, the scenario in this study was designed to specially assess hazard detection, risk assessment, impulsiveness and decision making ability (Bedard, et al., 2010; Elvik & Vaa, 2004). Traffic situations that are known to be affected by PD, such as driving at high speeds, turning corners, overtaking, merging and complex city intersections were included (Stolwyk, et al., 2006; Radford, et al., 2006). For example, during the scenario, a recorded verbal instruction told each participant to overtake three slow moving trucks whilst avoiding oncoming traffic. A similar process was used in a study by Amick et al., (2007) as they researched cognitive indicators of poor driving performance of drivers with PD. Driving Performance Assessment Guidelines was tabulated in Table 4.

2.4 Data analysis

Data was analysed using the Statistical Package for Social Sciences (SPSS) (SPSS Inc. 2009). Demographic information of participants was presented using descriptive statistics. The difference in total run time and driving performance score between groups was analysed using t-tests; whereas a Chi squared test and Fisher's Exact test was used to analyse ordinal variables, such as gender and number of collisions and infringements. A stepwise Multiple Linear Regression Model was used to analyse the driving performance and E-Prime scores; the driving performance score was the dependent variable and E-Prime (correct answers, time taken and participant group) were the independent variables. The psychometric assessments and the components of the Driving Performance Score were analysed using the non-parametric Wilcoxon 2-sample test. A repeated measure regression analysis was performed using the driving score as a dependent variable and the results of the psychometric assessments, simulator trial run number and group identifier (drivers with PD or control group) as independent variables. The least significant variables were then removed, one at a time, until the p-value associated with each of the remaining variables was less than 0.05. Prior to the analysis, normality of data and the assumptions of the statistical tests were checked to ensure that there were no violations.

3. Study results

3.1 Participant demographics

Seventeen people in the control group and 11 drivers with PD were assessed and their demographic data was tabulated in Table 5. In exploring the characteristics of the participants, it was identified that the number of years of driving experience was different between the comparison groups (p=0.042). The drivers with PD group had driven on average 7 years and 8 months longer than the control group. The participants' age, gender, employment status and education level were found to be not significantly different between groups.

Assessment Component	Definition of Required Behaviour/Skill	Assessment Frequency and Scoring Procedure
Frequency of Appropriate Use of Mirrors	- Driver checked left and right mirrors immediately before slowing down, turning or diverging.	- Assessed at 25 locations/events. One point deducted for each omission per mirror
Smooth Manoeuvring around Obstacles	- Driver smoothly manoeuvres around obstacles and maintains a safety buffer around vehicle.	- Assessed at nine locations/events. Up to three points deducted depending on severity of error
Frequency of Appropriate Stopping Distance	- Driver stops at an appropriate distance from traffic lights, stop signs and obstacles.	- Assessed at 20 locations/events. Up to four points deducted depending on severity of error
Maintains Appropriate Vehicle Speed	- Driver maintained vehicle within 9kms of the appropriate speed limit.	- Assessed at 23 locations. Points deducted for excess speed as per national guidelines.
Maintains Correct Lane Position	- Driver stays within the lane markers or to the left on unmarked roads.	- Number of deviations recorded by stimulator. One point deducted for each instance.
Maintains Control of Vehicle on Turns	- Driver kept vehicle stable and adjusted speed as required around turns and on winding roads	- Number of deviations recorded by simulator. One point deducted for each time.
Appropriate Behaviours to Avoid Hazards	- Driver had sufficient room to react, was alert and aware of environment and in control of vehicle	- Number of sudden braking incidents recorded by stimulator. One point deducted for each omission
Appropriate Use of Indicators	- Driver appropriately used indicators to give warning about future diverging movements.	- Assessed at 22 locations/tasks. One point deducted for each omission.
Demonstrates Caution during Manoeuvres	- Driver did not overtake when unsafe, allowed adequate room and stopped at yellow traffic lights.	- Assessed at 27 locations/tasks. Up to three points deducted depending on severity of error
Qualitative Feedback (Bedard, et al., 2010; Elvik & Vaa, 2004)	- Participants comments were recorded verbatim. Clinical observations regarding participant's affect were recorded.	- Information gathered to compliment quantitative data. No points were deducted for clinical observations and feedback

(Bedard, et al., 2010; Bryer, et al., 2006; Elvik & Vaa, 2004; National Road Transport Commission, 2003).

Table 4. Driving Performance Assessment Guidelines

Variable	Drivers with PD n=11 Mean (SD)	Control n=17 Mean (SD)	p-value
Age	68.2 (5.3)	65.6 (8.8)	0.427#
Gender			
– Female	6 (55%)ˇ	7 (41%)ˇ	0.489^
Weekly hours driving			
– Minimum	8.0 (8.5)	13.7 (9.9)	0.162#
– Maximum	9 (8.6)	14.7 (11.3)	0.204#
Years of Driving Experience	50.6 (5.5)	42.9 (9.2)	0.042*
Number of Collisions in last 2 years	0	3 (28%)	0.526+
Number of Infringements in last 2 years	0	2 (12%)	0.515+
Education Level			-
– Tertiary Study	4 (36%)ˇ	8 (47%)ˇ	-
– Year 12 High School	4 (36%)ˇ	6 (35%)ˇ	-
– No answer	3 (28%)ˇ	3 (18%)ˇ	
Disease Symptoms			-
– Tremors in legs	3 (28%)ˇ	-	-
– Tremors in arms	7 (63%)ˇ	-	-
– Mild Rigidity	4 (36%)ˇ	-	-
– Moderate Rigidity	4 (36%)ˇ	-	-
– Severe Rigidity	0	-	-
– Mild Fatigue	2 (18%)ˇ	3 (18%)ˇ	-
– Moderate Fatigue	7 (63%)ˇ	3 (18%)ˇ	-
– Severe Fatigue	0	0	

^ Chi squared test; # T-test; + Fisher's Exact test; *Results were statistically significant ($p<0.05$) and ˇ Categorical frequency (percentage)

Table 5. Results of Participant Demographic Data

The drivers with PD had on average a diagnosis of PD for approximately 8 years and 4 months. Medications that were prescribed to the participants with PD included: Sinemet, Madopar, Cabaser, Sifrol and Selgene. Some participants with PD reported experiencing tremors in arms and legs as well as mild to moderate rigidity and fatigue (refer to Table 5). Six of the control participants reported experiencing mild to moderate fatigue, which was not related to PD. All participants with PD reported they required only minimal assistance to complete self-care activities, whilst none of the participants in the control group required any assistance.

3.2 Psychometric assessment results

The results of four standardised, psychometric assessments and the E-Prime Assessment Tool are shown in Table 6. The only psychometric assessment tool that detected a difference between the groups was the Purdue Pegboard Both Hands subtest and Overall Score. These results indicate that there may be a difference in the speed and dexterity of upper limb movements between the two groups. There were no statistical differences between groups on the E-Prime Test, Symbol Digit Modalities Test, Digit Vigilance Test and Trail Making Test B.

Psychometric Test	Drivers with PD (n= 11) ** Mean (SD)	Control Group (n=15)** Mean (SD)	Wilcoxon Two-Sample Test) p-value
E-prime			
Correct Answers	12.6 (3.5)	12.7 (3.1)	0.96
Response Time/seconds	126,686 (45,463)	91,482 (34,344)	0.42
Symbol Digit Modalities Test	44.33 (5.63)	49.13 (8.46)	0.18
Digit Vigilance Test			
Page One	3.41 (0.63)	3.37 (0.69)	0.64
Page Two	3.57 (0.71)	3.46 (0.64)	0.87
Trail Making Test B	1.27 (0.65)	1.05 (0.45)	0.84
Purdue Pegboard			
Right Hand	11.75 (2.66)	13.71 (2.02)	0.20
Left Hand	11.25 (2.43)	12.79 (1.67)	0.17
Both Hands	16.25 (5.18)	21.50 (3.72)	0.04*
Assembly Task	12.88 (4.29)	17.43 (4.11)	0.07
Overall Score	39.25 (9.63)	48.00 (5.49)	0.06

*Results were statistically significant ($p<0.05$)
** 8 drivers with PD and 13 control group participants were assessed using the E-Prime Assessment.

Table 6. Participant Psychometric Assessment Results

3.3 Driving simulator results

Two participants, one control and one driver with PD requested additional practice in using the simulator. All other participants began the assessment trials immediately following the practice session. During the assessment process, three drivers with PD and four control participants experienced simulator-induced motion sickness and withdrew. Their partial data was included in the data analyse where appropriate. An Independent t-test was used to determine if there was a difference between each group on the Driving Performance Score and the Scenario Completion Time for each trial. The results are shown in Table 7. The parametric t-test was found to be appropriate for analysing these results as the pre-post nature of assessment doubled the data entries available for analysis; fulfilling the sample size requirements (Hedges, 2009). Of note is that the difference between scenario completion times for Trial 2 had a p-value of 0.014 (refer to Table 7).

This however does not represent a difference between groups as the baseline performance in Trial 1 was dissimilar for each group and this disparity affects the results of Trial 2. The results shown in Table 7 are displayed in two box-and-whisker plots. Figure 7 represents the change in Driving Performance Score between trials for both groups, whilst Figure 8 shows the change in Scenario Completion Time for each trial.

Variable	Drivers with PD (n=8) Mean (SD)	Control Group (n=13) Mean (SD)	Results p-value
Driving Performance Score			
Trial 1	82.7 (6.0)	76.5 (22.4)	0.36
Trial 2	59.2 (17.9)	67.4 (27.3)	0.47
Between Group Comparison	-23.5 (19.1)	- 9.2 (24.4)	0.17
Comparison between Trials			
- Drivers with PD			0.01*#
			0.02*^
- Control group			0.20#
			0.16^
Scenario Completion Time (seconds)			
Trial 1	864.8 (172)	782 (137)	0.21
Trial 2	776 (110)	674 (64)	0.02*
Between Group Comparison	-88.6 (73.0)	-107.5 (103.8)	0.66
Comparison between Trials			
- Drivers with PD			0.01*#
			0.01^
- Control group			0.01*#
			0.01^

* Results are statistically significant (p < 0.05)
^ Wilcoxon Two-sample Signed Rank Test
# Paired T-Test

Table 7. Driving Performance and Scenario Completion Time for Trial One and Two

3.3.1 Comparison between the driving performance of the groups

The Driving Performance Scores of both groups decreased in Trial 2. However, the extent of this decline was significantly greater for the drivers with PD (t-test p=0.01). These results were confirmed by Wilcoxon test (p=0.03) (refer to Table 7). Although the driving performance of the driver with PD was lower under time pressure, the driving performance was not unsafe or dangerous.

The control group had a greater variance in Driving Performance Scores compared with the drivers with PD in both trials, as shown by Figure 7. When under a time pressure, the variance in Driving Performance Scores of the drivers with PD increased.

3.3.2 Group comparison of scenario completion time

Figure 8 shows the difference within each group for the Scenario Completion Time for trial one and trial two. All participants in both groups, except one control participant, completed the second trial faster as required. In trial one, there were four outliers in the control group as shown by the dots in Figure 8. Both groups were able to significantly decrease their Scenario Completion Time; however the control group was able to decrease their score to a greater extent.

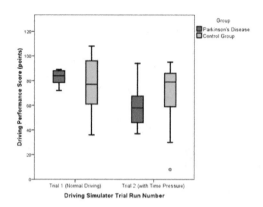

Fig. 7. Change in Driving Performance due to Time Pressure

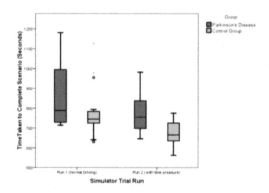

Fig. 8. Change in Scenario Completion Time for Trial One and Two

3.3.3 Group comparison of driving performance score components

As outlined in previous section, the Driving Performance Score comprised of 10 components representing important driving behaviours. Table 8 shows that in trial one, the drivers with PD had a low frequency of appropriate mirror use (p=0.014) and had more difficulty in maintaining the vehicle in a correct lane position (p=0.02). When under pressure, the drivers with PD continued to demonstrate a low frequency of appropriate mirror use (p=0.012) and they were less likely to stop the vehicle an appropriate distance from obstacles (p=0.02). The other components of driving were the same between groups (refer to Table 8).

3.4 Impact of decision making ability upon driving performance

To explore the relationship between decision making ability and driving performance, quantitative data and clinical observations that were gathered during Stage 1 and 2 of the study were analysed. A random effects regression model was adopted to analyse the results using the Driving Score as a dependent variable and the Psychometric Assessment Tests, Trial Run Number and group identifier (drivers with PD or control group) as the independent variables. All independent variables were originally included in the analysis,

Variable	Drivers with PD Mean Score n=8 Mean(SD)	Control Mean Score n=13 Mean (SD)	(Wilcoxon Two-Sample Test) p-value
Frequency of Appropriate Use of Mirrors			
Run 1	8.50 (2.67)	4.38 (3.43)	0.014*
Run 2	12.38 (5.95)	5.46 (3.02)	0.012*
Maintains Appropriate Vehicle Speed			
Run 1	6.25 (6.54)	8.08 (9.23)	1.00
Run 2	7.38 (6.50)	12.31 (9.07)	0.31
Demonstrates Caution during Manoeuvres			
Run 1	6.00 (2.98)	6.77 (3.98)	0.47
Run 2	7.00 (3.30)	7.46 (4.52)	0.91
Frequency of Appropriate Stopping Distance			
Run 1	4.50 (2.73)	4.00 (3.87)	0.43
Run 2	5.13 (4.36)	1.77 (2.35)	0.02*
Smooth Manoeuvring around Obstacles			
Run 1	3.50 (2.78)	3.46 (2.22)	1.00
Run 2	6.38 (2.56)	5.00 (2.24)	0.25
Maintains Correct Lane Position			
Run 1	8.13 (3.27)	14.23 (6.00)	0.02*
Run 2	14.50 (3.59)	13.38(6.78)	1.00
Maintains Control of Vehicle on Turns and Winding Roads			
Run 1	1.75 (2.25)	2.54 (2.30)	0.44
Run 2	3.38 (3.74)	3.46 (3.18)	0.83
Appropriate Behaviours to Avoid Hazards			
Run 1	1.75 (2.38)	1.08 (1.89)	0.39
Run 2	2.86 (3.67)	1.54 (2.07)	0.57
Appropriate Use of Indicators			
Run 1	4.63 (1.77)	6.38 (3.33)	0.15
Run 2	9.63 (3.96)	7.92 (5.20)	0.46
Number of Collisions			
Run 1	1.50 (0.53)	1.31 (1.03)	0.79
Run 2	1.25 (0.71)	0.92 (0.86)	0.41

* Results are statistically significant ($p < 0.05$)
Note: a higher score indicates poorer performance

Table 8. Analysis of Driving Performance Score Components

and then the least significant variables were excluded, one at a time, until the p-value associated with each remaining variable was less than 0.05 (refer to Table 9).

The independent variables that were found to be statistically significant were the Driving Simulator Trial Run Number, Purdue Pegboard Both Hands Score and Digit Vigilance Test Page 1 and Page 2. Confidence Intervals (set at 95%) show the reliability of the results by providing a range of scores that the true answer lies within (Hedges, 2009). As shown by the wide confidence intervals in Table 9, the reliability of these results was not convincing. A correlation between the psychometric assessment tools to driving performance therefore cannot be assumed. Due to the small sample size, it would be misleading to perform individual parametric analysis for each variable.

Variable	Least Squares Mean	Regression coefficient	95% Confidence Interval	p-value
Group				
- Control	76.2	13.0	-3.4 to 29.3	0.114
- Drivers with PD	63.3	0.0		
Trial Run Number				
- 1	76.8	14.2	3.2 to 25.2	0.014*
- 2	62.6	0.0		
Purdue Pegboard Both Hands test				
DVT Page1				
DVT Page2		-1.8	-3.5 to -0.1	0.049*
		-27.4	-51.1 to -3.8	0.025*
		30.2	7.5 to 52.9	0.012*

*Results were statistically significant (p<0.05)

Table 9. Multivariable Analysis of Driving Performance Score to Psychometric Assessment Results

3.5 Motion sickness

Three drivers with PD and four control participants experienced symptoms of motion sickness and withdrew from the study. Symptoms included mild dizziness, sweating, nausea and vomiting. The two participants who had requested additional driving simulator practice were amongst the participants who experienced motion sickness.

In all cases, the researcher ceased participation in the study as soon as mild symptoms of motion sickness were experienced. All participants except one driver with PD, recovered within half an hour without residual signs and symptoms of motion sickness. The exception was contacted the following day by the researcher, and reported no residual signs or symptoms.

4. Discussion

4.1 Participant demographics

Eight drivers with PD and 13 control participants were successfully assessed. The volunteer response rate was lower than anticipated. The recruitment process could have been affected by the stated reluctance of medical practitioners to refer clients due to potential legal implications. Legislation for the Compulsory Reporting of Medical Conditions came into effect in Western Australia only one year prior to the commencement of the study, which may have influenced the willingness of drivers with PD to volunteer. It was intended to match participants by gender, driving exposure per week and age, since these factors were identified by previous studies as having the potential to influence results (Bedard, et al., 2010). Although perfect matching of participants would have been ideal; age, gender and driving exposure per week were not found not to be significantly different between groups. These results concur with a Queensland study using 25 drivers with PD and 21 controls, which also found that age and gender did not appear to affect the results (Wood, et al., 2005).

The only difference between the groups was the number of 'Years of Driving Experience' as the drivers with PD had more experience. This difference may have potentially influenced the results in favour of the drivers with PD having an improved performance, compared with the control group. However, both groups had been driving for over 43 years and there was found to be no difference in the current exposure of the groups to driving. Therefore, the number of years of driving experience may have had a minimal or no impact upon the driving performance results. Elvik and Vaa (2004) investigated 42 different driving studies and found that the years of driving experience was not matched between study cohorts, implying that it is not common practice to do so.

4.2 Psychometric data

In the literature review, it was discussed that decision-making is a complicated process involving many areas of the brain. Dopamine plays an extensive role in enabling these areas to interact and allow a person to make accurate and timely decisions (Ernst & Paulus, 2005). Based upon the prevalence rates of cognitive impairment as discussed; between two and five of the 11 drivers with PD in this study may have had cognitive deficits (Adler, et al., 2000; Factor & Weiner, 2002). If this assumption holds, it was expected that PD-related cognitive deficits would cause drivers with PD to score lower on all of the psychometric assessment tools. The psychometric results however, indicated that there was no difference between the groups upon these decision making components. This may have been due to an inability to detect a difference between groups due to small sample size.

It is possible that a self-selection bias affected the results in favour of the drivers with PD sample performing better than the general population of people with PD. Anceaux et al. (2008) claimed that it is likely that only drivers, who are confident in their ability, tend to volunteer to undergo non-compulsory assessment for research purposes. Participants in the present study were volunteers, more confident drivers, are likely to have influenced the better result of the present study. Results from the Cognistat screening concur with this observation, further supported by the fact that the screening process did not exclude any potential participants due to severe cognitive deficits. Convenience sampling was chosen to recruit participants since a more stringent sampling process would not have been achievable within the time and budget constraints of the study, particularly for recruiting the PD participants (Anceaux, et al., 2008; Elvik & Vaa, 2004). Selection sampling bias due to either snowball or convenience sampling methods is a frequently identified issue in driving studies. Other driving studies, both on-road and using simulators, frequently experience difficulty in assessing large sample sizes due to high costs, the necessity of the participant travelling to the assessment area and high dropout rates (Elvik & Vaa, 2004; Innes, et al., 2009; Kulisevsky & Pagonabarraga, 2009).

A significant difference was found between the groups on the Purdue Pegboard subtest of Both Hand for coordination and speed of bilateral hand movements. The multivariable analysis of driving performance to psychometric assessment results also suggests that the 'Both Hand' subtest may be linked to driving performance. The results reflect findings from an on-road study with 25 PD patients and 21 age matched controls (Wood, et al., 2005).

However, when interpreting the results of the present study, caution should be used due to the wide confidence intervals. Additionally, Bonferroni's correction principle for multiple testing needs to be considered, as the other results, including the overall score on the Purdue Pegboard, were not different. Therefore, the significant results on the Both Hands subtest may be due to random effect and not due to the physical symptoms of PD. It is therefore uncertain if motor performance affected the psychometric assessment results. All of the psychometric tests required physical input of data through pushing a button or writing the answer, which required a physical motor movement. It is therefore worth investigating the validity of the Oral Symbol Digit Modalities test, as well as other motor free tests, on driving performance; especially as the written versions of these assessments are routinely used to assess drivers with PD.

4.3 Driving simulator data
4.3.1 Length of simulator practice time
As previously mentioned, two participants requested additional practice in using the driving simulator. It was noted that both of these participants later experienced motion sickness and withdrew from the study. Kennedy and Fowlkes (2000) found that increased exposure to simulated environments might increase the rate of motion sickness-related participant dropouts. Although this study cannot comment upon this phenomenon, additional research into a possible correlation of exposure time to motion sickness would be useful to provide guidelines for simulator scenario design, especially for older adults or people with PD.

4.3.2 Baseline driving performance
Drivers with PD had a higher mean driving performance than the control group at baseline driving. However this was not statistically different. As shown in Figure 7, all of the scores of the drivers with PD group fell within the interquartile range of the control group. This means that groups cannot be differentiated based upon overall driving performance scores alone. There was also no statistical difference in time to complete trial one; showing that baseline time of the groups was the same. The sub sections of the Driving Performance Score that varied significantly between groups were "Frequency of Appropriate Use of Mirrors" and "Driver Maintains Correct Lane Position". The present study results are similar to the findings of numerous other studies, both on-road and using simulators, that claim that drivers with PD have more errors in these particular aspects of driving (Radford, et al., 2004; Uc, et al., 2009; Uitti, 2009). The present study suggests that although the drivers with PD had a lower driving performance score; this does not necessarily mean that they are 'dangerous' drivers. Similar findings were reported by Uc et al. (2009). Although the 84 drivers with PD in their study committed more lane placement errors, they were still found to be safe drivers overall. Numerous other studies also claim that drivers with PD can be safe drivers (Bryer, et al., 2006; Radford, et al., 2004). The results of the other studies, as with the present study, may have been influenced by self-selection bias as these studies also used convenience sampling and had a small sample size. Therefore, it is possible that people with PD may be safe drivers and so licences should not be cancelled based purely upon having a diagnosis of PD.

4.3.3 Driving with time pressure
When a time pressure was implemented, the median driving performance of both groups decreased; with the drivers with PD experiencing a significant decrease in performance.

The median driving performance of the drivers with PD declined more than the control group, but none of the drivers with PD were found to be unsafe drivers. This indicates that when drivers with PD are under time pressure, they may not be able to compensate for the additional task demands as well as healthy drivers. As previously mentioned, self-selection bias may have affected the results. The drivers with PD in the study may be better or more confident drivers, suggesting that the difference between groups may be more substantial if comparing a more representative sample of drivers with PD to the control group. Findings support the results found by four other studies into PD (Devos, et al., 2007; Factor & Weiner, 2002; Radford, et al., 2004). These results should, however be taken with caution due to the possibility of self-selection bias influencing results. Both groups were able to decrease their individual Scenario Completion Time significantly when instructed to do so in trial two. In addition, it was found that the control group had a significantly greater decrease in driving completion time, compared with the drivers with PD. The difference in Scenario Completion Time does not mean that the drivers with PD are worse drivers. However, it is an interesting trend that has been noticed by other researchers. For example, an on-road study with 77 drivers with PD also found that drivers with PD were slower in completing the route than the control group (Uc, et al., 2009). Reasons for this trend and potential implications for on-road driving performance cannot be established based upon the results of the present study. The reason for the difference in time to complete the trial cannot be ascertained with complete certainty. It is possible that the drivers with PD were unable to increase driving speed whilst maintaining safe driving performance, due to either decision making deficits or other factors. Alternatively, the results could demonstrate that drivers with PD were more cautious and aware of their limitations; making them unwilling to take risks. This information confirmed the assertions made by the drivers with PD about their perception of driving performance since the onset of their PD symptoms. The observation that drivers with PD are more cautious in their driving was also concluded by numerous other studies (Adler, et al., 2000; Devos, et al., 2007). Whether behaviours undertaken by drivers with PD to self-regulate their driving are successful in maintaining safe driving performance is an important area for future research. The results indicate that drivers with PD may be capable of driving safely; showing that research projects such as this study are important in preventing capable drivers from having their licence cancelled, purely due to a diagnosis of PD. The finding that drivers with PD may be safe drivers is supported by other studies into PD and driving (Bryer, et al., 2006; Radford, et al., 2004).

4.4 Methodological considerations and limitations
4.4.1 Reliable protocol
The reliability of the study was improved by using instruction videos, the driving simulator and standardised psychometric assessment tools. Although filming the videos and constructing an appropriate driving scenario were time consuming, these tools increased the repeatability of the study, reduced risk of inter-rater error and can enable the protocol to be generalised to clinical settings in future (Bedard, et al., 2010). Additionally, if this research project were to be repeated on a larger scale, the setting up of the assessment process and training of another researcher could be quickly performed with ease.

4.4.2 Learning effect
It is possible that a learning effect influenced the results, as the participants would have been more familiar with the driving simulator and the scenario during the second trial. However,

this learning effect would have affected participants in both groups equally. Participants were not aware beforehand that they would undergo assessment on the same scenario twice and therefore would not have actively tried to memorise events and hazards during the first trial.

4.4.3 Motion sickness

Motion sickness is a common problem integral in driving simulator assessment (Kulisevsky & Pagonabarraga, 2009). Although the simulator presents a visual appearance of movement, the vestibular and proprioceptive systems do not detect presence of movement. The inconsistencies in sensory information may trigger feelings of nausea, dizziness or elevated temperature. This occurs more commonly in more experienced drivers and in people who have not regularly played computer and video games (Kulisevsky & Pagonabarraga, 2009). The drop out due to motion sickness experienced in this study (25%) was within the range reported by other studies using driving simulators, from 9% (Lee, et al., 2003) to 57% (Kennedy & Fowlkes, 2000), with older drivers being more susceptible to motion sickness. Kulisevsky and Pagonabarraga (2009) found that participants who experienced motion sickness in simulated driving did not have a reduced performance during on-road assessment and suggested that incidence of motion sickness is related to factors other than driving ability.

Potential reasons for the increased rate of motion sickness may include the larger size of the main simulator screen, the addition of side screens, the increased period of exposure and complexity of the driving scenario. The driving scenario in the present study included, right hand turns, driving at high speeds, winding roads, over taking and complex intersections, which were not used in the previous studies (Cordell, et al., 2008; Lee, et al., 2003). These particular elements are known to increase the risk of motion sickness; however, they are also highlighted as driving situations that are known to be challenging for drivers with PD (Kennedy & Fowlkes, 2000). Bedard and colleagues recommended that drivers should be assessed in challenging situations to ensure the detection of poor driving performance. The side screens are smaller than the main screen and consequently, the scenario images do not match up with complete accuracy in real life driving. This discrepancy in scenario images has been found in other studies to increase rates of motion sickness (Kennedy & Fowlkes, 2000). However, Kennedy and Fowlkes (2000) concluded that motion sickness occurs even on very expensive simulators with motion platforms and so purchasing a more expensive simulator will not necessarily be sufficient to address this issue.

Length of exposure to the simulator has been found to increase the risk of motion sickness, particularly among older adults and people with cognitive impairments (Kennedy & Fowlkes, 2000). Good ventilation, low lighting, herbal ginger tea and/or ginger supplements and a gradual introduction to the simulator over a three-day period can also assist to reduce the risk of motion sickness (Kennedy & Fowlkes, 2000).

4.5 Recommendations for future research

It is important to continue to research the cognitive deficits of drivers with PD; particularly decision making ability, as both the complexity of traffic situations, and the prevalence of PD increases (Uitti, 2009). Duplicating study designs of research projects investigating cognitive deficits amongst people with dementia may assist in improving research protocols for drivers with PD (Elvik & Vaa, 2004). A repeat of this study using a larger sample size and including drivers with PD recruited from driving assessment centres is recommended to answer the research question. When using a driving simulator to assess drivers with PD, the researcher needs to consider the implications of potential motion sickness when planning the research methodology.

Elvik and Vaa (2004) suggest that older drivers could be disadvantaged during driving assessment, since their last assessment may be as long as 50 years previously. The stress and anxiety of assessment could potentially affect driving performance, meaning that the assessment results may not represent actual ability (Elvik & Vaa, 2004). In the present study, the average time since participants had had a driving assessment varied from one to 61 years, with 35 years being the average. Participants in the present study commented that having to undergo driving assessment was stressful. As previously discussed, regular on-road assessment is impractical due to long waiting periods and high costs. There is currently no funding available for drivers with PD to undergo neither driving assessment nor driving training. Therefore, the driving simulator could potentially be used as a low cost method to assist drivers with PD to adapt to the assessment process, or to screen for people who may need an on-road review assessment of driving (Lee, et al., 2003).

4.6 Conclusions

This study aimed to explore the impact of impaired decision making ability upon the driving performance of people with PD. There was no difference between the decision making abilities of the groups as measured on the psychometric assessment tools. At normal baseline driving, the drivers with PD used their side mirrors less frequently, had poorer lane placement and took longer to complete the route.

When instructed to finish the scenario faster, both groups were able to have a significant reduction in the scenario completion time. The time pressure also caused a significant reduction in the driving performance scores of the drivers with PD, particularly in their stopping distance from obstacles. However, both groups were able to navigate the driving scenario safely under a time pressure. It is not possible to determine if the difference in completion time was due to the drivers with PD being unable to complete the route faster, or being unwilling to do as they self-regulated their driving. It is important to note, that although there was a difference in driving performance, the drivers with PD were not found to be dangerous or unsafe drivers. As the psychometric assessment results of the groups were the same, the impact of decision making ability upon driving performance cannot be determined at this stage. Information from the chapter is valuable in providing recommendations for further research projects into driving, Parkinson's disease and simulator use.

5. References

Access Economics. (2010). *Federal policy initiatives: a new approach to Parkinson's disease.* Retrieved September 2, 2010, from http://www.parkinsonsnsw.org.au/assets/attachments/media/PA_NewPolicy Initiative.pdf

Adler, G., Rottunda, S., Bauer, M., & Kuskowski, M. (2000). The older driver with Parkinson's Disease. *Journal of Gerontological Social Work, 34*(2), 39 - 49. doi:10.1300/J083v34n02_05

Allen, R. W., Rosenthal, T. J., & Park, G. (2003). Assessment and training using a low cost driving simulator. In *Tenth International Conference on Human-Computer Interaction* (pp. 57-61). Crete, Greece: Systems Technology Inc.

Amick, M. M., Grace, J., & Ott, B. R. (2007). Visual and cognitive predictors of driving safety in Parkinson's disease patients. *Archives of Clinical Neuropsychology, 22*, 957-967. doi:10.1016/j.acn.2007.07.004

Anceaux, F., Pacaux, M. P., Halluin, N., Rajaonah, B., & Popieul, J. C. (2008). A methodological framework for assessing driving behaviour. In L. Dorn (Ed.), *Driver behaviour and training* (Vol. 3, pp. 203 - 213). Hampshire, England: Ashgate Publishing, Ltd.

Arias-Carrión, O., & Pöppel, E. (2007). Dopamine, learning and reward-seeking behaviour. *Acta Neurobiologiae Experimentalis, 67*(4), 481-488. Retrieved from http://www.ncbi.nlm.nih.gov/pubmed/18320725

Australian Bureau of Statistics. (2004). *The health of older people in Australia, 2001*(Catalogue No. 4827.0). Canberra, Australian Capital Territory: Commonwealth of Australia. Retrieved from http://www.abs.gov.au/AUSSTATS/abs@.nsf/DetailsPage/4827.0.55.001200

Australian Bureau of Statistics. (2008). *Causes of death in Australia, 2008* (Catalogue No. 3303.0). Canberra, Australian Capital Territory: Commonwealth of Australia. Retrieved from http://www.abs.gov.au/ausstats/abs@.nsf/mf/3303.0

Australian Bureau of Statistics. (2009). *Motor Vehicle Census in Australia, 2009* (Catalogue No. 9309.0). Canberra, Australian Capital Territory: Commonwealth of Australia. Retrieved from http://www.abs.gov.au/ausstats/abs@.nsf/mf/9309.0/

Austroads. (2000). Model license re-assessment procedure for older and disabled drivers. Sydney, NSW: Austroads Incorporated.

Bedard, M., Parkkari, M., Weaver, B., Riendeau, J., & Dahlquist, M. (2010). Assessment of driving performance using a simulator protocol: validity and reproducibility. *American Journal of Occupational Therapy, 64*, 336-340. doi:10.5014/ajot.64.2.336

Betz, M. E., & Fisher, J. (2009). Trail making test B and driver screening in emergency departments. *Traffic Injury Prevention, 10*(5), 415-420. doi:10.1080/15389580903132819

Bryer, R. C., Rapport, L. J., & Hanks, R. A. (2006). Determining fitness to drive: neuropsychological and psychological considerations. In J. M. Pellerito (Ed.), *Driver Rehabilitation and Community Mobility: Principles and Practice* (pp. 165-181). St. Louis, Missouri: Elsevier Mosby.

Busemeyer, J. R., & Stout, J. C. (2002). A contribution of cognitive decision models to clinical assessment: decomposing performance on the Bechara gambling task. *Psychological Assessment, 14*(3), 253-262. Retrieved from http://www.ncbi.nlm.nih.gov/pubmed/12214432

Cools, R., Barker, R. A., Sahakian, B. J., & Robbins, T. W. (2001). Enhanced or impaired cognitive function in Parkinson's disease as a function of dopaminergic medication and task demands. *Cerebral Cortex, 11*, 1136-1047. doi:10.1093/cercor/11.12.1136

Cordell, R., Lee, H. C., Granger, A., Vieira, B., & Lee, A. H. (2008). Driving assessment in Parkinson's disease: a novel predictor of performance. *Movement Disorders, 23*(9), 1217-1222. doi:10.1002/mds.21762

Corrigan, J. D., & Hinkeldey, M. S. (1987). Relationships between parts A and B of the trail making test. *Journal of Clinical Psychology, 43*(4), 402-409. Retrieved from http://www.ncbi.nlm.nih.gov/pubmed/3611374

De Winter, J. C., deGroot, S., Mulder, M., Wieringa, P. A., Dankelman, J., & Mulder, J. (2008). Relationships between driving simulator performance and driving test results. *Ergonomics, 28*, 1-24. doi:10.1080/00140130802277521

Devos, H., Vandenberghe, W., Nieuwboer, A., Tant, M., Baten, G., & De Weerdt, W. (2007). Predictors of fitness to drive in people with Parkinson's disease. *Neurology, 69*(14), 1434-1441. doi:10.1212/01.wnl.0000277640.58685.fc

Elvik, R., & Vaa, T. (2004). Concepts of road safety research. In R. Elvik, A. Høye, T. Vaa & M. Sørensen (Eds.), *Handbook of Road Safety Measures* (pp. 15-33). Oslo: Elsevier.

Ernst, M., & Paulus, M. P. (2005). Neurobiology of decision-making: a selective review from a neurocognitive and clinical perspective. *Biological Psychiatry, 58,* 597-604. doi:10.1016/j.biopsych.2005.06.004

Factor, S. A., & Weiner, W. J. (2002). Driving. In S. A. Factor & W. J. Weiner (Eds.), *Parkinson's disease: Diagnosis and Clinical Management* (pp. 647-703). London: Demos Medical Publishing.

Hedges, L. V. (2009). Statistical Considerations. In H. M. Cooper, L. V. Hedges & J. C. Valentine (Eds.), *The handbook of research synthesis and meta-analysis* (pp. 37-50). New York: Russell Sage Foundation.

Heikkila, V. M., Turkka, J., Korpelainen, J., Kallanranta, T., & Summala, H. (1997). Decreased driving ability in people with Parkinson's Disease. *Journal of Neurology Neurosurgery and Psychiatry, 64*(325-30). Retrieved from http://www.ncbi.nlm.nih.gov/pmc/articles/PMC2170019/

Innes, C. R. H., Jones, R. D., Anderson, T. J., Hollobon, S. G., & Dalrymple-Alford, J. C. (2009). Performance in normal subjects on a novel battery of driving related sensory-motor and cognitive tests. *Behaviour Research Methods, 41*(2), 284-894. doi:10.3758/BRM.41.2.284

Jankovic, J. (2007). Pathophysiology and clinical assessment. In R. Pahwa & K. E. Lyons (Eds.), *Handbook of Parkinson's Disease* (4th ed., pp. 49-76). Kansas City, Missouri: Informa Healthcare.

Kalis, A., Mojzisch, A., Schweizer, T. S., & Kaiser, S. (2008). Weakness of will, akrasia, and the neuropsychiatry of decision making: An interdisciplinary perspective. *Cognitive, Affective & Behavioural Neuroscience, 8*(4), 402-417. doi:10.3758/CABN.8.4.402

Kelland, D. Z., & Lewis, R. F. (1996). The digit vigilance test: reliability, validity, and sensitivity to diazepam. *Archives of Clinical Neuropsychology, 11*(4), 339-344. Retrieved from http://www.sciencedirect.com/science/article/B6VDJ-3Y2G16K-8/2/f4ed9a85da96e69b69ff7be

Kennedy, R. S., & Fowlkes, J. E. (2000). Duration and exposure to virtual environments: sickness curves during and across sessions. *Presence, 9,* 463-472. doi:10.1162/105474600566952

Kiernan, R. J., Mueller, K., Langston, J., & Van Dyke, C. (1987). The neurobehavioural cognitive status examination: a brief but differentiated approach to cognitive assessment. *Annals of Internal Medicine, 107,* 481-485. doi: http://www.annals.org/content/107/4/481.short

Kulisevsky, J., & Pagonabarraga, J. (2009). Review of cognitive impairment in Parkinson's disease: tools for diagnosis and assessment. *Movement Disorder Society, 24*(8), 1103-1110. doi:10.1002/mds.22506

Lafayette Instrument Company. (1985). *Instruments and normative data for the Model 32020, Purdue Pegboard.* IN: Lafayette Instrument Company.

Lee, H. C., Cameron, D., & Lee, A. (2003). Assessing the driving performance of older adult drivers: on-road versus simulated driving. *Accident Analysis & Prevention, 35*(5), 797-803. Retrieved from http://www.sciencedirect.com/science/article/B6V5S-47K2G65-/9309ee8116ccc84a88849d985bb715bc

Lotfipour, S., Patel, B., Grotsky, T., Anderson, C. L., Carr, E. M., Ahmed, S. S., et al. (2010). Comparison of the visual function index to the Snellen visual acuity test in predicting older adult self-restricted driving. *Traffic Injury Prevention, 11,* 503-507. doi: 10.1080/15389588.2010.488494

Meindorfner, C., Körner, Y., Möller, J. C., Stiasny-Kolsterm, K., Oertel, W. H., & Kruger, H. P. (2005). Driving in Parkinson's disease: mobility, accidents and sudden onset of sleep at the wheel. *Movement Disorder, 20*(7), 832-842. Retrieved from http://onlinelibrary.wiley.com/doi/10.1002/mds.20412/pdf

Michon, J. A. (1985). A critical review of driver behaviour models: what do we know, what should we do? In L. Evans & R. C. Schwing (Eds.), *Human Behaviour and Traffic Safety* (pp. 485-520). New York: Plenum.

Molnar, A., Marshall, H. L., & Man-Son-Hing, K. (2006). Clinical utility of office based cognitive predictors of fitness to drive in persons with dementia: a systematic review. *Journal of American Geriatrics Society, 54,* 1809-1824. doi:10.1111/j.1532-5415.2006.00967.x

National Road Transport Commission. (2003). *Assessing fitness to drive* (3rd ed.). Sydney, NSW: Austroads Incorporated.

Nieoullon, A. (2002). Dopamine and the regulation of cognition and attention. *Progress in Neurobiology, 67,* 52-83. doi:10.1016/S0301-0082(02)00011-4

Psychology Software Tools, I. (2010). E-Prime 2: selected publications and other works. Retrieved October, 12, 2010, from http://www.pstnet.com/eprimepublications.cfm

Radford, K. A., Lincoln, N. B., & Lennox, G. (2004). The effects of cognitive abilities on driving in people with Parkinson's disease. *Disability and Rehabilitation, 26*(2), 65-70. doi:10.1080/09638280310001629633

Ranzini, M., Dehaene, S., Piazzaa, M., & Hubbard, E. M. (2009). Neural mechanisms of attentional shifts due to irrelevant spatial and numerical cues. *Neuropsychologia, 47*(12), 2615-2624. Retrieved from http://www.ncbi.nlm.nih.gov/pubmed/19465038

Smith, A. (2007). *Symbol digit modalities test* (10 ed.). Los Angeles, CA: Western Psychological Services.

Stolwyk, R. J., Charlton, J. L., Triggs, T. J., Lansek, R., & Bradshaw, J. L. (2006). Neuropsychological function and driving ability in people with Parkinson's disease. *Journal of Clinical and Experimental Neuropsychology, 28*(6), 898 - 913. Retrieved from http://www.informaworld.com/10.1080/13803390591000909

Systems Techonology Inc. (2010). System techonology software. Retrieved September, 3, 2010, from http://www.systemstech.com

Tröster, A. I., & Woods, S. P. (2007). Neuropsychological aspects. In R. Pahwa & K. E. Lyons (Eds.), *Handbook of Parkinson's disease* (4th ed., pp. 109-130). New York: Informa Healthcare.

Uc, E. Y., Rizzo, M., Johnson, J. E., Dastrup, E., Anderson, S. W., & Dawson, J. (2009). Road safety in drivers with Parkinson's disease. *Neurology, 73,* 2112-2119. Retrieved from http://www.neurology.org/cgi/content/abstract/73/24/2112

Uitti, R. J. (2009). Parkinson's disease and issues related to driving. *Parkinsonism & Related Disorders, 15S3,* S122-125. Retrieved from http://www.sciencedirect.com.dbgw.lis.

Wood, J. M., Worringham, C., Kerr, G., Mallon, K., & Silburn, P. (2005). Quantitative assessment of driving performance in Parkinson's disease. *Journal of Neurology, Neurosurgery and Psychiatry, 76,* 176-180. doi:10.1136/jnnp.2004.047118

Cognitive Rehabilitation in Parkinson's Disease Using Neuropsychological Training, Transfer Training and Sports Therapy

I. Reuter[1], S. Mehnert[1], M. Oechsner[2] and M. Engelhardt[3]
[1]Dept. of Neurology, Justus-Liebig University, Giessen, Germany
[2]Neurologisches Rehabilitationszentrum, HELIOS Klinik Zihlschlacht AG,
[3]Dept. of Orthopedic Surgery, Klinikum Osnabrück,
[1,3]Germany
[2]Swiss

1. Introduction

1.1 Cognitive impairment in Parkinson's disease

Idiopathic Parkinson`s disease (PD) is a neurodegenerative disorder characterized by basal ganglia dysfunction frequently being associated with frontostriatal dysfunction and cognitive impairment. The prevalence of PD increases with age and is estimated at 100-200/100000 people (Chen et al., 2001; Schrag et al., 2000) worldwide. The clinical hallmarks of PD are akinesia, rigidity and tremor (Douglas et al., 1999; Hughes et al., 1992). In the past PD has been considered as a pure movement disorder, but in recent years the presence of non-motor symptoms in PD has been recognized. Non-motor symptoms include a variety of autonomic dysfunctions such as orthostatic hypotension, postural tachycardia, bladder dysfunction, sleep disturbances, psychiatric symptoms, i.e. depression, hallucinations or psychosis and cognitive impairment. Non-motor symptoms such as pain, depression or sleep disturbances might precede the onset of motor symptoms in PD and are sometimes even more disabling than motor deficits. For many years cognitive impairment and the occurrence of dementia have been considered as not typical for IPD. James Parkinson (Parkinson, 1817) wrote in his essay on the shaking palsy " the senses are not disturbed". However, there is now enough evidence in the literature that dementia might occur in up to 40% of PD-patients (Emre et al., 2004). PD dementia is the third most common reason for dementia. Dementia in PD has been associated with reduced quality of life, greater sensitivity to medication, higher risk of developing psychosis, shortened survival (Levy, 2002), increased caregivers stress and frequent transfer to nursing homes (Aarsland et al., 2000) compared to PD-patients without dementia. In contrast to dementia mild cognitive impairment might occur early in the course of the disease. Approximately, a quarter of PD-patients without dementia have mild cognitive impairment (PD-MCI) and 20% might have MCI at the time of diagnosis (Aarsland et al., 2011). The cognitive deficits in PD are specific and include executive dysfunction, attentional and visuospatial deficits. Executive functions include control, manipulation, and cognitive flexibility (Funahashi et al., 2001; Lezak, 1995) and is part of working memory (Carpenter et al., 2000). The executive system is thought to be involved in handling new situations outside the domain of automatic psychological processes (no reproduction of learned schedules or set behaviours). The theoretic model of the executive system has been modified several times over the years. Crucial contributions to the concept of executive functions came from Norman (1980, 2000), Shallice (1982), Baddeley (1986) and Miller & Cohen (2001). In summary, executive functions involve planning and decision making, influence our handling and the processing of information. Furthermore, they are involved in error corrections or troubleshooting, in situations which require new sequences of actions. Components of the executive systems are attention (focusing on relevant information), selective visual attention, inhibition (inhibition of irrelevant information)(Smith & Jonides, 1999), overcoming of strong habitual responses or resisting temptation (Burgess & Shallice, 1996), task and time management, monitoring and coding of information for processing in the working memory, flexibility, set maintenance and set shifting. The executive system can be viewed as a manager enabling the adaptation of the perceptive, cognitive and motor system to new tasks. Some authors have claimed that cognitive control is the primary function of the prefrontal cortex (Miller & Cohens, 2001). Cognitive control is implemented by increasing gain of sensory or motor neurons that are involved in task or goal relevant actions (Miller & Cohen, 2001).

Patients with impaired executive functions face many difficulties in everyday life. They have a low attention span, difficulties in problem solving and decision making, in dual tasking, in set shifting, in visuoconstructive tasks, in adaptation to new tasks and even in verbal learning and delayed recall. Thus, PD-patients with impairment of executive functions have difficulties in simultaneously driving a car and searching for a street or in preparing a meal for several people. They also have difficulties in keeping appointments. Relatives report that patients avoid difficult tasks and retreat from social life. Executive dysfunctions also affect the social components and the interaction with other people (Smith & Jonides, 1999). Patients are reported of being more irritable and having difficulties in suppressing inadequate behaviour.

It has been proposed that executive dysfunction underlies all manifestations of cognitive impairment in PD (Lewis et al., 2005) as part of the 'frontal-executive brain syndrome' (Godefroy, 2003). In accordance Colman et al. (2009) found that executive dysfunction also underlies the performance of PD-patients on verb production.

Pathophysiologically (Leverenz et al., 2009) cognitive impairment in PD might be either associated with catecholaminergic or indolaminergic neurotransmission or with Alzheimer´s disease (AD) related pathology. While the first form manifests mainly with non amnestic features like impaired EF, and might be correlated with Lewy related pathology in limbic and neocortical regions. The second type of CI manifests in amnestic CI and might derive from processes of AD intersecting with PD. 40% of patients develop dementia (Emre et al., 2004).

1.2 Pathophysiology of cognitive impairment in PD

Decline of cognitive performance in PD might result from rupture of nigro-striatum-thalamus cortical circuit interconnecting the striatum to the prefrontal cortex, cholinergic deficits through the differentiation of neurons in the nucleus basalis of Meynert and the pedunculopontine-lateral dorsal tegmental neurons (Calabresi et al., 2006).

In PD the production of dopamine (DA) in the substantia nigra (SN) is decreased. DA is a major neurotransmitter of the basal ganglia, contributing seriously to the development of frontal-executive dysfunction. Dopaminergic frontal systems play a major role in working memory and executive function (Goldman-Rakic et al., 1992), especially the dorsolateral prefrontal lobe. However, dopaminergic medication has not shown to have a substantial effect on cognitive problems in PD (Fournet et al., 2000; Lewis et al. , 2005,). So far, medical treatment has not been effective enough to prevent PD dementia and restore executive dysfunction.Acetylcholine esterase inhibitors improve cognitive functioning only in some patients.

Furthermore, there is a large body of studies on animals and humans in the literature showing a positive effect of exercise and sports on cognition (Abbott et al., 2004; Colombe et al., 2003a, 2003b, 2006; Laurin et al., 2001; Rolland et al., 2010). Several studies suggest an enhancement of cortical plasticity by exercise. It is assumed that physical exercise mediates increased expression of neurotrophic factors as glial-derived neurotrophic factor (GDNF), basic fibroblast growth factor (FGF-2) , or brain-derived neurotrophic factor (BDNF) (Kleim et al., 2003). BDNF is a member of the neurotrophin family of growth factors vital for trophic support of neurons within both the peripheral and central nervous system. BDNF signals through tyrosine kinase receptor B and through the p75 receptor. Both are expressed by dopamine neurons. Postmortem studies in PD have shown that PD is associated with reduced BDNF levels in the SNC (Howells et al., 2000)

1.3 Treatment options for cognitive decline in PD

Executive functioning was found to be improved by aerobic endurance exercise (Colcombre & Kramer, 2003; Kramer et al., 1999). Motor training was reported to improve cortical plasticity and cortical reorganisation (Nelles 2004; Shepherd 2001). Physical exercise also was found to improve the quality of daily living (Baatile et al., 2000, Reuter et al., 1999) in PD-patients. Furthermore, Hausdorff et al (2005) have shown that higher cognitive functions correlate with gait variability while Ble et al. (2005) reported a close correlation between executive functions and tasks of the lower extremities.

Since patients with mild cognitive impairment have a higher risk to develop dementia, intervention at an early stage of cognitive decline is desirable. Patients who complain of cognitive problems suffer more often from cognitive deficits than patients without complaints (Dujardin et al., 2010). Therefore, these patients should be offered neuropsychological testing and treatment. However, according to our experience, it is difficult to convince patients to participate in cognitive training programmes. PD-patients noting declining cognitive performance are often anxious and ashamed of having cognitive problems. They rather deny their problems and try to avoid situations which make their problems obvious to other people. On the other hand the majority of PD-patients is very interested in exercise- and sport-programmes focusing on improvement of motor skills and mobility. Considering the correlation between cognitive function and motor tasks, it might be possible to improve cognitive function by physical training. Furthermore, achievements in cognitive training performed at a writing desk are often difficult to transfer into daily life. Therefore, we have chosen a comprehensive approach and designed a study using a multimodal cognitive training to improve cognitive functions.

The aim of the present study was to compare the effect of a multimodal cognitive training regime including paper and pencil tasks combined with transfer tasks and a psychomotor training with a cognitive training performed at a writing desk and a cognitive training consisting of various tasks requiring executive functions combined with transfer tasks.

2. Methods

2.1 Subjects

240 patients with idiopathic Parkinson`s disease according to the UK brain bank criteria (Hughes et al., 1991) and complaints about cognitive problems were recruited for the study at the Parkinson clinic Bad Nauheim. Exclusion criteria were severe concomitant diseases, which limit physical performances, and a second neurodegenerative disease. All patients were assessed by a movement disorder specialist. Medical treatment was optimised prior to the study. It was aimed at keeping medication stable during the study. Demographic data included age, body mass index (BMI), duration of disease, weekly sports activity, smoking habits, medication and concomitant diseases (hypertension, chronic obstructive pulmonary disease, thyroid disease, diabetes mellitus, hypercholesterinaemia, osteoarthritis).

2.2 Design

The study was divided into two phases, the first part consisted of a 4-week in-patient stay on a rehabilitation unit with a supervised cognitive training conducted by physiotherapists, occupational therapists and two neuropsychologists.

Patients were randomly allocated to one of the three training groups. Randomisation was conducted by using a computer-generated sequence. All groups received a cognitive training regime using paper and pencil material and a multimedial PC-training. Group A received cognitive training only, while group B took part in a transfer training and a cognitive training. Group C conducted a cognitive training, transfer- and psychomotor training. Patients of group A and B had relaxation training in addition to compensate for the additional training times and occupational therapy without translation training. (Fig. 1) The ethical committee of the Justus-Liebig University has approved the study and all patients gave informed consent. At the baseline visit a medical history was taken and all patients underwent a neurological assessment. Severity of disease was assessed by using the Unified Parkinson`s Disease rating scale (UPDRS).

Demographic data included information about education, profession, family, onset and severity of disease, medication, history of psychosis and impairments in daily living. Patients kept an activity log one week prior to the training programme and one week prior to the third assessment. Sports activities and time spent sitting, doing light, moderate, heavy work were recorded.

2.2.1 Scales used for neurological and neuropsychological assessment of PD

2.2.1.1 UPDRS

For the assessment of the longitudinal course of the disease the Unified Parkinson`s disease rating scale (UPDRS) was applied. The UPDRS is the most frequently used outcome measure in clinical trials in Parkinson`s disease (Fahn et al., 1987). The UPDRS has four subscales: part 1, which has 4 questions on mentation, behaviour and mood (range 0-16 points), part 2, which has 13 questions on activities of daily living (ADL) (range 0-52 points); part 3, which has 14 questions on motor functions (range 0-108 points); and part 4, which has 11 questions on motor and other complications of advanced disease (0-23 points). The UPDRS-Sum score ranges from 0 to 199 points, with a higher score indicating greater problems.

Study design

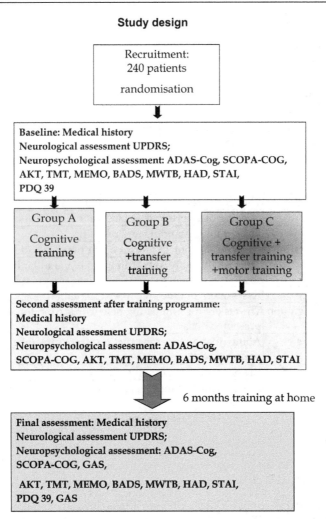

Fig. 1. Study design: First phase of the study: randomisation into three treatment arms, in-patient treatment; second phase of the study: training at home

Posture, postural stability, alternating movements and leg agility were assessed by using the single items of the UPDRS motor scale. The score of each item ranges between 0 to 4 points.

2.2.1.2 Goal attainment scale

The Goal Attainment Scaling (GAS) allows individualisation of realistic and feasible goals according to patient needs and expectations. All patients identified a task they want to improve by the training programme. In this study, GAS was measured using a 6-point scale, where −3 represented function that is worse than at the start of treatment, −2 was no change, −1 represented some improvement but did not meet the expected goal, 0 represented goal achievement and +1 or +2 represented over-achievement or exceeding the defined therapeutic goal (Royal College of Physicians, 2008).

2.2.1.3 Neuropsychological tests:

For neuropsychological assessment all patients underwent a detailed cognitive test battery at the beginning of the study including the ADAS-Cog subscale and the SCOPA-COG as outcome measures.

A: ADAS-Cog (Alzheimer Disease Assessment Scale-Cognition)

Although the ADAS-Cog is not a specific test for cognitive impairment in Parkinson`s Disease the scale was chosen as primary outcome measure in the current study, because it was the primary outcome measure in earlier trials assessing effects of medication on cognitive function in PD (Tab.1).

No	. Task	Characteristics	Score
1	Word recall	The recall task of frequent, easily to imagine words	0-10p
2	Naming	Naming of 12 presented objects and fingers on a hand	0-5p
3	Commands	Task of understanding and fulfilling	0-5p
4	Constructional	Drawing 4 geometric forms using praxis a pattern	0-5p
5	Ideational	The task of ability to perform praxis a familiar but complex sequence of actions	0-5p
6	Orientation	Assessment of time and space orientation	0-8 p
7	Word recognition	The task of discriminating new words from the already presented ones	0-12p
8	Instructions	Ability to remember instructions from remembering the previous recognition task	0-5p
9	Spoken language	Assessment of the quality of patient.s age ability speech	0-5p
10	Word finding	Assessment of patients ability to difficulty communicate verbally	0-5p
11	Comprehension	The patients ability to understand the spoken speech	0-5p

Table 1. Structure of ADAS-Cog scale.

The ADAS-Cog scale was the primary outcome measure in many clinical trials (Rosen WG et al., 1984). The conceptual framework underlying the ADAS-Cog identifies three reproducible factors: memory, language, praxis (Talwalker et al., 1996). The ADAS-Cog score ranges in total from 0 to 70 points with higher scores indicating greater impairment. Language ability is tested by naming objects and fingers, observer rated comprehension of spoken language, expressive language and word finding (range 0-25 points; memoryis tested by recall of instructions, word list recall and recognition (range 0-27 points), test of praxis (range 0-10 points) consists of constructional praxis (copying geometric figures) and ideational praxis (preparing envelope to send to oneself), orientation is assessed for time and space orientation (range 0-8points).

B: SCOPA-COG(Scales for Outcome of Parkinson`s disease-Cognition)

The SCOPA-COG is an instrument which was designed to assess the specific cognitive deficits found in Parkinson`s disease (Marinus et al., 2003). The scale consisting of 10 items covers the domains: memory and recall (verbal recall, digit span backward, indicate cubes), attention (counting backward, months backward), executive function (fist-edge-palm, semantic fluency, dice), visual-spatial functions (assembly pattern) and memory (delayed recall). The score ranges from 0 to 43 points with higher scores reflecting better performance.

Further tests requiring executive and memory functions for assessment of cognitive performance of the PD-patients at baseline, second and final assessment were conducted.

C: Mini Mental test (MMSE)

The Mini mental state examination (Folstein et al., 1975) was used as screening tool for dementia. The test assesses orientation, registration, attention, calculation, recall, language, writing and copying. The maximum score is 30 points; high scores indicate good performance. The cut off criteria for an abnormal result are 24 points and below. Dementia was assumed for less than 20 points.

D: Alters-Konzentrationstest

For assessment of attention the Alters-Konzentrationstest (Gatterer et al., 1989) was applied. Patients are asked to mark specific figures out of other figures alike the target. Time to complete the test, number of correctly marked figures, number and type of mistakes are recorded.

E: Paced auditory serial addition test (PASAT)

The Paced Auditory Serial Addition Test (Gronwall et al., 1977) assesses auditory information processing speed and flexibility and ability to calculate. Single digits are presented either every 3 seconds (trial 1) or every 2 seconds (trial 2). The patient has to add each new digit to the one immediately prior to it. The maximal possible score adds up to 60, the individual test score is equal to the total number of correct sums in each trial. In the current study the slower speed was used.

F: Trail making test

The trail making test (Reitan, 1958) assesses visual attention and task switching. Numbers from 1 to 30 are spread over a sheet, the patient is asked to connect the numbers in ascending order. Time and errors are recorded.

G: MEMO-Test

The MEMO-Test (Schaaf et al., 1994) assesses short-term verbal memory. Ten words are read to the patient. Five trials are performed. Patients are asked to repeat the words immediately, after each trial the words left out are read again. The following assessments are performed: UR: all words produced by short-term memory, ALZS: all words recalled from long term memory, UR + ALZS: all words recalled; KALZS: all words permanently recalled from long term memory; NKALZS: all words inconsistently recalled from long term memory; LZS: all words recalled from long term memory; delayed recall after 15 min..

H: Behavioural assessment of the dysexecutive syndrome (BADS)

The BADS (Wilson et al., 1998) is a battery of tests assessing executive function and comprises several subtests. In this study the Rule Shift Card test was applied to identify perseverative tendencies and mental flexibility, the Zoo Map test assessing was used the ability to plan and the Modified Six Element test, a test of planning, task scheduling and performance monitoring, were applied.

I : Mehrfach-Wortschatz-Test (MWT-B) Multiple choice word test

The MWT-B (Lehrl, 1989) serves as a control factor. A list consisting of 37 rows with 5 words is shown to the patient. Only one of the five words has a real meaning the others are fantasy words. The patients should mark the word with the meaning. The correct answers are added up to the sum-score. Each score is related to a standard score (z) which estimates the IQ of the patient.

K: Hospital anxiety and depression scale

The Hospital anxiety and depression scale (Zigmond & Snaith, 1983) was applied for exclusion of significant depression and anxiety. The scale consists of two subscales, an anxiety scale and a depression scale ranging from 0 to 21 points respectively. Patients are asked to choose one response from the four given for each question. Patients were strongly encouraged to respond promptly. Questions related to anxiety are marked with A and to depression with D. Depression and anxiety are scored separately. On each scale 0 to 7 points indicate a normal, 8 to 10 points a borderline abnormal and 11 or more points an abnormal result.

L: State Trait anxiety inventory (STAI)

The STAI scales (Spielberger et al., 1970) assess the trait anxiety (X2) and the anxiety in a specific situation (X1). Each scale consists of 20 items. Both scales present the answers on a 4 point Likert scale. Both scales range from 20 to 80 points with high scores indicating a high anxiety level.

M: Parkinson`s disease Questionnaire 39 (PDQ 39)

For assessment of health related quality of life patients filled in the PDQ 39 (Jenkinson et al., 1997, Peto et al., 1995). It consists of 8 subscales: subscale 1 mobility (max. 40 points); subscale 2 activities of daily living (max. 24 points), subscale 3 emotional well being (max. 24 points), subscale 4 stigma (max 16 points), subscale 5 social support (max 12 points), subscale 6 cognition (max.16 points), subscale 7 communication (max.12 points), subscale 8 bodily discomfort (max. 12 points) . The sum score of raw data ranges from 0 to 156 points, with high scores indicating lower health related quality of life. For better comparison of the results raw data were transformed and expressed in percentages of maximal possible sum score.

2.2.2 Training programmes

A: Cognitive training

The cognitive training content was individually tailored to patients` requirements based on the results of the baseline tests. Four individual (one to one) lessons took place each week each lasting 60 min. All patients received at least 14 cognitive training sessions.

The training included training of attention, concentration, biographical work, reasoning, memory, working memory, social rules, anticipation, cognitive information speed, prospective memory, cognitive estimation, problem solving, sequencing and planning, associations and coping with disease.

For the training programme a set of tasks requiring executive and memory functions were chosen from a variety of specific tests. Executive tasks of the BADS, which were not used for baseline tests were included in the training. Simple patterns of the "Raven`s Progressive Matrices" were used to establish problem solving strategies in the patients. Picture arrangement tasks, picture completion tasks, block design, and object assembly were adapted from the "Wechsler Intelligence test for children". For improvement of verbal fluency patients were encouraged to tell short stories or discuss short text-passages. Photos were used for training of working memory. Tasks including visual search, rule finding were practised by using a PC-based programme. The training methods were designed to improve the various cognitive deficits, diagnosed at baseline and focused on the executive functions. Task difficulty was adapted to the individual performance level of the patients.

B: Transfer tasks

The aim of the training was to support patients to manage better their daily life and to become more self-confident. Therefore, patients were asked to practise competence in tasks of daily routines. The transfer training programme was composed according to the baseline test results. Special preferences of the patients were considered. The transfer training included a training of concentration, use of mnemonics, strategy (planning), navigational skills, impulse control, decision processes, listening training and memory, behaviour, calculating, handling of money, summarising of articles read or heard and decision making. Typical tasks were to find the way to the supermarket or to prepare a meal, to go to the bank, pay a bill and to use mnemonics. For better evaluation of the training tasks were allocated to different categories: concentration, strategy, improvement of orientation, planning, use of mnemonic devices. The training took place 3 times a week each lasted 90 min. Patients received at least 10 sessions of transfer training.

C: Motor training

Group C performed a motor training resembling psychomotor training lessons applied in children. Psychomotor training (Golubović et al., 2011; Oswald et al., 1996) reflects a relationship between cognitive functions and physical movements. It includes training of co-ordination, strength, speed, perception and orientation. Patients should discover their body and their feelings. The therapeutic approach is multidimensional and based on individual capabilities and needs. The aim of the training was to practise motor sequences, dual tasking (walking and bouncing or throwing a ball, orientation in a space, walking through a parcours to improve anticipation. In summer the training was conducted partly outdoors with inclusion of Nordic walking. Thus, the training combines aerobic and psychomotor components. The training included at least 10, maximal 12 sessions each lasting 60 minutes.

2.2.3 Education of caregivers

A long lasting training effect depends on continuing training. Thus, cognitive training and exercises need to be adapted to the home environment. Consequently, the caregivers most often the patients` family were included in the programme. The education for the caregivers consisted of 5 modules (information about Parkinson`s disease, psychological aspects and the role of a caregiver, information about help aids, information on care instructions, assessment of individual problems, support in cognitive (all groups) and transfer training (group A and B), NW and psychomotor training). Course instructors were a specialist nurse, physiotherapist and a psychologist.

2.2.3.1 Phase II Continuing training

Corresponding to the allocation to the training groups patients got lessons for the cognitive training, transfer training and physical exercises for the training at home. Caregivers were advised how to organise the training but the hospital staff did not organise the training at home.

2.2.3.2 Evaluation of the training

All patients were tested using a neuropsychological test battery: prior to the training and prior to discharge to assess the short term effect and 3 months after the training to assess the long-term effect.

Caregivers were asked regarding their own well being and regarding the cognitive competence of the patients in daily living. Patients and caregivers kept a diary to record training lesions. The diaries were collected and analysed at the 3rd. assessment.

2.3 Statistical analysis

Statistical analysis was conducted using IBM SPSS Statistics 18.0 (IBM, Somers, USA) statistical software. Formal power analysis was performed prior to the study. The power analysis was based on an improvement of the ADAS-Cog by 3 points. The results indicated that a sample size of 60 subjects per group was sufficient. Since comprehensive training programmes including several assessments imply drop outs, a drop out rate of 20% was taken into account. Demographic data on ordinal level were analysed by using a non-parametric test (Kruskall-Wallis). The Kruskall-Wallis test was also applied for the analysis of depression and the BADS subscales. Continuous data were analysed by using a One – way-ANOVA. The repeated measure analysis provides information about "between and within subjects" effects. Within subject effects give information about training effects over the assessment period. Linear trends were extracted by orthogonal polynomials and analysed for days and for trials (Memo test). Linear trends showed if there was a systematic change of training effects over time. The interaction between groups and the linear trend of days yielded information about difference in the rate of improvement between groups. The between subject factor compared the overall treatment effect between the groups. Post hoc analysis was done using Bonferroni tests. Parametric data were tested for normal distribution by using the Kolmogorov-Smirnov test. Significance level was set at 0.05.

		Group A (N = 71)		Group B (N = 75)		Group C (N = 76)	
gender		F=35	M = 36	F = 36	M = 39	F = 36	M = 40
Duration of PD (months)		98± 8		95 ± 9		100 ± 6	
Stage (Hoehn & Yahr)	II	8		6		10	
	III	55		59		58	
	IV	9		10		8	
Medication	L-Dopa	Yes = 68		Yes = 64		Yes = 59	
	Dopamine agonist	Yes = 53		Yes = 56		Yes = 59	
	MA0 inhibitor	N = 43		N = 38		N = 43	
	COMT inhibitor	N = 33		N = 31		N = 34	
	Antidepressants	N = 7		N = 8		N = 8	
	Neuroleptic drugs	N = 5		N = 8		N = 7	
Formal education (years)		10 ± 1.2		11 ± 0.6		11 ± 1.0	
Marital status m = married, s = single, c = partner		m = 58	s = 9	p = 5 / m = 61	s = 11	p = 3 / m = 63	s = 9	p = 4
Home (own home, renting)		Own = 40	Renting = 32	Own = 43	Renting = 32	Own = 40	Renting= 36
BMI		27.5 ± 4		26.8 ± 7		27.2 ± 3	
Smoking		Yes = 7	No = 65	Yes = 10	No = 65	Yes = 9	No = 67
Sports activities (min)		∅ 155 ± 17		∅ 163 ± 25		∅ 147 ± 17	
Comorbidity	Coronary Heart disease	N = 7		N = 6		N = 8	
	Hypertension	N = 32		N = 33		N = 36	
	Diabetes mellitus	N = 7		N = 10		N = 8	
	COPD	N = 5		N = 6		N = 9	
	Thyroid disease	N = 12		N = 10		N = 11	
	Hypercholesteriaemia	N = 36		N = 32		N = 27	
	Osteoarthritis	N = 27		N = 31		N = 34	

Table 2. Demographic data

3. Results

3.1 General results, demographic data and accomplishment of the training

In total 222 patients (97.1%) completed the programme, 71 patients in group A, 75 patients in group B and 76 patients in group C.

The patients were on average 64 ± 4 years old and c. 8 years diagnosed with PD. The patients did not differ significantly in demographic data (Tab. 2). There was no difference in PD specific impairment and in the progress of PD between the groups.

The physical activity of the patients did not differ significantly either.

Patients of group A reported to perform 8.5 ± 2.6 hours very hard work per week, while patients of group B and C reported of 9.2 ± 2.8 and 9.8 ± 2.1hours very hard work respectively. Group A managed 15.2 ± 4.5, Group B 14.9 ± 5 and Group C 15.1 ± 5.5 hard work.

The neuropsychological baseline assessment did not reveal any differences between the groups. The multiple choice word test (MWT-B) was conducted as a measure for premorbid intelligence, the groups did not differ significantly, either. Thus the randomisation process was successful.

A: Cognitive Training:

The groups differed in time of practising concentration tasks and sequencing and planning tasks (F = 3.60; df = 2; p < 0.03). Group A and B spent 12% respectively 15% of the training with concentration training, group c only 8%. In contrast group C spent 22% of the training time with sequencing and planning tasks while group A 16% and group B 17%. The other training areas did not differ significantly between the groups (Fig. 2).

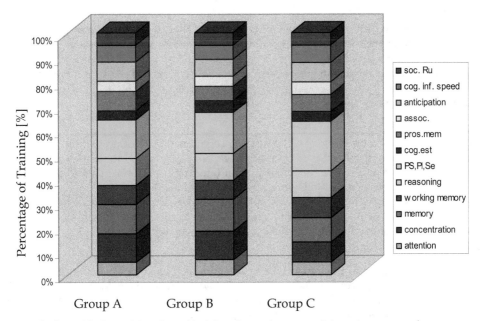

Soc.Ru= social rules; cog.inf.speed= cognitive information speed, assoc.=association; pros.mem= prospecive memory

Fig. 2. Group C spent more time of the training with sequencing and planning tasks, while group A spent more time with concentration tasks.

B: Transfer training

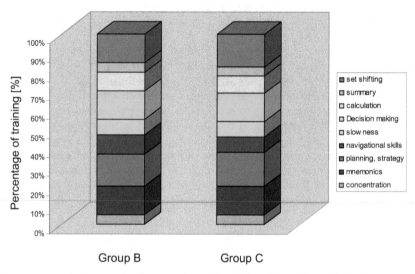

Fig. 3. There was no difference in the quantity and quality of transfer training between group B and C.

C: Motor training

Patients had many difficulties to cope with the tasks. They struggled to find strategies to solve the tasks on their own. The type of tasks and exercises were new to the majority of patients. The character of the tasks challenged the patients since PD-patients have both, deficits in proprioception and in perception of stimuli. The lessons were conducted as individual lessons. It was not possible to conduct group lessons. About 40% of the training took place outdoors, 60% in the gym.

D: Training at home

60% of patients of group A continued practising cognitive tasks 3 times a week, while 40% conducted the training only once or twice per week. All patients of group B tried to continue the transfer tasks learnt during the rehabilitation but further assessment showed that only 60% performed transfer tasks following a regular schedule. 90% of the patients practised cognitive tasks 3 times a week. Patients of Group C spent more time practising cognitive and transfer tasks than the other both groups. Patients conducted the physical training programme most often together with their spouses and very regularly.

E: Assessment of the training by the patients

Patients were asked to evaluate the training programme. Patients of group A felt that the cognitive training was arduous at times. Some patients perceived the training as stressful. Patients of group B and C were asked to compare the training programmes. Patients of group C preferred the motor training to transfer training and cognitive pencil and paper tasks. 80% of patients judged the training as strenuous and felt sometimes exhausted. 30% of patients reported of being frustrated at times but did not ask for help or further explanations.

F: Assessment of the training programme by the caregivers

Caregivers felt more relaxed and competent to handle difficult situation, while patients accepted the guidance of their care, felt more confident and thought that the caregivers were more understanding. Both, patients and caregivers felt competent to continue the training at home.

3.2 Neuropsychological results

Test	Baseline	T1	T2	Significance between groups
MMST				
Group A	27.36 ± 1.76	n.d.	26.4 ± 1.8	
Group B	27.6 ± 1.89	n.d.	27.1 ± 1.7	n.s.
Group C	28.14 ± 1.81	n.d.	28.5 ± 1.8	
ADAS-Cog				
Group A	21.51 ± 2.27	20.81 ± 2.77	20.5 ± 3.6	
Group B	21.37 ± 4.11	18.33 ± 3.67	18.5 ± 4.2	p< 0.001
Group C	22.92 ± 4.02	17.98 ± 2.76	17.4 ± 2.5	
SCOPA-COG				
Group A	29.07 ± 3.8	27.21 ± 3.6	26.86 ± 3.32	
Group B	29.68 ± 2.87	31.32 ± 3.24	30.71 ± 2.9	p< 0.001
Group C	31.83 ± 3.21	39.15 ± 2.9	39.29 ± 2.72	
TMT				
Group A	34.23 ± 16.87	31.7 ± 13.79	32.6 ± 14.5	
Group B	34.19 ± 15.6	32.0 ± 14.5	31.4 ± 13.5	p < 0.001
Group C	33.98 ± 15.8	26.2 ± 13.4	23.12 ± 9.8	
AKT (time)				
Group A	40.76 ± 15.2	42.85 ± 15.2	42.3 ± 14.2	
Group B	44.96 ± 16.5	41.67 ± 16.4	42.5 ± 15.3	n.s.
Group C	41.36 ± 15.23	40.98 ± 16.3	41.3 ± 16.3	
BADS Zoo (profile)				
Group A	2.5 ± 0.95	3.0 ± 1.2	2.4 ± 1.2	T1:
Group B	2.4 ± 0.9	2.8 ± 1.1	2.6 ± 1.1	Chi-square:
Group C	2.6 ± 0.98	3.54 ± 0.82	3.43 ± 1.0	49.31; p < 0.001 T2: Chi-square: 14.421; p > 0.001
BADS instruction				
Group A	2.8 ± 1.3	3.3 ± 1.1	2.9 ± 0.8	T1:
Group B	2.6 ± 1.3	2.9 ± 1.2	3.2 ± 1.1	Chi-square: 7.1;
Group C	2.7 ± 1.1	3.5 ± 1.1	3.8 ± 0.9	p < 0.03 T2: Chi-square: 9.1 p > 0.01

BADS 6 elements				
Group A	2.8 ± 1.2	3.14 ± 0.89	3.1 ± 0.9	T1:
Group B	2.9 ± 1.2	3.0 ± 1.2	2.9± 1.1	Chi-square: 39.4;
Group C	3.0. ± 0.7	3.55 ± 0.8	3.6 ± 0.9	$p < 0.001$ T2: Chi-square: 25.3 $p > 0.01$
PASAT				
Group A	29.94 ± 14.32	32.8 ± 14.83	32.5 ± 13.87	
Group B	31.00 ± 13.32	37.43 ± 12.72	39.57 ± 13.65	$p < 0.001$
Group C	30.4 ± 12.98	46.5 ± 11.5	49.2 ± 13.4	
TKS (points)				
Group A	10.1 ± 2.4	11.2 ± 2.2	11.2 ± 2.1	
Group B	10.7 ± 2.5	11.2 ± 2.1	11.24 ± 2	$p < 0.01$
Group C	11.0 ± 2.5	12.5 ± 2.2	12.8 ± 1.9	
STAI X1				
Group A	44.8 ± 10.9	39.62 ± 10.56	38.98 ± 10.4	
Group B	44.42 ± 11.43	42.43 ± 11.2	38.65 ± 9.87	n.s.
Group C	43.53 ± 9.8	38.76 ± 9.8	36.87 ± 10.0	
STAI X2				
Group A	42.68 ± 10.42	40.03 ± 10.2	41.2 ± 10.1	
Group B	41.84 ± 10.44	39.8 ± 9.8	40.2 ± 9.8	n.s.
Group C	40.72 ± 9.98	38.8 ± 9.6	38.2 ± 10.2	

Table 3. Summary of neuropsychological test results

3.2.1 Primary outcome measure

A: ADAS-Cog

All groups improved on the ADAS-Cog significantly shown by a significant linear trend (F_{lin} [1, 220] = 150; p< 0.001. Group C improved most indicated by a significant interaction between groups and days ($F_{groups \times days}$ [1, 220] = 27.26; p < 0.001) and a significant group difference (F [2,220] = 7.7, p < 0.001). Further analysis showed that 78% of the patients showed some improvement at the second assessment, 51% of patients of group A, 85% of patients of group B and 96% of patients of group C. 50% of the patients reached a reduction of the ADAS-Cog score of 3 or more points, 18% of group A, 54% of group B and 76% of group C. Six months after discharge of the rehabilitation unit 35% of patients (50% of patients of group A, 31% of patients of group B and 28% of group C) showed a deterioration compared to the assessment at the end of the in-patient training programme. Further improvement was observed in 21% patients of Group A, 37% patients of group B and 50% patients of group C.

B: SCOPA-COG

In accordance the SCOPA-COG test showed a significant difference between the groups (Fig. 4). All groups improved, indicated by the linear trend of days (F_{lin}[1, 220) = 46.09; p <

0.001). Group C improved most resulting in a significant difference between the groups (F[2, 220] = 31.4, df = 2; p < 0.001). Since the slopes of the improvements differed between the groups, a significant interaction between days and groups occurred (F [2, 220] = 65.63; p< 0.001). Post hoc tests revealed a significant difference between all groups (p< 0.001). Patients of Group A reached 28.8 ± 3.7 points, Group B 30.3 ± 2.7 points and group C 37.6 ± 3.4 points. After completion of the in-patient training programme 31% of group A, 64% of group B and 88% of group C had shown a significant improvement on the SCOPA-COG, six months later at the final assessment 70% of patients of group A, 80% of patients of group B and 94% of patients of group C had been able to keep their level of performance.

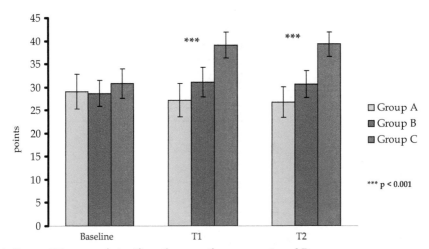

Fig. 4. Group C improved significantly more than group A and B

C: GAS

The GAS was performed on the final assessment. Group C reached more often the main goal than the other groups (Chi-square: 57.1; p < 0.001). The detailed analysis of the results is shown in table 4 and 5.

The main cognitive impairments reported by the patients could be attributed to the following domains: dual tasking, planning of complex and sequential tasks, decision making, rule recognition and rule shifting problems with delayed recall, difficulties in finding misplaced items. The patients based the selection of the goals on their individual main impairment. Table 4 shows the goals patients had chosen and if they were obtained.

More patients of group A compared to group B and C did not obtain the chosen goal or deteriorated compared to baseline while 27.6% of patients of group C obtained the goal and 39.4% exceeded the expectations mildly and 7.6% substantially.

D: Concentration

In the Alterskonzentrationstest (AKT) no difference between the groups was detected. Patients did not differ in attention span neither at baseline nor at the final assessment.

E: Information processing

In the ZVT no difference between the groups was detected at baseline assessment. The time to complete the test decreased in all groups after the training (F_{lin} [2,220] = 17.71; p< 0.001).

Groups	Goal	Goals chosen		Goals obtained	
		Total number	Percentage [%]	Total number	Percentage [%]
A N = 71	Dual tasking	15	21.1	3	20
B N = 75		14	18.7	9	6.4
C N = 76		15	20	10	67
A N = 71	Planning of complex tasks	15	21.2	3	20
B N = 75		16	21.3	9	56.3
C N = 76		17	22.4	10	58.9
A N = 71	Decision making	10	14.1	4	40
B N = 75		11	14.7	6	54.5
C N = 76		14	18.4	10	71.4
A N = 71	Rule recognition and rule shifting	13	18.3	4	30.8
B N = 75		16	21.3	7	43.8
C N = 76		14	18.4	10	71.4
A N = 71	Delayed recall	12	16.9	3	25
B N = 75		12	16	7	58.3
C N = 76		11	14.5	9	82
A N = 71	Search strategies	6	8.5	4	67
B N = 75		6	8	5	83.3
C N = 76		5	6.6	4	80

Table 4. Goals chosen by the patients

Group C was superior to group A and B (p < 0.003) while group A and B did not differ resulting in a significant group difference (F[2,220] = 7.81; p< 0.001).

In the PASAT test the groups produced on average 50% correct answers at the baseline assessment, group A improved only marginally. Group B and C benefitted from the training programme shown in a significant linear trend for days (F_{lin} [1, 154] = 63.71; p < 0.001). Since

GAS	Group A N = 71		Group B N = 75		Group C N = 76		Total	
	Total	Percent	Total	Percent	Total	Percent	Total	Percent
-3	12	16.7	6	8	2	2.6	20	8.9
-2	10	13.8	5	6.7	3	3.9	18	23.7
-1	28	40.3	21	28	18	23.6	67	30
0	13	18.1	19	25.3	23	30.2	55	24.7
1	8	11.1	24	32	24	26.3	56	25,112
2	0	0	0	0	6	7.9	6	2.7
	71		75		76		223	

Table 5. Results of the GAS

the improvement of the groups differed there was also a significant interaction between days and groups (F [2, 154] = 18.99; p < 0.001). Group C improved significantly more than group B (p < 0.03) and A (p< 0.001) (F [2, 154]= 15.46; p< 0.001).

Only 157 patients (Group A: 50, Group B: 53, Group C: 54) managed the PASAT test on the first assessment and were included in the statistical model. The other patients did not succeed in finding a strategy to cope with the task. On the second and third assessment 56 patients of group A, 64 of group B and 71 of group C scored on the test.

F: Memory

In the MEMO-Test the recall of words improved in all groups over the trials as well as over the assessment days. The subscales of all words permanently stored in the long-term store (F[2,220] = 2.95; p< 0.05).and the total number of words in the long-term store (F[2,220] = 3.27; p< 0.05) differed between the groups (Fig 4).

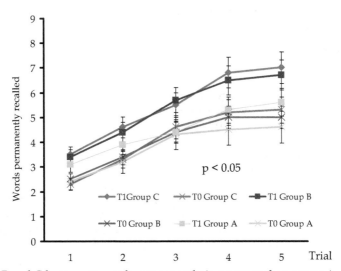

Fig. 5. Group B and C kept more words permanently in memory than group A.

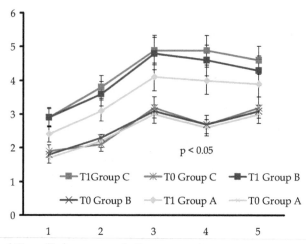

Fig. 6. Group B and C recalled more words than group A.

G: Executive function

The subtests of the BADS (rule shift cards, zoo map, modified 6 elements test) showed the following results:

The baseline scores of the rule shift cards did not differ between the groups. There was a mild but significant difference between the groups at the second assessment (Chi-square = 7.1; p < 0.03) and final assessment (Chi-square = 9.1;   p< 0.01).

At baseline assessment Group C showed a tendency to better performance on the BADS Zoo Test. The mean profile scores of all groups were higher at the second assessment, but significant more patients of group C improved compared to group A and B. There was a clear group difference at the second (Chi-square = 49.31; p < 0.03) and third assessment   (Chi-square = 14.42; 0.001)

There was no difference in the performance in the 6 elements test or set shifting test. All groups showed an increase of the average profile scores leading to significant group differences at the second (Chi-square = 39.3; p< 0.001) and third assessments (Chi-square = 25.3; p< 0.001).

H: TKS

The competence in cognitive estimation did not improve in Group A but in group B and C resulting in a significant difference between groups (T1:Chi square = 11.98; df = 2; p < 0.03; T2: Chi square = 22.153; df= 2; p < 0.002:

3.2.2 Assessment of mental state

15% of the patients in group A, 20% of group B and 18% of patients of group C reported to suffer from depression and received medication. The results on the HADS depression scale indicated in 20% of patients of group A and group C respectively and in 25% of patients of Group B the presence of a mild to moderate depression. The anxiety level was assessed by using the Hamilton anxiety scale and did not differ between the groups. The additional assessments of the current anxiety level at the time of assessment (STAI X1) and of the personality trait anxiety (STAI X2) did not reveal differences between the groups. The anxiety at the time of the assessments decreased mildly from baseline to the final assessment.

3.2.3 PD specific impairment

The PDQ39 shows that patients of group C rated their health related quality of life higher than the other groups. 13.8% of patients of group A, 38% of patients of group B and 52% of patients of group C reported less impairment due to PD. (Fig. 7)

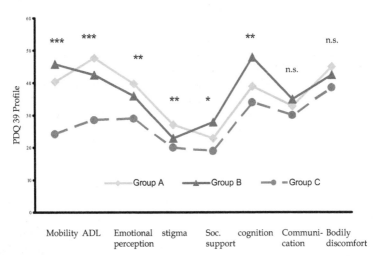

Fig. 7. PD-patients of group C reported less PD-specific impairment at the final assessment.
*** p < 0.001; ** p < 0.01; * p < 0.05

The UPDRS score showed a mild improvement in all groups at the final assessment but there was no significant difference between the groups indicating that cognitive improvement was not an unspecific effect resulting from general physical improvement. (Tab. 5)

	Group A N=71	Group B N = 75	Group C N = 76
Baseline			
UPDRS Motor scale	38.56 ± 12.44	37.53 ± 10.76	38.4 ± 11.78
UPDRS Sum-Score	59.20 ± 12.4	60.3 ± 12.4	61.5 ± 12.8
Final assessment			
UPDRS Motor scale	34.1 ± 11.4	34.2 ± 11.2	35.2 ± 12.4
UPDRS Sum-Score	55.4 ± 12.4	56.3 ± 11.5	57.2 ± 11.4

Table 6. UPDRS

3.2.4 Performance in daily living

The patients of Group C reported that they had adapted a more active life style, felt more confident in activities of daily living and had taken over some more chores. They perceived their partners and caregivers as being helpful. They enjoyed the participation of their partners in conjoint sports activities.

Patients of Group B also regarded the training programme as helpful but reported of having still problems with activities of daily living. Patients of group A had more difficulties with transfer of skills into daily life and the carry over effect was smaller than in the other groups.

Sports activities were with 300min/week higher in Group C than in group B (196min/week) and A (176 min/ week).

Patients of group A reported to perform 7.4 ± 3.1 hours very hard work per week, while patients of group B and C reported of 10.4 ± 2.2 and 11.5 ± 2.7 hours very hard work respectively. Group A managed 14.2 ± 3.9, Group B 16.1 ± 4.3 and Group C 17.9 ± 4.1 hard work

In accordance with the patients` reports 65% of the caregivers of patients in Group C found competence and cognition of the patients improved. In group B 54% of caregivers and in group A 49%of caregivers confirmed an improvement. A deterioration of the performance in daily living was reported in 11% of group C, 17% of group B and 25% of group A. In summary patients who conducted a multimodal cognitive rehabilitation programme improved most and continued coping with daily tasks. Patients of group C were more active in daily living and took more often part in sports activities.

4. Discussion

In summary 90 % of patients of group A, 93.8% of patients of group B and 95% of patients of group C completed the training. Data of patients who did not continue with the programme were not included into the statistical analysis. Although patients complained of a lack of concentration, they performed well on the AKT. The second and third assessment did not reveal further improvement. The lack of improvement might be due to a ceiling effect since the performance on this test at baseline was good in all groups. The same might apply for the MMST which did not differ significantly between baseline and follow-up assessments. The training programme did not affect the mood of the patients.

At the baseline assessment patients of all three groups had shown deficits mainly in tests addressing executive functions. Consecutively, the performance of the patients was worse on the subtests of the SCOPA-COG semantic fluency, LURIA, dice and assembly pattern of the SCOPA-COG, Zoo test of the BADS, PASAT and cognitive estimation. The memory tasks such as immediate and delayed word recall were only mildly disturbed. All groups showed some improvements at the assessment immediately after completion of the training programme in the following tests: TMT, BADS Rule shift cards, zoo map, modified 6 elements test, PASAT and TKS. The mean scores of the ADAS-Cog and SCOPA-COG test in group A were not significantly better compared to the baseline assessment although 18% of the patients reached an improvement of 3 or more points on the ADAS-Cog. The findings were similar for the SCOPA-COG test. 31% of the patients showed an improvement on the SCOPA-COG test. Clear differences between the groups were found for the following tests: TMT, BADS zoo map, BADS rule shift cards, BADS 6 elements, PASAT, TKS, 2 subtests of the Memo Test.

At the second outcome assessment, 6 months after completion of the training programme, 21% of the patients of group A showed a further improvement on the ADAS-Cog, on the other hand 50% of patients of group A deteriorated, 31% of patients of group B and 28% of patients of group C within the 6 months after discharge from the rehabilitation unit. Most of the patients of group B and C were able to keep their performance level between the second and third assessment on the SCOPA-COG, while group A deteriorated. Further improvements between the second and the final assessment were obtained in group B and C on the TKS, PASAT and MEMO test.

The BADS subscales especially the zoo map is a very demanding task requiring excellent planning skills. Even patients of group A and B with previously shown improvement on the BADS subscales lost most of that. Only patients of group C managed to keep their level of performance. The performance of group B and A dropped nearly to baseline level. Thus, Group C has been superior to group B and A immediately after completing the training programme and at the second assessment six months later.

The difficulties patients experienced while solving the tasks have been in accordance with the results of other studies (Lewis et al., 2003, 2005). Most improvement has been observed in the LURIA, dice, assembly pattern, MOSAIC test of the SCOPA-COG. Mild improvement has been observed in the ZOO map and the PASAT-test. The pattern of improvement did not differ between the groups but the percentage of subjects showing an improvement differed significantly as well as the speed of recovery. The UPDRS – score improved in all groups slightly. There were no significant differences between the groups and no significant change of medication. Accordingly, the improvement in the neuropsychological tests cannot be referred to a better physical condition of one group and can be attributed to the training programme.

90% of patients of group C pursued the training at home with the same quantity and intensity while only 75% of group B and 50% of group A did so. Patients of group C conducted a motor training programme three times/week and practised cognitive tasks twice a week for 45 min. Patients of group B and C continued with some tasks resembling the transfer tasks they had performed during the training programme. The partners of the patients of group B and C managed to support the patients in practising transfer tasks, they asked them to prepare a meal or to do the shopping. The majority of the spouses of patients of group C joined their partners in the sports programme. The support of the spouses alleviated the home training significantly. As known from a questionnaire sent to the patients social aspects are very important for PD- patients. It is difficult to decide whether the further improvement of cognitive performance which occurred in some tests was due to the quantity of training or the content of the training. However, group C was already superior to the other groups at the second assessment. Since patients were compliant with the programme during the in-patient stay and received the same quantity of training, the different performance might rather be due to the content of the training than to the quantity. The performance of the patients differed between the tasks suggesting that the different training schedules between the groups affect the training outcome. For example the BADS zoo map a very challenging test as mentioned above requires various training approaches to achieve an improvement. As a result only patients of group C obtained an improvement on this test. Depression might also influence the performance in neuropsychological tests. Klepac et al. (2009) had found that depression preceding PD motor signs might favour poorer cognitive abilities. However, there was no significant difference between the groups regarding the percentage of patients being depressed and the onset of depression. Thus, an influence of depression and anxiety on cognitive performance could be ruled out.

Assessment bias in favour for one treatment can be excluded because the movement disorder specialists conducting the tests were blinded to the treatment arms.

Thus, the findings of the study suggest that PD patients benefit from a specific cognitive training and that a multimodal training might be most suitable for improving cognitive performance in PD. As already shown in a previous study (Hullmann et al., 2004) the cognitive training needs to be specific. Therefore, we had chosen an individual approach based on the Patients` results in the neuropsychological test battery. The specificity of the training for executive functions is also shown in the fact that an other functional domain such as attention was not influenced by the training. Home based cognitive exercises were sufficient to keep the performance of the second assessment in patients of group C. However, patients of group B and C were able to keep some improvements as well. Home based cognitive training without transfer and physical training as performed by group A was less attractive for the patients. However, the poorer results of group A were not due to fewer training lessons since the performance of group A was already poorer on the second assessment. During the in-patient stay the quantity of training lessons were similar in all groups, only the percentage of specific training differed. Thus, the content of the training might be responsible for the different performance of the groups. The superiority of group B compared to group A suggests the efficacy of the transfer tasks. The psychomotor training helps the group C to improve further, especially in the challenging executive tasks regarding rule cognition, set shifting and decision making. However, it is not clear whether patients of group B and C could also cope better with completely new situations.

In contrast to a study by Paris et al. (2011), the present study suggested a translation of improved cognitive performance on the neuropsychological tests into daily living. Group C scored much higher on the PDQ 39 than the other groups. Thus, health related quality of life was improved markedly in these patients. The patients` caregivers also reported an improved competence in real life. In addition the goal attainment scale had been used in the present study. The patients picked the goals according to the cognitive problems they experienced in daily living. Most often the cognitive problem, they suffered most of, was chosen as goal. Half of the patients managed to obtain the goals agreed on prior to the training programme. Patients of group C reached significantly more often the goal than the patients of group B or A

The cognitive training performed in the study of Paris et al. (2011) resembled the training of group A in the current study. Only 29% of patients of group A obtained the goal compared to 69.8% of group C.

Some goals seemed to be more difficult to achieve (see Table 4). Patients faced more difficulties in attaining goals regarding rule generation and rule shifting while goals like dual tasking and memory improvement were easier to obtain. Group C was more successful to achieve an improvement in planning of complex tasks, rule generation and decision finding than group B and C.

Goebel et al. (2010) compared the ability of PD-patients to internally initiate a strategy with their ability to utilize an externally provided strategy in a simple Numerosity judgement task. The data of the study showed a general slowdown after strategy instruction. Furthermore, some patients reported difficulties in applying the strategies. The authors referred the findings to a failure in metacognition. Inferior utilization of metacognitive memory strategies seems to induce problems of PD-patients in real-life situations (Johnson et al., 2005, Shimamura, 2000). External instruction might activate metacognitive control processes and slow down the system. However, when PD-patients had sufficient time to solve the tasks there was no general deficit in the ability to internally generate a cognitive strategy in PD. Patients of group C had sufficient time during the psychomotor training to work out strategies to solve tasks and had time to initiate internal strategies. The combination of the psychomotor training with the transfer training provided the patients with some guidance and instructions to solve the tasks. However, the guidance was not too restrictive, there was enough time to find individual solutions. Additionally, the training was less standardised and strongly tailored to the patients` needs.

Our results are in accordance with the authors` conclusions (Goebel et al., 2008): "Adding training time and scheduling repetitive, cue-initiated learning trials may further improve training effects. Such a procedure may lead to more automated, implicit strategy application that demands less executive control (e.g., Baddeley,1998; Norman & Shallice, 1986; Sammer et al., 2006) whereas instruction alone bears the risk of increasing working memory load".

This is in accord with a work of Sinforiani et al (2004) who showed a significant improvement at verbal fluency, logic memory and Raven's matrices tests after a 6- week cognitive rehabilitiation training including cognitive and physical training. After the completion of the training a carry-over effect has been observed and the authors referred the effects to the combination of a cognitive and physical training. The authors suggested that the cognitive rehabilitation training exerts its positive effects by reinforcing cognitive strategies with improvement of frontal lobe functions.

Therefore, emphasis should be placed on the reduction of cognitive load in psychological training programmes. The combination of cognitive training at the writing table with transfer tasks and a physical training is recommended.

Research over the last decade has shown that cognitive deficits affect motor performance. Patients with cognitive deficits had more difficulties in motor tests than patients without cognitive deficits (Goldmann, 1998). Hausdorff et al (2005) have found a close correlation between walking and executive functions. Yogev et al. (2005) have shown that gait variability in dual tasking is closely associated with the performance in neuropsychological tests of executive tasks.

Therefore, one might speculate that motor functions might affect cognitive performance as well. There is a huge body of literature suggesting a prevention of cognitive decline by life long exercise or even an improvement of cognitive deficits by physical activity. Executive functions may be selectively maintained or improved in people with better physical condition provided by physical training (Churchill et al., 2002). The importance of aerobic physical exercise on cognitive functions, especially on executive functions has been shown (Kramer 1999, Colcombe et al., 2003, 2004, 2006). The studies have been mainly conducted in healthy elderly or patients with dementia. Tanaka et al. (2008) have shown that older people with PD can benefit their executive functions in the same way, as do their peers without PD. The results of some studies have shown that brain areas undergoing biological aging benefit most from endurance sports. Even structural changes have been observed (Colcombe et al., 2006). Exercise is thought to enhance brain plasticity. Neuroplasticity might be supported by BDNF release, which is exercise regulated. Physical exercise increases the release of growth hormone (GH) which represents the main stimulus for the release of insulin growth factor (IGF-1). IGF-1 is involved in processes regulating learning,, memory, neurogenesis and amyloid degradation (Holzenberger et al., 2003, Carter&Ramsey, 2002). The release of IGF-1 is closely related to the release of BDNF. Several responses of the brain to exercise have been described. In animal studies comparing young and old animals a difference was shown in the location of the BDnF mRNA upregulation in the hippocampus. Young animal showed an increase of BDNF mRNA in dendate gyrus, hilus and Ca3 region, old animals in the Ca1 and Ca2 region. Long term potentiation which is relevant for memory and learning was also found. LTP was correlated with increased expression of mRNA of the NR2B receptor unit of the NMDA (N-methyl-D-aspertate) receptor. Increase of cerebral blood flow and reduction of cardiovascular risk factors might also contribute to the positive effects of sport on cognition. The reduction of cardiovascular risk factors does not play a role in the present study because of the short observation time. The release of dopamine by exercise might also play a role. An increase in the activity of antioxidant enzymes, and thus increases the capacity to defend against the stress of oxidation in the central nervous system (Rodák et al., 2001) might also support neuroplasticity.

It is not specified so far which type of exercise might be most promising for improving cognitive performance. The role of endurance training has been shown, whether a combination of aerobic training with a cognitive challenging physical training is of advantage needs further research. The physical training in the present study provided both, a training of strategies to solve tasks and an aerobic training. Since intermittent training schedules have been shown to be as effective as daily training, the frequency of training sessions should have been sufficient as well.

It is not clear so far how cognitive training at the writing table might improve cognitive performance. The destruction of the nigrostriatal dopaminergic pathways is often about 75% and involves the ventral tegmental area, which innervates the prefrontal cortex. Therefore, it is unlikely that cognitive training reconstructs the dopaminergic system.

The multimodal training of cognitive functions is time- consuming and put demands on resources. Due to the quantity and quality of the trainings sessions it will also be costly. On the other hand dementia is a risk factor for falls and transfer to nursing –homes, which increases the costs for the patients´ care substantially and jeopardizes the patients` quality of life. Considering the sequelae of dementia such as increased dependence on care givers, high morbidity and increased mortality it is justified to spend more time and effort into prevention of dementia. Therefore, provision of adequate financing is also required.

5. Limitations of the study

One might criticise that we compared three different treatment arms and did not include a control group without cognitive training in this study. Patients were enrolled into the study during their stay in a rehabilitation unit and complained of a deterioration of their cognitive performance. For this reason it was not possible to withhold treatment. Further, we had shown in a previous study (Hullmann et al., 2004) the superiority of a cognitive training compared to standard treatment in control subjects. Therefore, we compared three different treatment arms with increasing stimulus modality.

Another limitation is that there are no evidence based data for the transfer training. Further research is necessary to evaluate and validate which transfer exercises are useful tools. The psychomotor training has been used for many years in children and has been used in patients with dementia (Oswald WP, 1996). However, it has not been validated in PD-patients so far. The selection of tasks had been based on the clinical experience of the therapists and medical staff and the published data based on the work with children.

One might also argue which improvement might be clinically relevant. However, the scales we used are all validated and had been often applied in clinical studies. The clinical relevance of the improvements is also shown by the observed translation into real life. One might criticize that the patients were not tested regarding their performance in completely new situations. Patients, caregivers and the neurologist supervising the treatment agreed on certain goals at the beginning of the study. Hence, situations resembling the agreed goals were trained during the study.

Furthermore, due to the short follow up period of 6 months we cannot report on long-term results. However, studies assessing long-term results are very difficult to conduct since it is very difficult to keep the medication stable. A change in dopaminergic (Fournet et al., 2000) or antidepressant medication might influence cognitive performance. In order to correct for these confounders a larger sample of patients will be needed.

6. Strengths of the study

To our knowledge, the results of the current study show for the first time, that a multidisciplinary cognitive training in patients with Parkinson`s disease can lead to improvements of cognitive function which translate into everyday life and are not only shown by improvements on neuropsychological scales. We want to emphasize that a blinded randomised design and a standardised neuropsychological test battery were employed. Furthermore, the cohort of patients undergoing the study protocol was big and the dropout rate was low for this type of study. In addition the training of the caregivers guaranteed a supporting environment in all groups. We were able to keep the medication stable avoiding confounding effects by the change of medication.

7. Conclusion

In conclusion, we have shown that PD-patients with cognitive deficits benefit from a multidisciplinary cognitive training. A multimodal training is superior to a paper and pencil based cognitive treatment. We have shown a translation of improvements in cognitive tests into performance in real life. Although the multimodal training is time consuming and requires high motivation, it is worth to pursue the training considering the secondary diseases, loss of quality of life and the costs following the diagnosis of dementia. The role of the caregivers has also to be emphasized, the involvement of the family improves the compliance with the training at home.

8. Acknowledgement

We thank the Dr. Werner Jackstädt-Stiftung, the support made the present study possible.

9. References

Aarsland D, Larsen JP, Tandberg E. & Laake K. (2000). Predictors of nursing home placement in Parkinson`s disease: A population based prospective study. *J Am Geriatr Soc* , 48, pp. 938-942.
Aarsland D, Brønnick K, & Fladby T. (2011 Epub ahead). Mild cognitive impairment in Parkinson`s disease. Curr Neurol Neurosci Rep.
Abbott RD, White LR, Webster R, Masaki KH, Curb JD. & Petrovitch H. (2004). Walking and dementia in physically capable elderly men. *JAMA*, 292 (12), pp. 1447-1453
Baatile J, Langbein WE, Weaver F, Maloney C & Jost MB. (2000). Effect of exercise on perceived quality of life in individuals with Parkinson`s disease. *J Rehabil Res Dev*, 37, pp. 529-534
Baddeley AD (1986). *Working memory*. Oxford: Clarendon Press
Ble A, Volpato S, Zuliani G, Guralnik JM, Bandinelli S, Lauretani F, Bartali B, Maraldi C, Fellin R, & Ferrucci L.(2005). Executive function correlates with walking speed in older persons: the InCHIANTI study.*J Am Geriatr Soc*, 53(3), pp. 410-5.

Brand M, Kalbe E &Kessler J. (2002). Test zum kognitiven Schätzen (TKS). Göttingen: Hogrefe.

Burgess PW& Shallice T. (1996) Response suppression, initiation and strategy use following frontal lobe lesions. Neuropsychologia, 34(4), p.263-72

Calabresi P, Picconi B, Parnetti L &Di Filippo M. (2006). A convergent model for cognitive dysfunctions in Parkinson's disease: the critical dopamine-acetylcholine synaptic balance. Lancet Neurol, 5(11), p.974-83

Caradoc-Davies TH, Weatherall M & Dixon GS. (1992). Is the prevalence of Parkinson´s disease in New Zealand really changing? Acta Neurol Scand 86, p. 40-44

Carpenter PA, Just MA &Reichle ED. (2000). Working memory and executive function: Evidence from neuroimaging. Curr opinion in Neurobiol,, 10,p. 195-199.

Carter S & Ramsey MM. (2002). A critical analysis of the role of growth hormone and IGF-I in aging and lifespan. Trends genet, 18 (6), p. 295-301

Chen RC, Chang SF, Su CL, Chen TH, Yen MF, Wu HM, Chen ZY & Liou HH (2001). Prevalence, incidence and mortality of PD: A door-to-door survey in Ilna county, Taiwan. Neurol, 57, p. 679-1686

Churchill JD, Calvez R, Colcombe S, Swain RA, Kramer AF & Greenough WT. (2002). .Exercise, experience and the aging brain. Neurobiol of aging, 23,p. 941-955.

Colman KSF, Koerts J, Beilen M, Leenders KL, Post WJ& Bastiaanse R. (2009). The impact of executive functions on verb production in patients with Parkinson`s disease. Cortex 45, p. 930-942.

Colcombe S&Kramer AF. (2003). Fitness effects on cognitive function of older adults: a meta-analytic study. Psychol Sci , 14, p. 125-130

Colcombe S, Erickson KI&Raz N. (2003). Aerobic fitness reduces brain tissue loss in aging humans. J Gerontol A Biol Sci Med Sci 58A, p. 176-180.

Colcombe S, Erickson KI, Scalf PE, Kim JS, Prakash R, McAuley E, Elavsky S, Marquez DX, Hu L& Kramer AF. (2006). Aerobic exercise training increases brain volume in Aging Humans. J Gerontology 61A (11), p. 1166-1170.

Colcombe SJ, Kramer AF, Erickson KI, McAuley E, Cohen NJ, Webb A, Jerome GJ & Marquez DX. (2004). Cardiovascular fitness, cortical plasticity, and aging. Proc Natl Acad Sci 10(9), p. 3316-3321.

Colman KS, Koerts J, van Beilen M, Leenders KL, Post WJ & Bastiaanse R. (2009). The impact of executive functions on verb production in patients with Parkinson's disease.Cortex, 45(8), p. 930-42.

Douglas J. Gelb, Eugene Oliver, Sid Gilman (1999) Diagnostic Criteria for Parkinson Disease. Arch Neurol, 56, p. 33-39

Dujardin K, Duhamel A, Delliaux M, Thomas-Antérion C, Destée A & Defebvre L. (2010). Cognitive complaints in Parkinson`s disease. Its relationship with objective cognitive decline. J Neurol. 257 (1), p. 79-84

Elgh E, Domello¨ f M, Linder J, Edstrom M, Stenlund H & ForsgrenL. (2009). Cognitive function in early Parkinson's disease: a populationbased study. Eur J Neurol 16, p. 1278-1284.

Emre M, Aarsland D, Albanese A, Byrne EJ, Deuschl G, De Deyn PP, Durif F, Kulisevsky J, van Laar T, Lees A, Poewe W, Robillard A, Rosa MM, Wolters E, Quarg P, Tekin S& Lane R. (2004). Rivastigmine for Dementia associated with Pakinson`s disease. N Engl J Med, 351, p. 2509-18.

Fahn S, Elton RL and the members of the UPDRS Development Committee. (1987). Unified Parkinson`s Disease rating scale. In: Fahn S, Marsden CD, Goldstein M et al. Eds. Recent developments in Parkinson`s disease II. New York. McMillan; p. 153-163

Folstein MF& Folstein SE. (1975). "„Mini Mental State". A practical method for grading the cognitive state of patients for the clinician. *J Psychiat Res* 12, p. 189-198.

Fournet N, Moreaud O, Roulin J, Naegele B & Pellat J. (2000). Working memory functioning in medicated Parkinson`s disease patients and the effect of withdrawal of dopaminergic medication. *Neuropsychology*, 14, p. 247-253

Fitzpatrick R, Peto V, Greenhall R& Hyman N. (1997). The Parkinson`s diasease Questionnaire (PDQ 39): Development and validation of a Parkinson`s disease summary index score. *Age and Ageing*; 26, p. 1757-1769

Funahashi S. (2001). Neuronal mechanisms of executive control by prefrontal cortex. *Neuroscience Research*, 39,p. 147-165.

Gatterer G, Fischer P, Simany M& Danielczyk W. (1989). The A-K-T (Alters-Konzentrations-Test a new psychometric test for geriatric patients. FunctNeurol; 4 (3), p. 273-276

Goldman-Rakic PS, Lidow MS, Smiley JF & Williams MS. (1992) The anatomy of dopamine in monkey and human prefrontal cortex. *J of Transmission*, suppl. 36, p. 163-177

Godefroy O. (2003).Frontal syndrome and disorders of executive functions. *J Neurol*, 250 (1), p. 1-6.

Goebel S, Mehdorn HM& Leplow B. (2010). Strategy instruction in Parkinson's disease: Influence on cognitive performance.*Neuropsychologia*, 48(2), p. 574-80

Gronwall, D.M.A. (1977). Paced auditory serial-addition task: A measure of recovery from concussion. *Perceptual and Motor Skills*, 44, p. 367-373.

Hausdorff JM, Yogev G, Springer S, Simon ES & Giladi N. (2005). Walking is more like catching than tapping: gait in the elderly as a complex cognitive task. Exp Brain Res. 164 (4); p. 541-8.

Heinz-Martin S., Oberauer K., Wittmann WW, Wilhelm O. & Schulze R. (2002). Working-memory capacity explains reasoning ability and a little bit more. *Intelligence*; 30, p. 261-288.

Hoehn MM, Yahr MR, Parkinsonism: onset, progression and mortality. (1967). *Neurology*, 17,p. 427-442.

Holzenberger M, Dupont J (2000). IGF-I receptor regulates lifespan and resistance to oxidative exercise in mice. *Nature* 421 (6919), p. 182-187

Howells DW, Porrit MJ & Wong JY. (2000). Reduced BDNF mRNA expression in the Parkinson`s disease substantia nigra. *Exp. Neurol*; 166,p. 127-135

Hughes AJ, Daniel SE, Kilford L& Lees AJ. (1992). Accuracy of clinical diagnosis of idiopathic Parkinson`s disease. A clinicopathological study of 100 cases. *JNNP*, 55, p. 181-184

Hullmann K, Sammer G & Reuter I. (2004). Training of executive functions in Parkinson`s disease. *Medimont International Proceedings*, p. 143-148.

Johnson AM, Pollard CC, Vernon PA, Tomes JL& Jog MS. (2005) Memory perception and strategy use in Parlinson`s disease. *Parkinsonism Relat. Disord.* 2005; 1, p. 111-115

Kleim JA, Jones TA& Schallert T. (2003). Motor enrichment and the induction of plasticity before and after brain injury. *Neurochem Res*, 28, p. 1757-1769

Kramer AF, Hahn S, Cohen NJ, Banich MT, McAuley E, Harisson CR Chason J, Vakil E, Bardell L, Boileau RA & Colcombe A. (1999). Ageing, fitness and neurocognitive function. *Nature*, 400, p. 418-419

Kramer AF, Colcombe SJ, Erickson KI, Paige P. (2006). Fitness training and the brain: From molecules to Minds. *Proceedings of the 206 Cognitive Aging Conference*, Atlanta, Georgia Atlanta GA: Georgia Institute of Technology.

Larson EB, Wang L, Bowen JD, McCormick WC, Teri L, Crane P &Kukull W. (2006). Exercise is associated with reduced risk for incident dementia among persons 65 years of age or older. *Ann Intern Med*, 144, p. 73-81.

Laurin D., Verreault R., Lindsay J, MacPherson K& Rockword K. (2001). Physical Activity and Risk of Cognitive Impairment and Dementia in elderly persons. *Arch Neurol* ; 58, p. 498-504

Lehrl, S. (1989). Mehrfach-Wortschatz-Intelligenztest: MWT-B. Perimed Fachbuch-Verlagsgesellschaft mbH, Erlangen

Leverenz JB, Quinn JF, Zabetian C, Zhang Jing, Montine K S& Montine T J. (2009). Cognitive impairment and Dementia in Patients with Parkinson Disease. *Curr Top Med Chem*, 9,p. 903-912

Levy G, Tang MX, Louis ED, et al. (2002) The association of incident dementia with mortality in PD. *Neurology*, 59, p. 1708–1713.

Lewis SJG, SlaboszA, Robbins TW, Barker RA & Owen AM. (2005). Dopaminergic basis for deficits in working memory but not attentional set-shifting in Parkinson`s disease. *Neuropsychologica*, 43, p. 823-832

Lezak MF. (1995). Neuropsychological assessment. Oxford: Oxford University Press.

Logsdon RG, McCurry SM, &Teri L. (2005). A home health care approach to exercise for persons with Alzheimer disease. *Care Manage J*, 6 (2), p. 90-97

Norris, G. & Tate, R.L. (2000). The behavioural assessment of the dysexecutive syndrome (BADS): ecological, concurrent and construct validity. *Neuropsychological Rehabilitation*, 10 (1),p. 33-45.

Marinus J, Visser N, Verwey FRJ, Middelkoop HAM, Stiggelbout AM &van Hilten JJ. (2003). Assessment of cognition in Parkinson`s disease. *Neurology*, 61, p. 1222-1228

Mc Curry SM, Gibbons LE, Logsdon RG, Vitiello MV&Teri L. (2005). Nighttime Insomnia Treatment and education for Alzheimner`s disease: A randomised controlled trial. *J Am Geriatr Soc*, 53, p. 793-802.

Miller BT & D'Esposito M (2005). "Searching for "the top" in top-down control". *Neuron*, 48 (4),p. 535–8.

Miller EK & Cohen JD (2001). "An integrative theory of prefrontal cortex function". *Annu Rev Neurosci*, 24 (1), p. 167–202

Nelles G. (2004). Cortical reorganisation – effects of intensive therapy. *Restor Neurol Neurosci*; 22, p. 239-244

Norman DA,&Shallice T (2000). "(1980) Attention to action: Willed and automatic control of behaviour". In Gazzaniga MS. *Cognitive neuroscience: a reader*. Oxford: Blackwell

Parkinson J. An essay on the shaking palsy. 1817London: Sherwood Neely and Jones

Reitan, R. M. (1958) Validity of the Trail Making Test as an indicator of organic brain damage. *Perceptual and Motor Skills* 8. 271-276

Reuter I, Engelhardt M, Freiwald J& Baas H. (1999) Therapeutic value of exercise training in Parkinson`s disease. *Med & Sci Sports Exerc*. 9: 1544-1549.

Rodák Z, Kaneko T, Tahara S, Nakamoto H, Pucsok J& Sasvari M. (2001). Regular exercise improves cognitive function and decreases oxidative damage in the rat brain. *Neurochenmistry international* 38, 17-23

Rolland Y, v Khan GA & Vellas B. (2010) Healthy brain aging: Role of exercise and physical activity. *Clin Geriatr Med* 26,p. 75-87

Rosen WG, Mohs RC& Davis KL (1984): A new rating scale for Alzheimer's disease. *Am J Psychiatr* , 141, p. 1356-1364

Royal College of Physicians, the Intercollegiate Stroke Working Party. (2008). National clinical guideline for stroke. Third edition. London: RCP

Sammer, G, Reuter, I., Hullmann, K., Kaps, M., & Vaitl, D. (2006). Training of executive. functions in Parkinson's disease. *J Neurol Sci*, 248, p. 115–119.

Schaaf, A., Kessler, J., Grond, M.&Fink, G.R. (1994). Memo-Test. Hogrefe, Goettingen, Germany.

Schrag A, Ben-Shlomo Y& Quinn NP (2000). Cross sectional prevalence survey of idiopathic Parkinson´s disease and Parkinsonism in London. *BMJ*, 321, p. 21-22

Shepherd RB. (2001). Exercise and training to optimise functional motor performance in stroke: driving neural reorganisation. *Neural Plast* 8, p. 121-129

Shallice T. (1982). Specific impairments of planning. Philos Trans R Soc Lond B Biol Sci 25, 298 (1089), p. 199-209.

Shimamura, A. P. (2000). Toward a cognitive neuroscience of metacognition. *Consciousness and Cognition*, 9, 313–323.

Sinforiani, E., Banchieri, L., Zucchella, C., Pacchetti, C. & Sandrini, G. (2004). Cognitive rehabilitation in Parkinson's disease. *Archives of Gerontology and Geriatrics:* Suppl 9, p. 387–391.

Smith EE, Jonides J. (1999). Storage and executive processes in the frontal lobes. *Science*, 283, p. 1657-1661

Spielberger CD, Gorsuch RL, Lushene RE. (1970): STAI; Manual for the State-Trait-Anxiety-Inventory. Consulting Psychologist Press, Palo Alto.

Talwalker S.: Assessment of AD with the ADAS-cog.(1996) . *J. Geriatr. Psychiat. Neurol.*, 9, p. 39.46.

Teri L, Gibbons LE & McCurry SM (2003). Exercise plus behaviour management in patients with Alzheimer disease: A randomised controlled trial. *JAMA* 290 (15), p. 2015-2022

Trejo JL, Carro E, Torres-Aleman EL. (2001). Circulating insulin-like growth factor mediates exercise-induced increases in the number of new neurons in the adult hippocampus, *J Neurosci* 25, p. 1628-1634

Willis SL, Tennstedt S, Marsiske M.Ball K, Ekias J, Koepke KM, Morris JN, Rebok GW, Unverzagt FW, Stoddard AM Wright E, Active Study group. Long-term effects of cognitive training on everyday functional outcomes in elder adults. *JAMa,* ; 296, p. 2805-2814

Wilson BA, Evans JJ, Emslie H,Alderman N & P. Burgess. (1998). The development of an ecologically valid test for assessing patients with a dysexecutive syndrome. *Neuropsychol Rehabilitation 8 (3)*, p: 213–228.

Yogev G, Giladi N, Peretz C, Springer S, Simon ES & Hausdorff JM. (2005). Dual tasking, gait rhythmicity, and Parkinson`s Disease: which aspects of gait are attention demanding? *Eur J Neurosci*, 22(5), p. 1248-56.

Zigmond AS& Snaith RP. (1983). The Hospital Anxiety and Depression Scale. *Acta Psychiatr.Scand,* 67, p. 361-370

3

Mobile Systems as a Challenge for Neurological Diseases Management – The Case of Parkinson's Disease

Laura Pastor-Sanz, Mario Pansera, Jorge Cancela,
Matteo Pastorino and María Teresa Arredondo Waldmeyer
Life Supporting Technologies, Universidad Politécnica de Madrid
Spain

1. Introduction

Nowadays the importance of bio-medical engineering and mobile applications for healthcare is amazingly growing. During the last decades many devices and technological solutions have become available on the market and the interest in applying those technologies to the treatment of several kinds of pathologies has consequently increased. This chapter addresses the problem of continuous monitoring of patients affected by Parkinson's Disease (PD) and proposes a set of technologies to improve the following and management of such subjects.

PD is a neurodegenerative disorder of the central nervous system that affects motor skills and speech (Tolosa, 1998). The primary biochemical abnormality in PD is a deficiency of dopamine due to degeneration of neurons in the substantia nigra pars compact (D. G. Standaert & Young, 2001). The characteristic motor features of the disease include bradykinesia (i.e. slowness of movement), tremor, rigidity (i.e. resistance to externally imposed movements), flexed posture, postural instability and freezing of gait. Furthermore, PD is usually characterised by the loss of normal prosody of the speech (Darkins et al., 1988).

According to the World Health Organisation [WHO], 2002), there are more than six million people worldwide affected by PD. The syndrome typically appears around the age of 60. It affects Europeans and North Americans more often than Asians or Africans and it is more common in men than in women. PD affects about 2% of the population over the age of 65 years, figure that is expected to double by 2020 (de Lau & Breteler, 2006). For those reasons, PD poses a significant public health burden, which is likely to increase in the coming years. Annual medical care, including doctors' visits, physical therapies and treatment for co-occurring illnesses -such as depression- is estimated at $2,000 to $7,000 for people in early stages of the disease, and it is probably much higher for advanced stages. Surgical treatments for PD can cost $25,000 or more. As the disease progresses, institutional care at an assisted-living facility or nursing home may be required, and the related costs can exceed $100,000, per person annually.

Technology in general and specifically ICT might be an affordable alternative for PD's patients' treatment and management. The development of platforms for remote health status monitoring, the qualitative and quantitative assessment and treatment personalization for people suffering from neurodegenerative diseases is expecting to provide in the future a remarkable improvement in patients' management as well as a substantial cutting-off of the economic burden generated by the disease. New technologies allow monitoring the evolution of the disease through the employment of a wide range of wearable and user-friendly micro-sensors. Moreover, the last advances in data processing and data mining algorithms is bound to provide more accurate information about the diverse aspects of PD evolution. Finally, it is important to highlight the huge potential in costs reduction that such platforms could yield. Furthermore, it is worth mentioning that the reduction in costs of hospitalization and treatment represents an attractive asset for the market forces involved in the development of biomedical applications.

2. Treatment

Current clinical treatment of Parkinson's disease is performed through ersatz dopamine administration or by using Deep Brain Stimulation (DBS) (Singh et al., 2007).

2.1 Dopamine treatment

Current therapy is based on augmentation or replacement of dopamine, using the biosynthetic precursor levodopa or drugs that activate dopamine receptors. These therapies are effective at the beginning of treatment. However, after a variable period of time, this initially excellent response is complicated by the appearance of MRCs. Complications include wearing-off, the abrupt loss of efficacy at the end of each dosing interval and diskinesias (de la Fuente-Fernández et al., 2004). Wearing off and dyskinesias produce substantial disability and frequently interfere with medical therapies (A.E. Lang & A.M. Lozano, 1998). Usually, motor fluctuations appear first, as a shortening of the initially smooth and long lasting dopaminergic response. In the typical case, few hours after drug intake the patients start to realize the re-emergence of signs and symptoms of the disease. This is known as end of dose deterioration or wearing off. This may happen several times a day; therefore the patient may actually several hours per day in the off state (Lees, 1989).

2.2 Deep brain stimulation

DBS is a surgical treatment involving the implantation of a medical device called a brain pacemaker, which sends electrical impulses to specific parts of the brain (Vaillancourt et al., 2003). The introduction of DBS as a therapeutic tool for advanced PD has revolutionised the clinical management of this condition. Due to its safety profile and efficacy, DBS has evolved from a last-resort therapeutic option to a modality that is now routinely offered to patients. Over the years, surgical candidates and the outcome expected with this procedure has become well established (Deuschl et al., 2006). Overall improvement that might be expected with surgery is similar to that provided by levodopa without the associated involuntary movements (Group, 2001). As the diseases progresses, however, non-dopaminergic symptoms (gait, postural instability, sleep disorders and depression, among others) become more prominent, leading to a significant increase in morbidity. To overcome some of the problems, the use of different surgical targets has been advocated. Perhaps the most promising application of DBS on this regards involves the use of Pedunculopontine Nucleus (PPN) stimulation for the treatment of gait and postural instability (Mazzone et al.,

2005). Recent studies suggest that this procedure might be suited for the treatment of falls and freezing. In addition to motor symptoms, an improvement in rapid eye movement sleep in patient with PD treatment with PPN DBS has been reported (Lim et al., 2009). In the future, a tailored approach to patient's specific symptoms may be possible (Lozano, 2009).

3. Assessment - state of the art

The assessment of PD can be performed through clinical and technological methods. Both types of solutions are reviewed.

3.1 Clinical solution

In Europe, each neurologist or general practitioner (GP) normally cares for 50 to 800 patients with PD. The range in workload is a result of diversity both in national health systems and in the availability of clinical resources across Europe. Even at 50 patients per clinician, this represents a serious challenge to homecare monitoring for specialised conditions. PD's patients normally visit their specialised clinician or GP every 4-6 months. As a result, any changes in the patient's conditions may not be recognised for several months, unless the patients themselves make contact (R. Greenlaw et al., 2009).

In clinical practice, information about motor fluctuations is usually obtained by asking patients to recall the number of hours of ON (i.e. when medications effectively attenuate tremor) and OFF time (i.e. when medications are not effective). This kind of self–report is subject to perceptual bias (e.g. patients often have difficulty distinguishing dyskinesia from other symptoms) and recall bias. Another approach is the use of patient diaries, which can improve reliability by recording symptoms as they occur, but does not capture many of the features useful in clinical decision making (Group, 2001).

Certainly for PD there is the additional complication of symptoms which vary throughout the day (swinging between ON and OFF states). During the short office visit in this neurologist the patient may appear very well and he misses to report symptoms of wearing off. As a result, treatment modifications are not undertaken in time. Besides, it is disempowering for the patient to be asked to present a true picture of their disease in a pre-scheduled one hour appointment (R. Greenlaw et al., 2009).

The actual emergence of dyskinesias throughout the day mainly depends on the intermittent dopaminergic drug intake, even in influence by timing and quantity of each individual dose of levodopa. While other phenomena, such as delayed response or no-response depends also on stress, food intake and many other factors. In this case, patients will greatly benefit from quantitative objective assessment of their motor status in daily life in relation to the dosing schedule.

In an attempt to solve these problems and to find more objective assessment, several rating scales have been designed and used. Among them, the Unified Parkinson's Disease Rating Scale (UPDRS) is the most widely used (Goetz et al., 2004). This rating tried to quantify selected symptoms and signs of Parkinsonism in a 5-points scoring system (with 0 for no signal and 4 for a marked severity of the sign). Unfortunately, the use of the UPDRS scale, like any other semi-objective rating scale presents some limitations like intra and inter observer inconsistencies. Besides, it can be time consuming and ca be biased by subjectivity issues related to historical information. Moreover, the pattern and severity of PD symptoms may vary considerably during the day, while clinical rating scales only provide moment-to-moment assessment; and finally, measurements of motor fluctuations made in the clinic may not accurately reflect the actual functional disability experienced by the patient at home.

The accurate assessment of speech quality is a major research problem that has attracted attention in the field of speech communications for many years. Subjective quality measures given by professional personnel who have received special assessment training are necessarily time consuming and costly (Lingyun Gu et al., 2005).

3.2 Technological solution: sensors for motion analysis

Over the past decades various technologies, methodologies and systems have been proposed for the monitoring and the assessment of the Parkinson's disease. A significant number of studies investigated various parameters of the gait of PD patients. Others focused on the evaluation and quantification of the patients' motor status and various disease symptoms by the use of computerized motion tests (e.g. handwriting, inserting pegs, and games). Table 1 describes some features of the human motion, as well as the characteristics which can be measured through the use of wearable sensors.

Features	Characteristics	Sensor
Gait	Speed of Locomotion	Motion sensor
	Variability of the gait	
	Rigidity of legs	
Posture	Trunk inclination	Motion sensor
Leg movement	Speed	Motion sensor
	Length of Step	Motion sensor
	Step Frequency	Motion sensor
	Stride	Motion sensor
Hand Movement	Speed	Motion sensor
	Angle Amplitude	Motion sensor
Tremor	Amplitude	Motion sensor
	Frequency	
	Duration	
	Asymmetry	
Fall	Fall detection	Motion sensor
Freezing of Gait	Leg movement analysis	Motion sensor
Levodopa-Induced Dyskinesia (LID)	Duration	Motion sensor
	Severity	
Bradykinesia	Duration	Motion sensor
	Severity	
	Asymmetry	
Aphasia	Pitch	Microphone
	EPE	

Table 1. Parkinson's disease – wearable sensors for human motion related measurements

The accuracy of measurements of the parameters above described depends on several technical features that are often in conflict with other needs such as usability, wearability, technical feasibility and the social acceptance of the devices used by the subjects. In Table 2 a description of these desirable properties along with their conflicts is presented.

Desirable properties	Conflict
Small sensor	The size of sensor is definitely an important factor, especially for portability and mobility matters. However, small sensors may not have enough room for long-lasting battery or storage capacity.
Smart sensor	Sensors possessing many characteristics are often bigger in size, expensive and consume more power
Sensor storage capacity	Due to a limit in storage capacity, sensors have to upload data frequently to the data personal server. So it is important to employ a good wireless communication technology that does not drain excessive power from the sensors.
Sensor processing capability	Because sensors do not often have large processing capability, they may not be able to process all data before the upload to the personal server. This means that large amount of raw data should be stored and eventually sent. Therefore it is important to have an efficient communication channel.
Sensor communication range	Whilst sensors are only able to communicate over short range, it is crucial to define a specific radius of action.

Table 2. Wearable sensors desirable properties & conflicts

3.2.1 Systems for Parkinson's disease monitoring

Most of the research work carried out in the field of PD monitoring focuses on the assessment of the motor status of PD's patients. During the last decade, many research groups have been trying to develop a system able to objectively quantify the severity of the motor disturbances using motion sensors (Patel et al., 2010; 2009; 2007). An important number of these studies is based on the study of various parameters of motor behaviour, in particular features related to the gait (R. Greenlaw et al., 2009; Salarian et al., 2007; 2004). Other studies focused on the identification of ON/OFF fluctuations through the assessment of tremor (Van Someren et al., 1993), dyskinesias (Keijsers et al., 2003; 2000) and bradykinesia (Papapetropoulos et al., 2010). Some groups are also committed to use electromyogram (EMG) or voice analysis (Kimura et al., 2007).

Additionally, in the literature there are examples of remote monitoring and patient management for PD (Tindall & Huebner, 2009), as well as the use of telematic services to facilitate the performance of motor tests remotely (Das, 2010; Dorsey et al., 2010; Giansanti et al., 2008; Westin et al., 2010).

Even though many advances have been done in the last years, it must be said that there is still a lack of an all-inclusive system able to provide reliable assessment of the status of PD patients being at the same time economically affordable. In particular it is crucial to provide:

- An effective evaluation of PD symptoms through monitoring and testing routines while not interfering with the patient daily life.
- A personalised profile of the patient allowing the correlation between those factors affecting the severity of symptoms (i.e. medication schedule and meals) and the evolution of the disease.
- The clinician with a system able to manage more efficiently the patient by providing timely indications on the effectiveness of the therapy and suggestions on therapy changes.

3.2.2 Available systems in the market/research

There are several products produced by certain research groups or commercially available for the assessment of PD. Some examples follow:

Cleveland Medical Devices

Cleveland Medical Devices Inc. commercialises Kinesia, a compact wireless system for monitoring the severity of PD motor symptoms. The system includes miniature motion sensors worn on the hand and it wirelessly transmits motor symptom information to a personal computer. Data is collected while patients follow computer based video instructions.

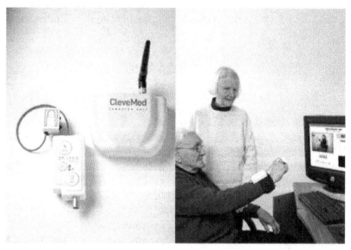

Fig. 1. Kinesia, Cleveland Medical Devices Inc. system for PD monitoring based on motor sensors (Jovanov et al., 2001)

Cleveland Medical Devices Inc. also commercialises Kinetisense, a compact wireless system for monitoring gait, posture or upper limb movement. The system integrates two channel Electromyography (EMG) and three orthogonal accelerometers and gyroscopes collecting data on three dimensional movements. The system is wearable and lightweight and is wirelessly connected to a computer for real-time data transmission. As alternative, data can be stored on a memory card for 12 hours recording and transmitted asynchronously. The system can be linked to different software tools for movement and posture analysis, detection of slips and falls and for the performance and monitoring of rehabilitation exercises.

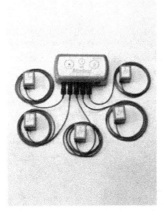

Fig. 2. Kinetisense, Cleveland Medical Devices Inc. system for PD monitoring based on motor sensors and electromyography (Jovanov et al., 2001)

Intel Corporation

Intel Corporation has developed a system called At home Telemonitoring Device (AHTD), based on nonlinear speech single processing methods around the use of discrete variational integrator. It could be used to perform speech analysis detect abnormalities and telemonitor neurological disorders with voice singles.

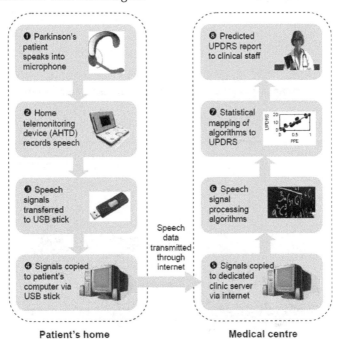

Fig. 3. At Home Telemonitoring Device (AHTD), Intel Corporation system for PD monitoring based on speech processing (Tsanas et al., 2010b)

Karolinska Institute

The Karolinska Institute, Sweden, has developed a prototype test battery for evaluating fluctuation motor symptoms in PD together with a decision support system as part of the Movistar TEVAL project (Westin et al., 2010). The system is based on a handheld device with built-in mobile communication, where combined patient diaries with on-screen motor tests are implemented. The data collected from the patient are transmitted to a central system where they are analysed through Artificial Intelligence methods. Besides, it originates alerts and advice via a web interface.

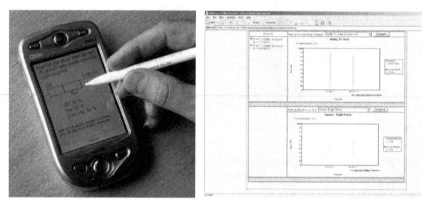

Fig. 4. TEVAL project prototype, Karolinska Institute, Sweden, based on patient diaries together with on-screen motor tests

Twente University

The University of Twente, Enschede, in the Netherlands, has developed a system called SensorShoe that is a mobile gait analysis tool. It is composed by a low-power sensor node equipped with movement sensors (3D accelerometers and 2D gyroscopes) connected to a PDA which provides immediate feedback to the patient while walking and suggest physical

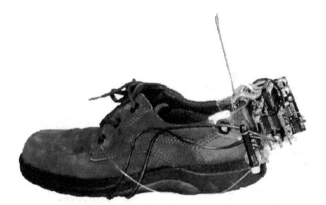

Fig. 5. Sensor Shoe, University of Twente, Enschede, The Netherlands. Gait analysis based on movement sensors (Kauw-A-Tjoe et al., 2007)

exercises based on the personal rehabilitation and training program defined for the patient and stored in the PDA. The system can connect to the hospital or to the physician through the PDA and transmit daily motion data, which can be analysed by physicians and be used to improve the physical therapy.

Federal Polytechnic School of Lausanne

The Federal Polytechnic School of Lausanne, Switzerland, has developed a system for motion monitoring based on a portable data-logger with three body-fixed inertial sensors.

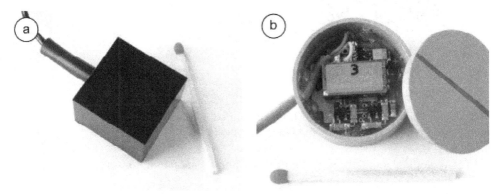

Fig. 6. a) The trunk sensor used for physical activity monitoring b) The uni-axial gyroscopes used for the gait analysis, The Federal Polytechnic School of Lausanne, Switzerland (Salarian et al., 2007).

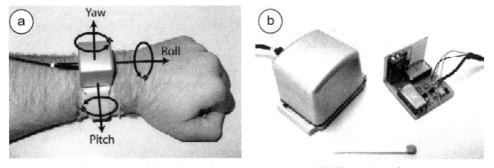

Fig. 7. a) Trunk sensor used for physical activity monitoring b) The uni-axial gyroscopes used for the gait analysis, The Federal Polytechnic School of Lausanne, Switzerland (Salarian, et al., 2007b)

Boston University

The Boston University National Institute of biomedical Imagining and Bioengineering has developed a wearable-sensor system for monitoring motor function. The system is composed by a device that can be worn unobtrusively by patients in their home to automatically detect the presence and severity of movement disorders associated with PD. The onset of the OFF status is based on the motor status of the patient that can be related to the motor status of the patient with the medications assumptions. The system involves electromyographic (EMG) and accelerometric (ACC) body worn sensors, whose signals are analysed by a system using Artificial Intelligence methods.

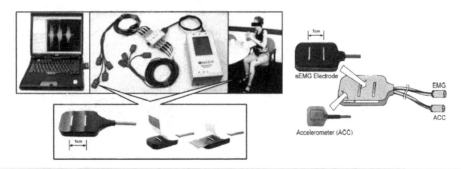

Fig. 8. Boston University National Institute of Biomedical Imaging and Bioengineering, PD monitoring system through motor and EMG sensors (UB, 2011)

3.3 Technological solution: non autonomous home based monitoring closed loop systems

Close loop systems are those in which stimulation parameters are adjusted according to recorded signals. Talking about neurodegenerative diseases such as PD, close loop systems imply that medication doses and timing is adjusted based on the measurement of certain biomedical signals. Some examples follow.

3.3.1 PERFORM project

A sophisticated multi-paRametric system FOR the continuous effective assessment and Monitoring of motor status in Parkinson's disease and other neurodegenerative diseases research project has developed an intelligent system that monitors several motor signals of the patients that are analyzed in a medical centre by a medical professional. The system is able to propose treatment changes, based on the clinical assessment. Further explanations are provided later in this chapter (Perform, 2008).

3.3.2 HELP project

The HELP project (Home-based Empowered living for Parkinson's Disease Patients) aims at developing a comprehensive system able to administer drug therapy without patient intervention, in either continuous or on-demand basis in order to manage disease progression and to mitigate PD's symptoms (Help, 2011).

It is based on inertial sensors that capture inertial information about the patient's motion and compute spatiotemporal properties and Parkinson's related symptoms. At the point of care remote supervision of the patient is performed, together with Verification of the infusion algorithm and possible modification of its parameters. An intraoral device continuously administrates dopamine agonists to the mucosa from the mouth. Besides, a subcutaneous pump receives commands adapting the infusion rate of apomorphine, a non-selective dopamine agonist.

4. PERFORM system

4.1 Introduction

PERFORM is a project partially funded by the European Commission under the Seventh Framework Program, aiming at providing an innovative and reliable tool that is able to monitor and evaluate motor neurodegenerative disease patients, such as PD patients.

The PERFORM project is based on the development of an intelligent closed loop system that seamlessly integrates a wide range of wearable micro-sensors constantly monitoring several motor signals of the patients. Data acquired are pre-processed by advanced knowledge processing methods, integrated by fusion algorithms to allow health professionals to remotely monitor the overall status of the patients, adjust medication schedules and personalize treatment. Personalization of treatment occurs through PERFORM's capability to keep track of the timing and doses of the medication and meals that the patient is taking.

4.2 The PERFORM medical and technological vision

The information gathered by the inertial sensors (accelerometers and gyroscopes) is processed by several classifiers. As a result, it is possible to evaluate and quantify the PD symptoms that the patient presents as well as analyze the gait of the patient. Based on this information, together with information derived from tests performed with tests devices (e.g. virtual reality gloves) and information about the medication and food intake, a patient specific profile is built. Next steep is to compare the patient specific profile with his evaluation during the last week and last month, checking whether his status is stable, improving or worsening. Based on that, the system analyses whether a medication change is needed-always under medical supervision- and in this case, information about the medication change proposal is sent to the patient.

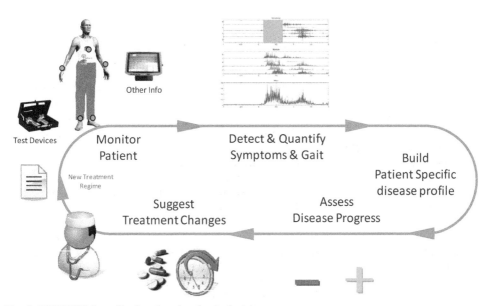

Fig. 9. PERFORM medical and technological vision

4.3 The PERFORM architecture

The system architecture proposed to meet the previously described medical and technological vision is presented in Fig. 10. It consists of two subsystems: the patient-side subsystem and the healthcare centre subsystem.

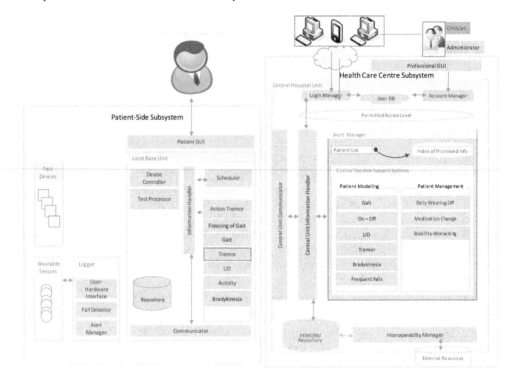

Fig. 10. PERFORM system architecture (R. Greenlaw et al., 2009)

The patient-side subsystem is responsible for the identification and quantification of the patient symptoms and the recording of other useful information for the evaluation of the patient status. The healthcare centre subsystem evaluates the disease progression and suggests appropriate treatment and changes, based on medical knowledge acquired from published medical guidelines.

The patient-side subsystem is composed by the following modules:

Continuous monitoring Module. It is used to monitor the patient motor status through the day. It consists of five accelerometers and a wearable device. The wearable device processes the recorded signals and detects patient falls in real time. The sensors position was hosen after careful examination and research on the targeted disease symptoms.

It is composed of four tri-axial accelerometers used to record the accelerations of the movements at each patient extremity, one accelerometer and gyroscope (on the trunk) used to record body/chest movement accelerations and angular body velocity during trunk and body turning, and a wearable device receiving all recorded signals. The sensors' position was chosen to allow all targeted symptoms detection and quantification with the minimum number of sensors.

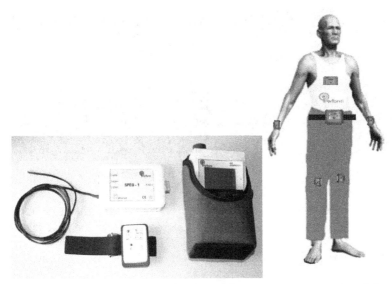

Fig. 11. PERFORM System prototype including accelerometers, gyroscope and data logger (left) System placement on the body (right)

All sensors transmit using Zigbee protocol to the wearable device which is located on the patients' waist thus making up a body sensor network. Special attention is given to the sensors usage and the easy set up by the patient and the caregivers. The sensor size is no bigger than a small matchbox. Sensors on the arms and legs are attached on specially designed elastic Velcro bands, which allow fixation to any wrist or ankle size. The sensors are placed inside an elastic pocket on the band, which secures it firmly on the patient body avoiding motion artefact due to cloth movement. The sensor on the trunk in placed within a zipped elastic pocket on a vest. The vest is also equipped with Velcro straps to firmly adjust the sensor on the patient chest. The selected design allows the easy wearing and attachment/detachment of sensors.

Test Module. It consists of a set of devices (such as virtual reality gloves, microphones or video cameras) used to record patient information, while the patient is performing specific tests, as normally done at the clinician's office during an examination. The patient wears the test devices and performs the tests as instructed from the visual interface of the Base Module (Local Base Unit). The test module records the performed activities and identifies any abnormalities, such as wrong sensor or patient position. Finally, it processes the recorded data and extracts the information about the number of taps and hand movements per second, the detection of hypophonia and neutral face expression.

Patient interface. Emphasis is given in designing an easy to use interface for the patient, considering the patient motor disabilities and limited computer familiarity. The designed interface inherits the feel and tough of the phone dialling pad, and all system choices are based on it. Patient use the interface to declare their subjective estimation of their own status, to gain access to relevant disease information, to receive instructions on life-style interventions, such as medication and good intake and on the execution of tests. Moreover, PD's patients declare medication intake information, which is useful for the patient status assessment.

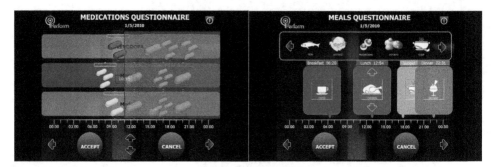

Fig. 12. PERFORM Patient Interface. Medication intake information (left). Food intake information (right)

Communication: the Base Module supports Bluetooth and Zigbee communication with the continuous monitoring system, and fixed line communication to the hospital centre over ISDN and xDSL.

Symptom Detection. This submodule processes received patient signals and detects the targeted patient symptoms (tremor, levodopa induced dyskinesia and off state). For each symptom dedicated submodule processes the relevant signals, detests the symptom episode and quantifies it into a severity scale from 1 to 4, according to the UPDRS scaling for PD patients (Cancela et al., 2010; Keijsers et al., 2000; Pansera et al., 2009). Other features such as duration, frequently and amplitude might also be provided for further clinician review and system evaluation.

The healthcare centre subsystem is composed of the following modules:

Patient Modelling Module. This module exploits the recorded patient information to build a patient symptom profile. For each main symptom (tremor, levodopa induced dyskinesia and on-off states), it produces a patient profile which describes the patient's common symptom features. When a new patient recording is processes, it is checked against the patient symptom profile. If significant differences are found, it might be due to two reasons: either a temporarily patient behaviour abnormality or a change to the patient profile. In the last case, the system checks whether a substantial number of similar situations are identified for the last time period for the specific patient and if that occurs, it creates an alert.

Patient Management Module. This module considers the detected symptoms and their characteristics, combines them with other recorded information and suggests appropriate treatment changes based on the accumulated specialists' knowledge on the management of PD.

Medical Interface: The system can be accessed either locally or remotely by the treating clinician and the general practitioner, using either a large screen access device (e.g. PC, laptop) or a small screen access device (e.g. PDA). Clinicians are directed to the home system screen, which presents the produced patient alerts to the patient specific screen, which provides the information needed to evaluate visually the patient condition. On request, the actual recorded signal and tests are downloaded from the patient-side to the healthcare centre for review. The focus is on the provision of an adequate visual description of the patient status within one screen, minimising the time spend by a clinician. Clinicians will access the system periodically to check patient status, but the option to be alerted when patient status changes are also available.

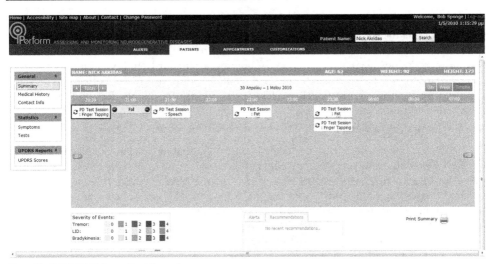

Fig. 13. PERFORM medical interface

Communication. All patient-side data (signal features and patient inserted information) are transmitted to the health-care subsystem once a day, through Internet.

4.4 Evaluation methodology

In order to test PERFORM system, several clinical trials have been arranged into 4 different phases, taking place between 2009 and 2011. Their description follows.

Phase 1: Data collection with SHIMMER

Eight subjects participated in this study, separated in two groups: four PD patients and four healthy subjects. The symptoms were rated by a professional neurologist with more than 20 years of experience with PD patients. Four accelerometers were placed on the right and left forearms and on the right and left calves, with a fifth accelerometer being placed on the trunk, at the base of the sternum. Motion data was collected using the SHIMMER platform (RealTime, 2011). SHIMMER is a small wireless sensor platform designed by Intel as a wearable device for health sensing applications. All sensors provide 3-axis accelerometer signals large storage, and low power-standards based communication capabilities. They also provide a Bluetooth protocol capability that allows SHIIMERs to stream the data to a computer. During the experiment, the accelerometry measurements were complemented by a reflective marker and a camera collection system. This complimentary analysis served as a support tool to validate the data used for this work.

Phase 2: Data Collection with ANCO first release trainer classifier

The data collection was performed with a network of wireless 3-axis ALA-6g sensors (Anco, 2011), located on the limbs, trunk and belt of the patient. During this phase, data were collected during tests with patients in a supervised environment, with the collaboration of the clinic's medical staff. Patients involved in this phase were required to be aged between 18 and 85 years old, suffering from PD, capable of complying with study requirements, receiving dopaminergic treatment and experiencing motor fluctuations. Dementia, Psychosis and significant systemic diseases (such as cancer) were the exclusion criteria applied when selecting participants. The data set used in this study included trials with twenty PD patients, ten in Navarra (Spain) and ten in Ioannina (Greece). In order to comply with ethical requirements, all procedures were carried with the Clinic Institutional Review Board's permission. Data were collected following a standard clinical protocol in which patients carried out daily basic activities (i.e. walking, lying, sitting, etc.) during two cycles of on-off oscillations in response to levodopa during the same day and under the supervision of a clinician.

Phase 3: Long time recording

Data collection of phase 3 was performed with an updated version of the devices that includes a wearable and programmable logger that gave a better mobility to the patient and new ALA-6g accelerometers sensors equipped with an external battery allowing longer data collection session. Data were collected in a supervised environment and with the collaboration of the medical staff. Furthermore, patients involved in this phase, fulfilled with the age and medical specifications of the previous phase. The data were recorded with twenty-four PD patients, twelve in Navarra and twelve in Ioannina. Data were collected during a six-hour daily session in which patients carried out their normal daily activity. Moreover, four standard clinical protocol sessions were performed during two cycles of on-off oscillations in response to levodopa treatment and under the supervision of a clinician. At the end of the day, data were processed using the train set computed in the previous phase and the output were checked with the results provided by the clinicians

Phase 4: Final system testing

From March 2011, the integrated and final PERFORM system will be introduced to a new group of patients that will perform the final evaluation. The patient group will be constituted by 20 PD patients for regular tests and 4 PD patients for mid-term tests, all recruited from the Neurology Department from the Azienda Unita' Sanitaria Locale di Modena hospital in Modena, Italy.

4.5 Results

PERFORM project has released promising results in patients monitoring and status assessment. Due to the short-term nature of the clinic trials that have been carried out it is difficult to determine the future impact on patient treatment; however it is possible to at least provide a quantification of the performances of the modules of the Patient –Side Subsystem. It is designed to assess the motor status of the patients and establish a direct connection with the physician. Its basic functions are:

- to determine the activity of the subject
- to provide a quantification of symptoms severity based on the UPRDS scale and present such an information to the physician through remote communication
- to gather information about the daily life of the patient

The validation has proved that the first prototype of the Patient Side Subsystem is able to provide a very reasonable assessment of the daily activity of the patients using data classification techniques based on accelerometers. More specifically, the algorithms are able to discriminate activities such as walking, standing, laying or sitting with an accuracy of nearly 99%. The activity recognition is the base information needed to evaluate the symptoms related to movement. Besides, the clinical trials have proved that the algorithms are able to classify with an acceptable degree of accuracy the main symptoms of PD. General body bradykinesia is quantified with a classification accuracy within the range of 70%-86% (depending on the number of sensors used in the measurements) compared to medical evaluation. Dyskinesia and tremor classification accuracy are respectively 93.6% and 97%. Those results are quite good in comparison with the subjective medical evaluation, with accuracy around 95%. The gait module has also proved to release useful information with acceptable level of accuracy. The gait analysis system provides a measure of stride length with a 7.3% of average error and a measurement of the complexity of movement through an analysis of the entropy of the walking.

Phase IV of the pilots is expected to provide a more accurate validation with long-term recording data.

4.6 Comparison with SoA systems

Compared to Kinesia system, a sophisticated multi-paRametric system FOR the continuous effective assessment and Monitoring of motor status in Parkinson's disease and other neurodegenerative diseases (PERFORM) presents the advantage of integrating other data from patient's monitoring, such as data from normal daily activity Kinesia monitors only upper extremity motor symptoms, while PERFORM is able to monitor the entire motor disorder, involving walking and moving in general, including freezing, falls risks, etc. The system is based on proprietary software and raw data may not be available.

In relation to Kinetisense commercial product, PERFORM links motion monitoring data to other information such as medication assumption, stress situations and historic data of the patient, in order to draw a complete picture and not only a snapshot such as Kinetisense does. The system is based on proprietary software and raw data may not be available. PERFORM integrates more data from continuous monitoring rather than on e-diary and voluntary motion exercises as the TEVAL Movistar system does.

Compared with SensorShoe system, PERFORM provides link to medication and enables complex data interpretation and analysis. On the other hand, PERFORM system is also able to detect abnormalities in motion, which the prototype built by the École Polytechnique Federale de Lausanne is not detecting.

In comparison with the system proposed by Boston university, PERFORM manages data from more devices and is able to correlate different data input.

Finally, in comparison with the project HELP, PERFORM is able to provide an assessment for specific symptoms such as dyskinesia, bradykinesia, tremor and akynesia, delivering a quantification based on the UPDRS scale, which HELP is not taking into consideration. On the other hand, the system is not providing a feedback to adjust the medication directly on the patients. In other word, PERFORM is not closing the loop of monitoring/assessment/medication adjustment in an automatic way, that is what HELP project has tried to do.

5. Conclusions

This chapter has presented a SoA review of the main methods used to monitor and assess PD's patients. On one hand, clinical assessment is usually performed through annotations in diaries and self-reports from the patient during the short office visit in this neurologist the patient may appear very well and he misses to report some symptoms, as a result, treatment modifications are not undertaken in time. The UPDRS is a scale that tries to quantify selected symptoms and signs of Parkinsonism in a 5-points scoring system (with 0 for no signal and 4 for a marked severity of the sign). Unfortunately, the UPDRS like any other semi-objective rating scale has limitations like intra and inter observer inconsistencies, can be time consuming and ca be biased by subjectivity issues related to historical information.

On the other hand, technological solutions are able to provide quantitative objective information, including the use of motor sensors, electromyography, position transducers, and speech recognition systems.

This chapter has presented PERFORM, a project partially funded by the European Commission under the 7th Framework Program, aiming at providing an innovative and reliable tool that is able to monitor and evaluate motor neurodegenerative disease patients, such as PD patients.

The PERFORM project is based on the development of an intelligent closed loop system that seamlessly integrates a wide range of wearable micro-sensors, constantly monitoring several motor and signals of the patients. Data acquired are pre-processed by advanced knowledge processing methods, integrated by fusion algorithms to allow health professionals to remotely monitor the overall status of the patients and adjust medication schedules and personalize treatment. Personalization of treatment occurs through PERFORM's capability to keep track of the timing and doses of the medication and meals that the patient is taking. The system architecture has been presented. A comparison with available related systems has been performed.

The system has already been tested in hospitals in Navarra (Spain) and Ioannina (Greece). The integrated tests of the system will be performed in Modena (Italy) from March 2011.

Obtained results so far suggest an overall valid closed loop system, able to detect PD symptoms based on motor signals and additional information, evaluate with a high accuracy level the overall status of the patient and propose medication changes accordingly. However, to achieve more improvements especially in the automation of close-loop mechanism, further improvements are needed in order to provide a complete reliable assessment system for symptoms severity.

6. Acknowledgment

The authors thank PERFORM project Consortium for their valuable contribution to this work, and especially Prof. José Antonio Martín Pereda, Prof. Francisco del Pozo and Prof. Ana González Marcos from the Universidad Politécnica de Madrid for their collaboration and scientific support. PERFORM project (Contract Nr. 215952) is partially funded by the European Commission under the 7th Framework Programme.

7. References

Anco. (2011). Retrieved March 2011, Available from http://www.anco.gr/

Cancela, J, Pansera, M, Arredondo, M T, Estrada, J J, Pastorino, M., Pastor-Sanz, L., (2010). A comprehensive motor symptom monitoring and management system: the bradykinesia case. *Conference proceedings of Annual International Conference of the IEEE Engineering in Medicine and Biology Society*, pp. 1008-11. 2010, August 31 – September 4.

Darkins, A. W., Fromkin, V. A., & Benson, D. F. (1988). A characterization of the prosodic loss in Parkinson's disease. *Brain and Language*, 34(2), 315-327. ISSN 0093-934X.

Das, R. (2010). A comparison of multiple classification methods for diagnosis of Parkinson disease. *Expert Systems with Applications*, 37(2), 1568-1572. ISSN 0957-4174 .

Deuschl, G., Schade-Brittinger, C., Krack, P., Volkmann, J., Schöfer, H. & Bötzel, K., (2006). A randomized trial of deep-brain stimulation for Parkinson's disease. *New England Journal of Medicine*, 355(9), 896-908. ISSN 0028-4793.

Dorsey, E., Deuel, L. M., Voss, T. S., Finnigan, K., George, B. P. & Eason, S., (2010). Increasing access to specialty care: A pilot, randomized controlled trial of telemedicine for Parkinson's disease. *Movement Disorders*, 25(11), 1652-1659. ISSN 0885-3185.

Fuente-Fernández, R. de la, Sossi, V., Huang, Z., Furtado, S., Lu, J.-Q. & Calne, D. B., (2004). Levodopa-induced changes in synaptic dopamine levels increase with progression of Parkinson's disease: implications for dyskinesias. *Journal of neurology*, 127(Pt 12), pp. 2747-54. ISSN 1560-9545.

Giansanti, D., Maccioni, G., Cesinaro, S., Benvenuti, F., & Macellari, V. (2008). Assessment of fall-risk by means of a neural network based on parameters assessed by a wearable device during posturography. *Medical engineering & physics*, 30(3), pp. 367-372. ISSN: 1350-4533.

Giansanti, D., Maccioni, G., & Morelli, S. (2008). An Experience of Health Technology Assessment in New Models of Care for Subjects with Parkinson's Disease by Means of a New Wearable Device. *Telemedicine and e-health*, 14(5), 467-472. ISSN 1530-5627

Goetz, C. G., Poewe, W., Rascol, O., Sampaio, C., Stebbins, G. T., Counsell, (2004). Movement Disorder Society Task Force report on the Hoehn and Yahr staging scale: status and recommendations. *Movement Disorder*, 19(9), pp.1020-8. ISSN 0885-3185.

Greenlaw, R., Estrada, J., Pansera, M., Konitsiotis, S., Baga, D & Maziewski, P., (2009). PERFORM: Building and Mining Electronic Records of Neurological Patients Being Monitored in the Home. *Proceeding of World Congress on Medical Physics and Biomedical Engineering* (Vol. 25/9, pp. 533-535-535). Munich, Germany. September 7-12.

Group, P. S. (2001). Evaluation of dyskinesias in a pilot, randomized, placebo controlled trial or remacemide in advanced Parkinson disease. *Archives of Neurology*, 58, pp. 1660-1668. ISSN 0003-9942.

Help project (2011). Home Based Empowed Living for Parkinson Disease's Patients. Retrieved March 2011, from http://www.help-aal.com/HELP/

Jovanov, E., Raskovic, D., Price, J., Krishnamurthy, A., Chapman, J., & Moore, A. (2001). Patient monitoring using personal area networks of wireless intelligent sensors. *Biomedical Sciences Instrumentation*, 37, 373-378. ISSN 0067-8856.

Kauw-A-Tjoe, R. G., Thalen, J. P., Marin-Perianu, M., & Havinga, P. J. M. (2007). SensorShoe: Mobile Gait Analysis for Parkinson's Disease Patients. University of Innsbruck public document.

Keijsers, N L W, Horstink, M., Van Hilten, J. J., Hoff, J I, & Gielen, C. (2000). Detection and assessment of the severity of levodopa-induced dyskinesia in patients with Parkinson's disease by neural networks. *Movement Disorders*, 15(6), pp. 1104-1111. John Wiley & Sons. ISSN 0885-3185.

Keijsers, N L W, Horstink, M.W.I.M., & Gielen, S. C. A. M. (2003). Automatic assessment of levodopa-induced dyskinesias in daily life by neural networks. *Movement disorders*, 18(1), 70-80. ISSN 0885-3185.

Keijsers, N. L. W., Horstink, M. W. I. M., Hilten, J. J. van, Hoff, J. I., & Gielen, C. C. A. M. (2000). Detection and assessment of the severity of Levodopa-induced dyskinesia in patients with Parkinson's disease by neural networks. *Movement Disorders*, 15(6), 1104-1111. ISSN 0885-3185.

Kimura, F., Horio, K., Hagane, Y., Yu, W., Katoh, R., Katane, T., (2007). Detecting Perturbation Occurrence during Walking. *Conference proceeding of Towards sysnthesis of Micro-/Nano-systems: The 11th international conference on precision engineering (ICPE)*. Tokyo, Japan, 2007. August 16-18.

Lang, A.E., & Lozano, A.M. (1998). Parkinson's disease: First of two parts. *New England Jorunal of Medicine*, 339, 1044-1053. ISSN 0028-4793

Lau, L. M. L. de, & Breteler, M. M. B. (2006). Epidemiology of Parkinson's disease. *Lancet neurology*, 5(6), 525-35. ISSN 1474-4422.

Lees, A. J. (1989). The on-off phenomenon. Journal of Neurology, *Neurosurgery & Psychiatry*, 52(Suppl), 29. ISSN: 1359-5067.

Lim, A. S., Moro, E., Lozano, A M, Hamani, C., Dostrovsky, J. O., Hutchison, W. D., (2009). Selective enhancement of rapid eye movement sleep by deep brain stimulation of the human pons. *Annals of neurology*, 66(1), pp.110-114. ISSN 0364-5134.

Lingyun Gu, L., J.G, H., Shrivastav, R. M., & Sapienza, C. (2005). Disordered Speech Assessment Using Automatic Methods Based on Quantitative Measures. *EURASIP Journal on Applied Signal Processing*, 9 (pp.1400–1409).ISSN 1110-8657.

Lozano. (2009). Deep brain stimulation: current and future perspectives. *Neurosurgery Focus*, 27(1). ISSN 1092-0684

Mazzone, P., Lozano, A., Stanzione, P., Galati, S., Scarnati, E., Peppe, A., (2005). Implantation of human pedunculopontine nucleus: a safe and clinically relevant target in Parkinson's disease. *Neuroreport*, 16(17), 1877. ISSN 0959-4965.

Pansera, Mario, Estrada, Juan Jacobo, Pastor, L., Cancela, Jorge, Greenlaw, Reynold, & Arredondo, Maria Teresa. (2009). Multi-parametric system for the continuous assessment and monitoring of motor status in Parkinson's disease: an entropy-based gait comparison. *Conference proceedings of Annual International Conference of the IEEE Engineering in Medicine and Biology Society*, 2009, pp.1242-5. Minneapolis, USA. September 2-6.

Papapetropoulos, S., Heather, K., Scanlo, B. K., Guevara, A., Singer, C., & Levin, B. (2010). Objective Quantification of Neuromotor Symptoms in Parkinson's Disease: Implementation of a Portable, Computerized Measurement Tool. *Parkinson's Disease*, 010 (Article ID 760196), 6.

Patel, S, Buckley, T., Rednic, R., McClure, D., Shih, L., Tarsy, D., et al. (2010). A Web-Based System for Home Monitoring of Patients with Parkinson's Disease Using Wearable Sensors. *IEEE transactions on bio-medical engineering*, 58(3), 831-836. ISSN 0018-9294.

Patel, S, Lorincz, K, Hughes, R, Huggins, N, Growdon, J. H., Welsh, M, (2007). Analysis of feature space for monitoring persons with Parkinson's Disease with application to a wireless wearable sensor system. Engineering in Medicine and Biology Society,

2007. *Proceeding of EMBS 2007. 29th Annual International Conference of the IEEE* (pp. 6290-6293). Lyon, France, 2007. August 23-26.

Patel, Shyamal, Lorincz, Konrad, Hughes, Richard, Huggins, Nancy, Growdon, J., Standaert, D., (2009). Monitoring motor fluctuations in patients with Parkinson's disease using wearable sensors. *IEEE transactions on information technology in biomedicine*, 13(6), 864-73. ISSN 0018-9294.

Perform. (2008). *Perform Project*. Grant Agreement Nr. 215952.

RealTime. (2011). *Shimmer Research*. Retrieved March 2011, from http://www.shimmer-research.com/

Salarian, A., Russmann, H., Vingerhoets, F. J. G., Burkhard, P. R., & Aminian, K. (2007). Ambulatory monitoring of physical activities in patients with Parkinson's disease. *IEEE Transactions on Biomedical Engineering*, 54(12), pp. 2296-2299. ISSN 0018-9294.

Salarian, A., Russmann, H., Vingerhoets, F. J. G., Dehollain, C., Blanc, Y., Burkhard, P. R., (2004). Gait assessment in Parkinson's disease: toward an ambulatory system for long-term monitoring. *IEEE Transactions on Biomedical Engineering*, 51(8). ISSN 0018-9294.

Singh, N., Pillay, V., & Choonara, Y. E. (2007). Advances in the treatment of Parkinson's disease. *Progress in neurobiology*, 81(1),pp.29-44. ISSN 0301-0082.

Standaert, D. G., & Young, A. B. (2001). Treatment of CNS neurodegenerative diseases. In H. and Limbird (Ed.), *Goodman and Gilman's Pharmacological Basis of Therapeutics* (pp. 549-620). ISBN-10: 0071354697; New Your, Mc Graw-Hill.

Tindall, L. R., & Huebner, R. A. (2009). The Impact of an Application of Telerehabilitation Technology on Caregiver Burden. *International Journal of Telerehabilitation*, 1(1), 3-8.

Tolosa. (1998). *Parkinson's disease and movement disorders*. ISBN 0-7817-7881-6. Baltimore: Lippincott Williams & Wilkins Philadelphia.

Tsanas, A., Little, M. A., McSharry, P. E., & Ramig, L. O. (2010). Enhanced classical dysphonia measures and sparse regression for telemonitoring of Parkinson's disease progression. *Proceeding of Acoustics Speech and Signal Processing (ICASSP), 2010 IEEE International Conference on Biomedical Engineering* (pp. 594-597). Buenos Aires, Argentina, 2010. August 31 – September 4.

UB. (2011). Boston University National Institute of Biomedical Imaging and Bioengineering. Retrieved March 2011, from http://www.bu.edu/bme/

Vaillancourt, D. E., Sturman, M. M., Verhagen Metman, L., Bakay, R. A. E., & Corcos, D. M. (2003). Deep brain stimulation of the VIM thalamic nucleus modifies several features of essential tremor. *Neurology*, 61(7), pp.919-925. ISSN 0340-5354.

Van Someren, E. J. W., Van Gool, W. A., Vonk, B. F. M., Mirmiran, M., Speelman, J. D., Bosch, D. A., (1993). Ambulatory monitoring of tremor and other movements before and after thalamotomy: a new quantitative technique. *Journal of the neurological sciences*, 117(1-2),pp.16-23. ISSN 0022-510X.

Westin, J., Dougherty, M., Nyholm, D., & Groth, T. (2010). A home environment test battery for status assessment in patients with advanced Parkinson's disease. *Computer methods and programs in biomedicine*, 98(1), 27-35. ISSN 0169-2607.

Westin, J., Ghiamati, S., Memedi, M., Nyholm, D., Johansson, A., Dougherty, M., (2010). A new computer method for assessing drawing impairment in Parkinson's disease. *Journal of neuroscience methods*, 190(1), 143-148. ISSN 0165-0270.

WHO. (2002). Integrating prevention into health care. Retrieved 2011, from http://www.who.int/mediacentre/factsheets/fs172/en/index.html

4

Effects of a Multimodal Exercise Program on Clinical, Functional Mobility and Cognitive Parameters of Idiopathic Parkinson's Disease Patients

L.T.B. Gobbi, F.A. Barbieri, R. Vitório, M.P. Pereira and C. Teixeira-Arroyo
on behalf of the PROPARKI Group*
*UNESP – Univ Estadual Paulista, Rio Claro, SP,
Brazil*

1. Introduction

This chapter has as main objective to present the effects of a multimodal exercise program on major signs/symptoms, functional mobility and cognitive parameters of people with Parkinson's disease (PD). This program is developed to improve all functional capacity components (strength, balance, aerobic resistance, coordination and flexibility) in order to increase patients' independence, autonomy and quality of life. As main result, we found maintenance of clinical status and memory after the exercise program with an increase in functional mobility. These results can be attributed to neuro-protection mechanisms enhanced by exercise and to an increase in functional capacity.

Parkinson's Disease (PD) is the second most incident neurodegenerative pathology in subjects over 60 years old (Olanow et al., 2009). PD has been described to affect approximately 0.3% of the population and 1% to 2% of those older than 60 years (de Lau & Breteler, 2006). It is a neurodegenerative pathology characterized by progressive degeneration of the dopamine-producing neurons in the substantia nigra pars compacta. The neuromotor impulses in the subcortical to cortical pathways, responsible for accurate control of muscle activation, are compromised with the decreased amount of dopamine. As a consequence, people with PD show motor (e.g. resting tremor, rigidity, postural instability, mobility and others) and non-motor (e.g. executive functions, depression, memory, humor alterations, dementia and others) (Taylor et al., 1986; Chaudhuri et al., 2006; Martinez-Martin, 2006; Olanow et al., 2009) signs/symptoms. Clinical parameters of PD patients tend to get worse progressively (Karlsen et al., 2000) even though pharmacological interventions associated with non pharmacological therapies have shown some benefits to patients (Sage & Almeida, 2009, 2010).

Motor signs/symptoms related to PD can contribute to the decline in balance control and mobility (Christofoletti et al., 2006), which subsequently can lead to a reduction in functional

*A.P.T. Alves, R.A. Batistela, P.M. Formaggio, E. Lirani-Silva, L.C. Morais, P.H.S. Pelicioni, V. Raile, N.M. Rinaldi, P.C.R. Santos, C.B. Takaki, F. Stella and S. Gobbi

independence. As a consequence, individuals with PD experience an increase in both the difficulties in performing daily activities, such as rising from a chair or walking, that are directed related to impoverishment in balance control (Hong & Steen, 2007), and in the risk of falls (Grimbergen et al., 2004). Together with motor disturbances, cognitive deficits in PD are detectable in the early stages (Stella et al., 2007) and are evidenced primarily by impairments in executive functions, i.e., the ability to generate spontaneous action as well as to develop motor strategies in specific planning for the performance of a given task (Taylor et al., 1986; Chaudhuri et al., 2006). Although the people with PD have the ability to decode, store and consolidate new information preserved, they present difficulty in retrieving these information (Dubois & Pillon, 1997; Dujardin & Laurent, 2003; Costa et al., 2008). These tasks involve transient working memory (handling, maintenance and temporary activation of the memory) and episodic memory (conscious recollection of individual events, reported within a specific context of space and time) (Dujardin & Laurent, 2003). Executive functions are regulated by both the prefrontal areas and the frontostriatal circuitry (Dujardin et al., 2003; Owen, 2004). In the prefrontal cortex, the transmission of dopamine by the dopamine receptors (D1) plays an important role in the functioning of working memory and learning (Cropley et al., 2006; Rashid et al., 2007), while the frontostriatal circuitry is related to motor planning (Olanow et al., 2009).

One possibility for the treatment of PD is the pharmacological therapy, i.e., the administration of synthetic dopamine (levodopa). Studies in patients with early stage of the disease have shown antagonistic effects during the *on phase* of the medication. Positive effects have been observed in locomotor (Pieruccini-Faria et al., 2006) and cognitive (Cools, 2006; Pascual-Sedano et al., 2008) parameters. However, over the years as the disease progresses, the effect of drug decreases and higher doses are needed for treatment. As a result, patients start to present motor fluctuations and dyskinesias (involuntary movements), which are side effects associated with long-term drug treatment (Obeso et al., 2000). Associated with drug therapy, non-pharmacologic therapies related to PD, such as physical exercises and nutrition, helped to attenuate the disease's severity or reduce its progression (Hirayama et al., 2008; Morris et al., 2009). The regular practice of physical exercise is effective to provide improvements in quality of life of this group of patients (White et al., 2006; Hirayama et al., 2008). Forced aerobic exercise affected both the scores in motor sub-section of the UPDRS and the performance in manual skills (Ridgel et al., 2009) while the sensory focused exercise program improved functional mobility and the motor symptoms (Sage & Almeida, 2010) in people with PD. The physical exercise can act as a protector factor generating brain changes due to a greater cerebral oxygenation, such as neuroplasticity, brain repairing and an increase of the dopaminergic cells (Smith & Zigmond, 2003; Fox et al., 2006). Besides, when the exercise is introduced in the early stages of the disease, the disease progression can slow down (Fox et al., 2006).

Physical exercise is an important factor that can improve functional capacity in the elderly (Cyarto et al., 2008). Crizzle and Newhouse (2006), reviewing the literature, concluded that, through exercise, patients with PD improve their physical performance and the performance of activities of daily living. Recently, some evidences have been showed positive changes after the exercise program not only in balance and mobility (Gobbi et al., 2009; Hackney & Earhart, 2010) but also for the motor (Sage & Almeida, 2009; Sage & Almeida, 2010) and non-motor signs/symptoms (Tanaka et al., 2009) in PD patients. Therefore, systematic participation in physical exercise programs can help individuals with PD to maintain their motor repertories and their cognitive ability to perform daily living activities.

Effects of a Multimodal Exercise Program on Clinical, Functional Mobility and Cognitive Parameters of Idiopathic
Parkinson's Disease Patients

87

Any type of physical exercise is better than no exercise to improve the level of functional capacity (Brach et al., 2004). However, little is known about the effect of exercise on cognitive function in patients with PD. For healthy elderly, without PD, studies have shown positive results of exercise on cognitive functions, especially on memory (Chiari et al., 2010). Aerobic exercises are the more effective ones to improve memory parameters of older people when compared to cognitive exercises and the ones that combine aerobic and cognitive exercises (Fabre et al., 2002). The positive results found for the elderly population may suggest that people with PD also benefit from physical exercise practice. Physical exercise programs for people with PD that focus on improvements in functional capacity and mobility vary according to the type of proposed activity, whether it will be practiced individually or in a group, the program's duration, the frequency and duration of the weekly sessions, and the means of evaluation. Such programs include intensive sports training (Reuter et al., 1999), treadmill training with body weight support (Miyai et al., 2000), resistance training (Scandalis et al., 2001; Dibble et al., 2009), aerobic exercise (Bergen et al., 2002), alternative forms of exercise (Hackney & Earhart, 2009), home-based exercise intervention (Nocera et al., 2009), and the practice of movement strategies (Morris et al., 2009).

The results of our group, using a multimodal exercise program based on the improvement of the functional capacity components (strength, balance, aerobic resistance, coordination and flexibility) revealed a positive effect on the executive functions (Tanaka et al., 2009) and on the functional mobility and balance (Gobbi et al., 2009). Tanaka et al. (2009) analyzed the effects of an aerobic exercise program on executive functions in older people with PD. We found significant improvements in executive functions in people with PD after six months of participation in aerobic exercise program. Such benefits were expected to play an important role on independence, autonomy and quality of life of such population. Gobbi et al. (2009) investigated the effects of two intervention programs, a multi-mode exercise program and an adaptive program, on the mobility and functional balance in people with PD. We found that both the intensive and adaptive exercise programs improved balance and mobility in patients with PD.

Within this context, the purpose of this chapter is to demonstrate the effectiveness of a long-term multimodal exercise program in improving clinical parameters, functional mobility and cognitive function in people with PD. We analyzed the benefits of the long-term exercise interventions in motor and non motor signs/symptoms in a more holistic point of view, since this type of physical exercise intervention for people with PD have not been reported.

2. Methods

This study adhered to the guidelines of the Declaration of Helsinki, and was approved by the local Ethics Committee. All patients signed informed consent forms before involvement in the study.

2.1 Participants

Fifteen idiopathic PD patients were enrolled in the study. All had a diagnosis of idiopathic PD, with no other major neurological problems. Inclusion criteria were: disease in Stages I–III of the Hoehn and Yahr Rating Scale (H&Y; Hoehn & Yahr, 1967), independent walker, and no cognitive impairment, as judged by Brucki et al.'s (2003) suggestions for utilization of the Mini-Exam of Mental Status (MEMS; Folstein et al., 1975) in Brazil. Demographic data of PD patients are outlined in Table 1.

Subject	Gender	Age (years)	Body height (cm)	Body mass (kg)	H&Y (stage)	Years since diagnosis
A	female	66	162.2	85.5	1	3
B	female	60	163	56.7	2	2
C	female	67	153	47.5	1	3
D	female	59	154.4	67	1	2
E	female	60	142.8	57.5	1	2
F	female	82	153	71.7	3	4
G	female	65	151.8	39.5	1.5	4
H	female	60	162	70.4	1	3
I	male	75	176.5	62.5	1.5	4
J	male	64	161.8	85.1	3	19
L	male	69	174	69.7	1	3
M	male	59	165.5	88.7	1	2
N	male	78	165.5	88.7	2	1
O	male	65	163.3	77.9	1	1
P	male	73	165.5	91.6	1	4
Mean		**67**	**161.0**	**70.7**	**1.5**	**3.8**
SD		**7.28**	**8.74**	**15.87**	**0.7**	**4.33**

Table 1. Demographic characteristics of the participants.

2.2 Intervention

The aim of the multimodal exercise program was to develop the patients' functional capacity, cognitive functions, posture, and locomotion through a program that is primarily aerobic. It was composed of a variety of activities that simultaneously focus on the components of functional capacity, such as muscular resistance (specific exercises for large muscle groups), motor coordination (rhythmic activities), and balance (recreational motor activities). These components were selected because they seem to be those most affected by PD. The multimodal program took place over a six-month period (72 sessions, 3 times a week, and 60 minutes per session). Each session consisted of five components (warm-up, pre-exercise stretching, the main exercise session, cool-down and post-exercise stretching). All sessions were conducted in the morning, in the "on medication" state, between 1 and 1½ h after participants' first morning dose of medication. The program was designed in six phases and each phase was composed of 12 sessions and lasting approximately one month. At the end of each phase there was a progressive increase of load (Chart 1). Heart rate during the sessions remained between 60% and 80% of maximum heart rate (220 minus the participant's age in years), which characterizes training with aerobic predominance. The exercise program was supervised by at least three physical education professionals at any

Effects of a Multimodal Exercise Program on Clinical, Functional Mobility and Cognitive Parameters of Idiopathic Parkinson's Disease Patients

89

one time. Each participant was required to attend at least 70% of the sessions in order to be included in the data analysis. This protocol has been previously described by Tanaka et al. (2009).

Phases	Capacities		
	Coordination	Muscular Resistance	Balance
Phase 1	Upper and lower limbs movements.	Exercises without weights.	Recreational activities that stimulated the vestibular system.
Phase 2	Trunk movements were added to upper and lower limbs movements.	Light-weight equipment (hoops, ropes and batons).	Recreational activities that stimulated the visual and vestibular systems.
Phase 3	Trunk movements were substituted by head movements.	Heavier equipments (barbells, ankle weights, medicine balls).	Recreational activities that stimulated the visual and somatossensorial systems.
Phase 4	Head, trunk and upper and lower limb movements.	Load was again increased with heavier equipment for resistance training (increase of intensity) or increased repetitions (increased volume).	Recreational activities integrated the vestibular, visual and somatossensorial systems.
Phase 5	Four different movement sequences, two of which were the same for upper and lower limbs and two other sequences that alternated movements for upper and lower limbs in place and in movement.	Exercises were done with weights: leg press, pulley, seated cable rows, pecdeck, and bench press, in two series of 15 repetitions.	Recreational activities included static balance, dynamic balance, half-turn and complete turn (all with visual cues).
Phase 6	Four sequences of different movements, two sequences of alternating movement for upper and lower limbs and two sequences of different movement for upper and lower limbs, with or without trunk movement and equipment (balloons, balls, hoops and rope).	Series of 15 repetitions were added.	Recreational activities were composed of activities with tactile cues.

Chart 1. Designed phases of the 6-month intervention protocol with progressive increments on load and complexity for people with Parkinson's disease (adapted from Tanaka et al., 2009).

2.3 Evaluation protocol for the dependent variables

Participants were tested before commencing the multimodal program (pre-test), and upon completion (post-test). All assessments were carried out in the morning, in the "on medication" state, at least 1 h after participants' first morning dose of medication. The participants were evaluated by the same trained assessor (blinded as to the study purpose) under the same conditions in both moments (pre- and post-tests).

2.3.1 Clinical evaluation

A neuropsychiatrist performed a clinical assessment by means on the Unified Parkinson's Disease Rating Scale (UPDRS; Fahn & Elton, 1987), MEMS, and H&Y. Higher scores on the UPDRS and H&Y represent higher commitment levels of the disease. Conversely, higher scores on the MEMS indicate a more preserved cognitive function. For data analysis, scores on the UPDRS sub-sections I (Mentation, Behavior, and Mood), II (Activities of Daily Living), and III (Motor) were considered separately.

2.3.2 Functional mobility evaluation

Basic functional mobility was assessed by means of the Timed Up and Go Test (TUG; Podsiadlo & Richardison, 1991) and the Postural Locomotion Manual test (PLM; Steg et al., 1989).

i.   TUG: The task consisted of the participant to stand up from a sitting position in an armless chair with a seat height of 46.5 cm, walk a distance of 3 m, circumvent a cone, return, and sit back down in the chair. Participants were instructed to perform the test as quickly as possible, but without running. At least one practice trial was offered to the participants at the beginning of the procedure so that they could become familiar with it. Three trials were performed for testing purposes, and the time to perform the task was measured in seconds. Time was recorded from the instant the person's buttocks left the chair (standing up) until the next contact with the chair (sitting down). The mean value of the three attempts was considered for statistical analysis.

ii. PLM: This test measures postural control, locomotion and a goal directed reaching arm movement and the efficacy with which these movements compose a smooth dynamic action of the whole-person. To perform the PLM test, the participants were asked to move a small squared object (500 g), from a clearly marked starting place on the floor, to a stand located at eyes level, 1.82 m away in front of the starting place. Subjects had to deal with postural changes during the different phases of the test (to bend the upper body to pick up the object, walk forward and place the object on the stand). Time to perform the task was recorded from the "go" sign to the first contact of the object with the stand. The mean value of the three attempts was considered for statistical analysis.

iii. Since each subject performed three attempts of each task, we also compared these attempts (Attempt 1 vs Attempt 2 vs Attempt 3) before and after the training program.

2.3.3 Cognitive evaluation

The following tests were applied for cognitive function assessment:

i.   Executive Functions, by the Wisconsin Card Sorting Test – WCST (Heaton et al., 1993; Paolo et al., 1995). This test specifically assesses abstraction, mental flexibility and attention. It consists of 4 stimulus cards and 128 response cards that must be combined with the stimulus cards by following the hints "right" or "wrong" provided by the evaluator. From this hint, without pre-established rule, the participant must find the right combination (according to color, shape or number). Every 6 consecutive hits, the evaluator changes the mix and the participant must change his or her strategy. The test continues until the participant completes 6 categories of combinations or the 128 attempts. The WCST was chosen due to: a) its good construct validity for people with PD; b) it assesses three executive functions at the same time (abstraction, mental flexibility, attention) and; c) it does not require high level of schooling and this also

makes it appropriate for the population involved in our study. Within the executive
functions, mental flexibility was the variable of interest for this study. It was assessed
based on the number of perseverative errors made by patients.

ii. The subtest Logical Memory I and II, Wechsler Memory Scale Revised – WMS-R
(Wechsler, 1997) was used to measure the short-term memory (logical memory I) and
episodic declarative memory (logical memory II). In this subtest two stories are told
separately. Immediately after hearing each story, the patient states what was
remembered and the amount of linguistic units remembered is computed for logical
memory I. After 30 minutes, participants are asked to retell the two stories and the
points concerning linguistic units remembered are computed for logical memory II.

3. Results

Clinical, functional mobility and cognitive data from pre- and post-tests are outlined in
Table 2. The Wilcoxon test did not show significant differences between pre- and post-
intervention for H&Y, UPDRS-I, UPDRS-III, MEMS, perseverative errors and episodic logic
memory I. The multimodal exercise program was effective in improving UPDRS-II scores,
episodic declarative memory II, TUG and PLM.

Dependent variable	Pre-test	Post-test	P value
Clinical			
H&Y (stage)	1.47±0.72	1.53±0.72	0.157
UPDRS-I (score)	3.67±2.69	3.33±2.44	0.301
UPDRS-II (score)	11.07±6.36	9.73±6.04	0.022
UPDRS-III (score)	20.13±12.26	21±14.53	0.728
MEMS (score)	26.2±3.47	25.9±4.35	0.778
Functional mobility			
TUG (s)	10.37±4.54	8.41±2.27	0.002
PLM (s)	4.03±1.42	3.58±0.76	0.013
Cognitive			
Perseverative errors (errors)	6.87±6.83	5.13±7.52	0.151
Logic memory I (score)	14.8±5.02	17.07±5.93	0.132
Logic memory II (score)	8.6±5.95	13.8±6.38	0.005

Table 2. Means and standard deviations for each clinical dependent variable at pre and post-
test and P value.

Figures 1 and 2 show respectively times to complete all attempts of the TUG and the PLM
tests at pre- and post-intervention. The Friedman test showed a significant effect for
attempts on TUG at pre-test (p=0.019) and post-test (p=0.047; not confirmed by the
Wilcoxon test, p>0.05) and PLM at pre-test (p<0.001). Therefore, at pre-test a significantly
increase in time to complete TUG (Attemp1 vs Attempt 3 - Z=2.240; p=0.025) was observed.

During the PLM, patients reduced their time at pre-test (Attempt 1 vs Attempt 3 - Z=3.678; p<0.001), showing a learning effect. No differences were observed on Attempt 1 and Attempt 2 in all cases.

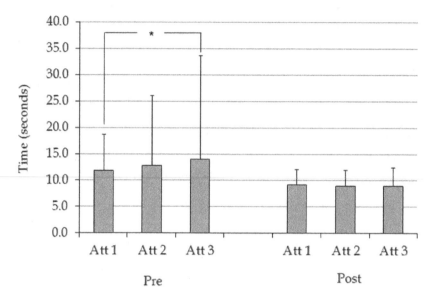

Fig. 1. Mean (+SD) time to complete attempts 1 to 3 (Att1 – Att3) of TUG test at pre- and post-intervention. * p<0.05

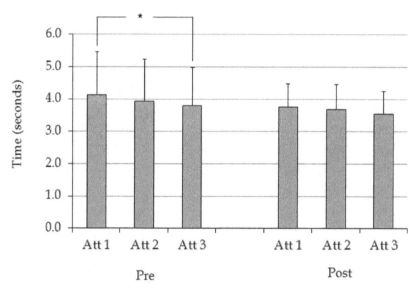

Fig. 2. Mean (+SD) time to complete attempts 1 to 3 (Att1 – Att3) of PLM test at pre- and post-intervention. * p<0.05

Effects of a Multimodal Exercise Program on Clinical, Functional Mobility and Cognitive Parameters of Idiopathic
Parkinson's Disease Patients

93

4. Discussion

The purpose of this chapter was to demonstrate the effectiveness of a long-term multimodal exercise program in improving clinical parameters, functional mobility and cognitive function in people with PD. Our results show a clear maintenance in the disease stage and severity with an increase on balance control and functional mobility. Also, the maintenance of both the executive functions and the short-term memory was observed.

Even with an expected increase in the disease stage and severity (H&Y scale), patients that were enrolled in our 6-moths multimode exercise program maintained their disease and motor impairments (Table 1). Since PD is a neurodegenerative and progressive disorder (Olanow et al., 2009) it would be expected that after the intervention period these patients would present a reduction in their motor performance as also observed by others (Hackney & Earhart, 2010). Alves et al. (2005) found an increase of 3.2% in the H&Y score for each year. However, as shown in Table 2, our multimode training program was successful to maintain both UPDRS I and UPDRS III sub-scores and to decelerate the increment in H&Y score, since it was observed only a 0.04% raise in 6-months.

In this way, we can speculate that exercise promotes at least in part, a protective role on dopaminergic neuronal loss and on the disease impairments. Several studies had pointed out a positive exercise effect on brain function, as neural growth (Zigmond et al., 2009), higher neurotransmissors use efficiency (Petzinger et al., 2010) and angiogenesis (Hirsch & Farley, 2009). According to Tajiri et al. (2010), exercise can enhance synaptic plasticity with a re-construction of cortical path network on PD induced rat models. Therefore we can suggest that exercise played some role, not yet fully understand (Hirsch & Farley, 2009), in the protection of dopaminergic neural loss.

The characteristics of the multimodal exercise program were responsible for increase stability of these patients. All exercises were focused on the patients' impairments, as bradykynesia, unbalance, difficulties to perform sequential movements and changing movement directions. Therefore, we can affirm that the 10-20% of reduction in time to complete TUG and PLM tests (Table 2) was due, at least in part, to the intervention features, such as the group sessions and long-term duration. The program effect was enough to approach the patients' performance to healthy elderly (8.8 to 9.1 seconds – Alfieri et al., 2010). The reduction presented by our subjects is highly superior to that observed on both healthy elderly (Alfieri et al., 2010: 8-12%; Arai et al., 2009: 8%) and people with PD (Sage & Almeida, 2009: 6-8%). In this way, our data are particularly important, since the improvement in balance control reduces the risk of falling and therefore, reduces patients' mortality and morbidity (Lee & Chou, 2006).

It is believed that physical capacities such as strength, flexibility, aerobic resistance and others were worked properly during our multimode exercise program, allowing subjects to improve functional capacity and decrease their time spent to perform the TUG and PLM tests. We can also suggest that aerobic resistance was also improved by our intervention program. Before the program, subjects presented an increase on time to complete TUG in different attempts, suggesting the presence of fatigue (Garber & Friedman, 2003). However, after the 6-months intervention period, this time was maintained during different attempts (Figure 1). Also, subjects performed TUG and PLM tests with a lower variability at post-test in comparison to pre-test (Figures 1 and 2), showing an improvement on stability.

The multimodal exercise program also improved the episodic declarative memory, despite the physical exercise did not change the executive function and short-term memory performance. However, studies have shown that the annual rate of clinical decline in people with PD is between 3.5% (Alves et al., 2005) and 11.2% (García-Ruiz et al., 2004). So, the maintenance of the scores in executive functions and short-term memory in the period of six months is also an important outcome for the patient.

The different memory systems depend on different anatomical structures. The short-term memory is located in the hippocampus and adjacent cortical areas of the temporal lobe, while episodic declarative memory is related to the medial temporal lobe, anterior thalamic nucleus, mammillary bodies, fornix, and prefrontal cortex (Robertson, 2002; Budson & Price, 2005). People with PD do report declarative memory loss but they do not report implicit memory loss, which suggests a problem of memorization strategy (Appollonio et al., 1994). To retrieve some information, people can use declarative memory, which requires conscious effort and attention, or implicit memory (typically unconscious), which is automatically accessed (Johnson et al., 2005). Due to degeneration of dopaminergic and cholinergic neurons in the nigrostriatal pathway in PD, cognitive behavior and the control of motor action are impaired. Therefore, the anatomical damages due to the disease can explain why episodic memory is the most affected (Calabresi et al., 2006). Our results showed that the episodic declarative memory (logical memory II) was more sensitive for the exercise. Perhaps, the exercise may achieve most impaired memory areas in PD patients.

As a study limitation we can not forget that all these results are applicable for subjects in the inital stages of the disease as those evaluated by our group. Also, it is important to remeber that a control group was not assessed and therefore there is a need to evaluate if some of these results were not related to learning or aging effects. However, our research group is already performing another study to fullfil this need.

5. Conclusion

As conclusion we can affirm that exercise as proposed by our group – a multimodal exercise program of long duration – plays an important role on the quality of life in people with PD by improving or maintaining their clinical parameters, functional mobility and cognitive function. This program has the capacity to decelerate the disease advance. This is particularly true when the disease stage and impairments are considered, as also seen in memory. These exercise effects are believed to be due to neuroprotection mechanisms no yet fully understudied and to an increase of all components of the functional capacity.

6. Acknowledgments

This study was supported in part by the PROEX/UNESP Univ Estadual Paulista and by the FAPESP – Fundação de Amparo à Pesquisa do Estado de São Paulo throughout scholarships (contract # 2010/07040-0, 2010/50532-0, 2009/02862-4 and 2007/06261-0).

7. References

Alfieri, F.; Riberto, M.; Ribeiro, C.; Lopes, J.; Santarém, J. & Battistella, L. (2010). Functional mobility and balance in community dwelling elderly submitted to multisensory versus strength exercises. *Clinical Interventions in Aging*, Vol. 5, pp.1810-185.

Alves, G.; Wentzel-Larse, T.; Aarsland, D. & Larsen, J. (2005). Progression of motor impairment and disability in Parkinson disease: a population-based study. *Neurology*, Vol. 65, pp. 1436-1441.

Appollonio, I.; Grafman, J.; Clark, K.; Nicheli, P.; Zeffiro, T. & Hallet, M. (1994). Implicit and explicit memory in patients with Parkinson's disease with and without dementia. *Archives of Neurology*, Vol. 51, No. 4, pp. 359-367.

Arai, T.; Obuchi, S.; Inaba, Y.; Shiba, Y. & Satake, K. (2009). The relationship between physical condition and change in balance functions on exercise intervention and 12-month follow-up in Japanese community-dwelling older people. *Archives of Gerontology and Geriatrics*. Vol. 48, pp. 61-66.

Bergen, J.; Toole, T.; Elliott III, R.; Wallace, B.; Robinson, K. & Maitland, C. (2002). Aerobic exercise intervention improves aerobic capacity and movement initiation in Parkinson´s disease patients. *NeuroRehabilitation*; Vol. 17, pp. 161-168.

Brach, J.; Simonsick, E.; Kritchevsky, S.; Yaffe, K. & Newman, A. (2004). The association between physical function and lifestyle activity and exercise in the Health, Aging and Body Composition Study. *Journal of the American Geriatrics Society*, Vol. 52, pp. 502-509.

Brucki, S.; Nitrini, R.; Caramelli, P.; Bertolucci, P. & Okamoto, I. (2003). Suggestions for utilization of the mini-mental state examination in Brazil. *Arquivos de Neuropsiquiatria*, Vol. 61, pp. 777–781.

Budson, A. E. & Price, B. H. (2005). Memory Dysfunction. *The New England Journal of Medicine*, Vol. 352, No. 7, pp. 692- 699.

Calabresi, P.; Picconi, B.; Parnetti, L. & Di Filippo, M. (2006). A convergent model for cognitive dysfunctions in Parkinson's disease: the critical dopamine–acetylcholine synaptic balance. *The Lancet Neurology*, Vol. 5, pp. 974-983.

Chaudhuri, K.; Healy, D. & Schapira, A. (2006). Non-motor symptoms of Parkinson's diseases: diagnosis and management. *The Lancet Neurology*, Vol. 5, pp. 235-245.

Chiari, H.; Mello, M.; Rezeak, P. & Antunes, H. (2010). Physical exercise, physical activity and the benefits of the memory of elderlys. *Revista Psicologia e Saúde*, Vol. 2, pp. 42-49.

Christofoletti, G.; Oliani, M.; Gobbi, L.; Gobbi, S. & Stella, F. (2006). Risk of falls among elderly people with Parkinson's disease and Alzheimer's dementia: A cross-sectional study. *Brazilian Journal of Physical Therapy*, Vol. 10, pp. 429-433.

Cools, R. (2006). Dopaminergic modulation of cognitive functionimplications for L-DOPA treatment in Parkinson's disease. *Neuroscience and Biobehavioral Reviews*, Vol. 30, pp. 1-23.

Costa, A.; Peppe, A.; Brusa, L.; Caltagirone, C.; Gatto, I. & Carlesimo, G. (2008). Levodopa improves time-based prospective memory in Parkinson's disease. *Journal of the International Neuropsychological Society*, Vol. 14, pp. 601-610.

Crizzle, A. & Newhouse, I. (2006). Is physical exercise beneficial for persons with Parkinson's disease? *Clinical Journal of Sport Medicine*, Vol. 16, pp. 422-425.

Cropley, V.; Fujita, M.; Innis, R. & Nathan, P. (2006). Molecular imaging of the dopaminergic system and its association with human cognitive function. *Biological Psychiatry*, Vol. 59, pp. 898-907.

Cyarto, E.; Brown, W.; Marshall, A. & Trost, S. (2008). Comparison of the effects of a home-based and group-based resistance training program on functional ability in older adults. *American Journal of Health Promotion*, Vol. 23, No. 1, pp.13-17.

de Lau, L. & Breteler, M. (2006). Epidemiology of Parkinson's disease. *The Lancet Neurology*, Vol. 5, pp. 525-535.

Dibble, L.; Hale, T.; Marcus, R.; Gerber, J. & LaStayo, P. (2009). High intensity eccentric resistance training decreases bradykinesia and improves quality of life in persons with Parkinson's disease: A preliminary study. *Parkinsonism and Related Disorders*, Vol. 15, No. 10, pp. 752-757.

Dubois, B. & Pillon, B. (1997). Cognitive deficits in Parkinson's disease. *Journal of Neurology*, Vol. 244, pp. 2-8.

Dujardin, K. & Laurent, B. (2003). Dysfunction of the human memory systems: Role of the dopaminergic transmission. *Current Opinion in Neurology*, Vol. 16 (Suppl. 2), pp. S11-S16.

Dujardin, K.; Defebvre, L.; Krystowiak, P.; Degreef, J. & Destee, A. (2003). Executive function differences in multiple system atrophy and Parkinson's disease. *Parkinsonism and Related Disorders*, Vol. 9, pp. 205-211.

Fabre, C.; Chamari, K.; Mucci, P.; Massé-Biron, J. & Préfaut, C. (2002). Improvement of cognitive function by mental and/or individualized aerobic training in healthy elderly subjects. *International Journal of Sports Medicine*, Vol. 23, No. 6, PP. 415-421.

Fahn, S.; Elton, R. & Members of the UPDRS Development Committee. (1987). Unified Parkinson's disease rating scale. In: Fahn S, Marsden CD, Calne DB, Goldstein M, editors. *Recent Developments in Parkinson's Disease*. Florham Park, NJ: Macmillan Health Care Information, pp. 153-63.

Folstein, M.; Folstein, S. & McHugh, P. (1975). Mini-mental state: a practical method for grading the cognitive state of patients for the clinician. *Journal of Psychiatric Research*, Vol. 12, pp. 189-198.

Gobbi, L.; Oliveira-Ferreira, M. D.; Caetano, M. J.; Lirani-Silva E.; Barbieri, F.; Stella, F. & Gobbi, S. (2009). Exercise programs improve mobility and balance in people with Parkinson's disease. *Parkinsonism and Related Disorders*, Vol. 15, pp. S49-52.

Grimbergen, Y.; Munneke, M. & Bloem, B. (2004). Falls in Parkinson's disease. *Current Opinion in Neurology*, Vol. 17, pp. 405-415.

Hackney, M. & Earhart, G. (2009). Health-related quality of life and alternative forms of exercise in Parkinson disease. *Parkinsonism and Related Disorders*, Vol. 15, No. 9, pp. 644-648.

Hackney, M.. & Earhart, G.. (2010). Effects of dance on gait and balance in Parkinson's disease: a comparison of partnered and nonpartnered dance movement. *Neurorehabilitation and Neural Repair, Vol.* 24,No. 4, pp. 384-392.

Heaton, R.; Chelune, G.; Talley, J.; Kay, G. & Curtiss, G. (1993). *Wisconsin card sorting test manual*. USA: Psychological Assessment Resources.

Hirayama, M.; Gobbi, S.; Gobbi, L. & Stella, F. (2008). Quality of life (QoL) in relation to disease severity in Brazilian Parkinson's patients as measured using the WHOQOL-BREF. *Archives of Gerontology and Geriatrics*, Vol. 46, pp. 147-160.

Hirsch, M. & Farley, B. (2009). Exercise and neuroplasticity in persons living with Parkinson's disease. *European Journal of Physical and Rehabilitation Medicine*, Vol. 45, No. 2, pp. 215-229.

Hoehn, M. & Yahr M. (1967). Parkinsonism: onset, progression and mortality. *Neurology*, Vol. 17, pp. 573–581.

Johnson, A. M.; Pollard, C.; Vernon, P.; Tomes, J. & Jog, M. (2005). Memory perception and strategy use in Parkinson's disease. *Parkinsonism and Related Disorders*, Vol. 11, pp. 111-115.

Karlsen, K.; Tandberg, E.; Arsland, D. & Larsen, J. (2000). Health related quality of life in Parkinson's disease: a prospective longitudinal study. *Journal of Neurology, Neurosurgery and Psychiatry*, Vol. 69, pp. 584–589.

Lee, H. & Chou, L. (2006). Detection of gait instability using the center of mass and center of pressure inclination angles. *Archives of Physical and Medicine Rehabilitation*, Vol. 87, pp. 569-575.

Miyai, I.; Fujimoto, Y.; Ueda, Y.; Yamamoto, H.; Nozaki, S.; Saito, T. & Kang, J. (2000). Treadmill training with body weight support: its effect on Parkinson's disease. *Archives of Physical Medicine and Rehabilitation*, Vol. 81, pp. 849-852.

Morris, M.; Iansek, R. & Kirkwood, B. (2009). A randomized control trial of movement strategies compared with exercise for people with Parkinson's disease. *Movement Disorders, Vol. 24*, pp. 64-71.

Nocera, J.; Horvat, M. & Ray, C. (2009). Effects of home-based exercise on postural control and sensory organization in individuals with Parkinson disease. *Parkinsonism and Related Disorders*, Vol. 15, No. 10, pp. 742-745.

Obeso, J.; Olanow, C. & Nutt, J. (2000). Levodopa motor complications in Parkinson's disease. *Trends in Neurosciences*, Vol. 23, pp. S2-S7.

Owen, A. (2004). Cognitive dysfunction in Parkinson's disease: the role of frontostriatal circuitry. *Neuroscientist*, Vol. 10, pp. 525-537.

Olanow, C.; Stern, M. & Sethi, K. (2009). The scientific and clinical basis for the treatment of Parkinson disease. *Neurology*, Vol. 72, No. 4S, pp. S1-S136.

Paolo, A.; Troster, A.; Axelrod, B. & Koller, W. (1995). Construct validity of the WCST in normal elderly and persons with Parkinson's disease. *Archives of Clinical Neuropsychology*, Vol. 10, No. 5, pp. 463-473.

Pascual-Sedano, B.; Kulisevsky, J.; Barbanoj, M.; García-Sánchez, C.; Campolongo, A.; Gironell, A.; Pagonabarraga, J. & Gich, I. (2008). Levodopa and executive performance in Parkinson's disease: A randomized study. *Journal of the International Neuropsychological Society*, Vol. 14, pp. 832-841.

Petzinger, G.; Fisher, B.; Van Leewmen, J.; Vucovik, M.; Akopian, G.; Meshul, C.; Holschneider, D.; Nacca, A; Walsh, J. & Jakowec, M. (2010). Enhancing neuroplasticity in the basal ganglia: the role of exercise in Parkinson's disease. *Movement Disorders*, Vol. 25, p. S141 – S145.

Pieruccini-Faria, F.; Menuchi, M.; Vitório, R.; Gobbi, L.; Stella, F. & Gobbi, S. (2006). Kinematic parameters for gait with obstacles among elderly patients with Parkinson's disease, with and without Levodopa: a Pilot Study. *Brazilian Journal of Physical Therapy*, Vol. 10, No. 2, pp. 233-239.

Podsiadlo, R. & Richardison, M. (1991). The Timed "Up & Go": A Test of Basic Functional Mobility for Frail Elderly Persons. *Journal of the American Geriatrics Society*, Vol. 39, pp. 142–148.

Rashid, A.; So, C.; Kong, M.; Furtak, T.; El-Ghundi, M.; Cheng, R.; O'Dowd, B. & George, S. (2007). D1-D2 dopamine receptor heterooligomers with unique pharmacology are coupled to rapid activation of Gq/11 in the striatum. *Proceedings of the National Academy of Sciences of the United States of America*, Vol. 104, No. 2, pp. 654-659.

Reuter, I.; Engelhardt, K. & Baas, H. (1999). Therapeutic value of exercise training in Parkinson's disease. *Medicine and Science in Sports and Exercise*, Vol. 31, pp. 1544-1549.

Ridgel, A.; Vitek, J. & Alberts, J. (2009). Forced, not voluntary, exercise improves motor function in Parkinson's disease patients. *Neurorehabilitation and Neural Repair*, Vol. 23, pp. 600-608.

Robertson, L. T. (2002). Memory and the brain. *Journal of Dental Education*, Vol. 66, No. 1, pp. 30-42.

Sage, M. & Almeida, Q. (2009). Symptom and gait changes after sensory attention focused exercise vs aerobic training in Parkinson's disease. *Movement Disorders*, Vol. 24, pp. 1132-1138.

Sage, M. & Almeida, Q. (2010). A positive influence of vision on motor symptoms during sensory attention focused exercise for Parkinson's disease. *Movement Disorders*, Vol. 25, pp. 64-69.

Scandalis, T.; Bosak, A.; Berliner, J.; Helman, L. & Wells, M. (2001). Resistance training and gait function in patients with Parkinson's disease. *American Journal of Physical Medicine and Rehabilitation*, Vol. 80, pp. 38-43.

Steg, G.; Ingvarsson, P.; Johnels, B.; Valls, M. & Thorselius M. (1989). Objective measurement of motor disability in Parkinson's disease. *Acta Neurologica Scandinavica*, Vol. 126, pp.67-75.

Stella, F.; Gobbi, L. T. B.; Gobbi, S.; Oliani, M. M. & Tanaka, K.; Pieruccini-Faria, F. (2007) Early impairment of cognitive functions on Parkinson's disease. *Arquivos de Neuropsiquiatria*, Vol. 65, pp.406-410.

Tanaka, K.; Quadros Jr, A. C.; Santos, R.; Stella, F.; Gobbi, L. & Gobbi, S. (2009). Benefits of physical exercise on executive functions in older people with Parkinson's disease. *Brain and Cognition*, Vol. 69, pp. 435-441.

Taylor, A.; Saint-Cyr, J. & Lang, A. (1986). Frontal lobe dysfunction in Parkinson's disease: The cortical focus of neostriatal outflow. *Brain*, Vol. 109, pp. 845-883.

Wechsler, D. (1997). *The Wechsler Memory Scale – III Revised (Manual)*. Santo Antonio Texas: Psychological Corporation.

White, D.; Wagenaar, R. & Ellis, T. (2006). Monitoring activity in individuals with Parkinson's disease: a validity study. *Journal of Neurological Physical Therapy*, Vol. 30, No. 1, pp. 12-21.

Zigmond, M.; Cameron, J.; Leak, R.; Mirnics, K.; Russell, V.; Smeyne, R. & Smith, A. (2009). Triggering endogenous neuroprotective processes through exercise in models of dopamine deficiency. *Parkinsonism and Related Disorders*, Vol 15, No S3, pp. S42-S45.

5

Rehabilitation of Patients Suffering from Parkinson's Disease by Normotensive Therapy

Gilles Orgeret
Regional Hospital,
Poissy/Saint Germain en Laye,
France

1. Introduction

Neurodegenerative injuries lead to disabilities, such as sensory and motor disturbances, with patients often losing their balance, and falling as a consequence. Moreover, capsulo-ligamentary adhesions often occur, which create stiffness and secondary retractions due to the lack of mobilization of the periarticular structures. These complex clinical pictures, when interlinked, are even more important when simultaneously the patients suffer from recurrent diseases, such as degenerative rheumatism.

Parkinson's disease, this public health issue, is evaluated through clinical criteria, as there are as many forms of Parkinson's disease as there are various cases. Personalized and adaptable physiotherapist option is therefore necessary. The syndrome associated with Parkinson's disease is characterized by a motor disorder, an akinesia combined with one of the following symptoms: extra pyramidal stiffness, tremor and postural instability. A depressive syndrome, a cognitive decline, and more or less disabling pain, come on top of the clinical picture. The patients frequently suffer from cramps or painful contractions, which mainly affect (74%): calves, neck, lumbar rachis, and which are more or less combined with dystonia. Comorbidities make the treatment even more complex. And it is always difficult to know, when considering the symptoms and their origin, whether it is Parkinson's or other illnesses which are to blame. These comorbidities should always be taken very seriously, and be properly treated, as they have an influence on the patient's mobility fluctuations (1).

Normotensive Therapy reinitiates the movement, it treats stiffness, pain, and lack of mobility. 68% of patients, whatever the stage of the disease they are in, suffer from concomitant illnesses such as: arthritis which can affect shoulders and knees and make the postural syndrome even worse, undefined chronic pain, arterial hypertension or heart pathologies. Unfortunately taking drugs often triggers rheumatism symptoms, and either contributes to their development, or keeps them going and makes them worse (2). The drugs intake is, on top of that, one of the main risk factors of fall among the elderly, and therefore complicates the rehabilitation. These drugs intake is a real risk factor whatever the patient's residence, autonomy and independence level are, as it underlines poor health condition and pre-existent fragility. The drugs classes which are mostly to blame are :

psychotropic substances (most of the time the first to be cited), as well as hypnotic, sedative, antihypertensive, antalgic and opiate drugs (3).

Mepronizine, a treatment for accidental insomnia, is to be avoided in the elderly, especially when over 75 years old, as it may cause falls and intoxications. At the opposite, some other drugs like Dopamine might help the patient suffering from Parkinson's disease, especially at the beginning of the illness as it has a protective role, which is not so obvious when the illness is more developed.

An increase in the L-Dopa dose, the first intention drug, might lead to motor fluctuations after a two year treatment, such as diskinesia and akinesia.

Furthermore, the end of dose of L-Dopa is to be taken into account versus akinesia (4). A well trained Normotensive Therapy physiotherapist will consider the stage of the patient's illness before making his choice among the different maneuvers. Should the Physiotherapist consider a maneuver for the patient, if it proves inadequate, he would easily switch to another one. For example, he could switch from an active exercise which involves the patient's participation to a passive and gentler manoeuver. The NT (Normotensive Therapy) is a very adaptable physiotherapist option, but it requires the patient's total acceptance, in order to avoid situations of conflict which might cause confusion and/or diskinesia. The NT must be carried out at fixed time, so that the patient is physically and mentally well prepared, and available (never disturb a family visit for instance, wait until toilet is over). The NT will be more effective in favorable conditions: correct heating of the room, well adapted clothes and shoes. The after-meal times should be avoided as the digestion might disturb the course of the exercises. Abrupt exercises are to be avoided.

2. Successive stages of the illness

Parkinson's disease takes on three different main stages: the honeymoon period, the stage when the illness gets settled, and the dependency stage.

In the initial phase of the illness, the symptoms are usually mild and the NT attempts to keep and reinforce the patient's balance, while trying to improve the pain and functional impotency resulting from degenerative rheumatism. Back pain is frequently shown as the main preexisting handicap, often disturbing the thoracic amplitude and therefore the cardiorespiratory system.

In the second phase, and during the "on" period, the patient's balance will be improved by exercising on the Klein balloon, wearing an elastic bandage for other specific exercices, and by foot-stimulation with TENS (Transcutaneus electro-neuro-stimulation) as described further on (new treatments). The patient will be encouraged to keep a straight and upright position as long as possible, and the NT will help the joints to stay supple and the breathing to keep its former amplitude thanks to anti-kyphosis and anti-flessum NT maneuvers.

During the "off" period, the postural, articular, and muscular pain increase, due to motor deficit, depressive syndrome, and medication (5) . That is why it is very important to keep using the Klein balloon during that period (under supervision) while the patient's physical movements are usually limited. The physiotherapist will try to make the muscles relax in order to facilitate the movements and the NT maneuvers will deaden the pain.

In the third phase, when the dependency becomes complete, the physiotherapist will try to prevent the patient from becoming utterly bedridden, in carrying on NT maneuvers (relaxing maneuvers), and the pain treatment. An appropriate use of the Klein balloon in handicapped patients, will be encouraged under strict supervision.

3. The *Normotensive Therapy*: An alternative method to reinitiate the movement

NT is not a medicine, although it depends on a personalized morpho-staturo-dynamic examination. It is based on a medical diagnosis, and is carried out in close collaboration with the medical staff (general practitioner, psychologist, nutritionist, occupational therapist, speech therapist, relaxation therapist). NT is not symptomatic and treats the whole body, focusing on zones which seem essential to treat, even if these zones have not been mentioned by the consultant.

Two main poles of intervention :

1. Atraumatic manual normalization of the tissues which should correct stiffness and allow mobility to be restored without any pain.
2. Control and correction of the posture thanks to specific exercises.

The NT is a manual atraumatic therapy with no articular thrust beyond physiological amplitude. It is an important source of somesthetic afferences, as the patient suffering from Parkinson's is particularly receptive to the neuro-informational sensory component of this kind of specific massage.

The word "Normotensive" is a contraction of two words: "normalization and tension". It is a myofascial and neurosensorial therapy which doesn't imply hooking the tendons. During the session, the patient is kept in an active postural activity all the time, the passive maneuvers on the tissues being carried out before and after the exercises. In the Parkinson's case, NT helps restore scapulothoracic mobility, reduce kyphosis, improve ventilation often disturbed by thoracic tightening, and improve the functional clinical picture: postural reactions, balance, walking. It treats the pain due to bad postures, or the after-effects of concomitant disorders such as degenerative rheumatism. No excess stress or fatigue can arise from NT, as it is quite a soft therapy.

The manual normalization of the tissues depends on two maneuvers: *the triggering touch* and the *relaxing touch*.

These maneuvers are not to be carried out in case of inflammation or injuries whether superficial or deep.

3.1 The triggering touch

It is a sustained vibrating proprioceptive therapeutic maneuver, which is less than one minute long, and can be manual (most of the time) or instrumental, according to two distinct methods. In the Parkinson's, the plastic hypertonia expresses itself in a resistance to the passive stretching of the muscles. It is therefore essential to control the muscular contraction, so that it is more effective, and the *triggering touch* is part of it, being a soft stretching method encouraging the muscular relaxation. Indeed, in central neurology, the response to the vibrations is more easily recognized than some other finer tactile perceptions.

The *triggering touch* is based on two methods:

The first maneuver called *static triggering touch*, aimed at the soft tissues. It is a long lasting transcutaneous vibration under soft traction of the dysfunctional myofascial structure.

The vibratory intensity is modulated according to the local thickness of the teguments, to the more or less deep situation of the above-mentioned soft tissues, and to the wish not to be algogenic.

The second maneuver called *dynamic triggering touch*, aimed at the joints. The physiotherapist will give the regarded joint a soft passive vibratory movement of limited amplitude (flexion-extension, rotation, or adduction-abduction, according to the contingent possibilities). If possible this gesture is backed up by a very gentle segmental traction-decoaptation.

Tissue traction

In order to properly understand the interest of the superficial tissue traction, let's cite *Rabishong:* "the identification of rachidial posture and position is made by tractions on the skin". This traction gives to the central nervous system a feeling of muscular stretching. Then, the vibration made on highly tendinous zones, makes the treated muscle relax by activation of the antagonist (Sherrington Law).

Besides, the Golgi tendon organs, neuronal endings surrounded by a connective capsule, are situated at the junction between the smooth muscle fibers and the tendinous tissue. The Golgi tendon organs, could help monitor muscle strengths in order to fight gravity. Mechanoreceptors, Ruffinian corpuscles, Golgi corpuscles, are situated inside the articular capsules and the ligaments. And this is precisely where the NT is efficient.

Vibrations

Vibrations have been used since antiquity as therapeutic means. Transcutaneous mechanoreceptors are very sensitive to transcutaneous vibrations. These vibrations result in a mainly sensorimotor neuronal message, facilitate the sliding plans, relieve the pain, and reinforce the *gate control* (6). The primary endings of the neuromuscular spindles are activated too, especially when the source of the vibratory impact is close to the tendons. So, proprioceptive information can easily be rigged by a vibration, and this one, if its intensity and frequency are well adapted, leads to a modification in the information coming from the fibers Ia, and therefore will be read by the neuronal system as a muscular stretching (7, 8, 9). This misinterpretation from the central nervous system gives the illusion that the joint is moving, and that the vibrated muscle is contracting, which leads to a change in the patient's postural control. Using this information, several studies have analyzed the effect of a vibration upon the muscles of different joints on the postural control (10, 11, 12). Results show that the nervous system interprets the signal coming from the vibrated muscles differently according to its location. Applying a vibration to the pelvic limbs leads to corrective reactions from the whole body in an opposite direction of the perceived movement, whereas above the pelvis the reaction occurs in the same direction as the perceived movement. For some authors (13, 14, 15), this is due to the strong interaction between the vestibular and proprioceptive cervical informations while the information is being treated by the central nervous system, because of the necessity to know the relative position of the head and the trunk to use the vestibular information in a satisfying way. For other authors (16, 17, 18), it is due to the functional role of the proprioceptive messages coming from different body parts. For instance, it is possible to give a function of opposition to the destabilization of the body to the proprioceptive messages coming from the lower body, whereas they give the function of orientation of the body to the information coming from the cervical region. These items of scientific research help the Normotensive treatment determine how to correct the posture. They always involve a cephalocervical treatment.

3.2 The relaxing touch

It always takes place after the triggering touch and takes into consideration the fact that a disruption in the articular micro-movements leads to a loss of performance in great amplitude movements. The *relaxing touch*, according to two modes, will allow the tissue mobility to be restored and the pain to be soothed, by working on the *tensive lesions*, a few millimeters long pathogenic threadlike cords, or tight strings. In case of a skeletal muscle being contracted, they are very easily recognizable in a softer surrounding myofascial structure. It is explained by the comprehension of the myotatic reflex, and of the effect of the motoneurons. The alpha and beta motoneurons, are equipped with an inhibition system called recurrent inhibition. Golgi receptors which are scattered at the muscle-tendon or muscle-aponeurosis junction, are receptive to their stretching. They have a direct role in the control of the contraction and in the feed-back of the normal myotatic reflex. And this zone is precisely the one which interests the NT (19). Furthermore, about the nature of the collagen, the late Eric Viel used to describe an ogive shape which overlaps, with *cross-linkage* contacts between the fibers beams. These *cross-linkages* can turn into points which become hardened because of: an immobilization, an attitude syndrome, a trauma, or any deep or superficial injury. The great anatomist Xavier Bichat used to call these *cross-linkages* : "hardened tissues". The stiffness of the collagen tissue being a sign of ageing, and making the spine tissues harder. The physiotherapist fingers, used to the NT, can detect these points where collagen sticks, and set it free (20).

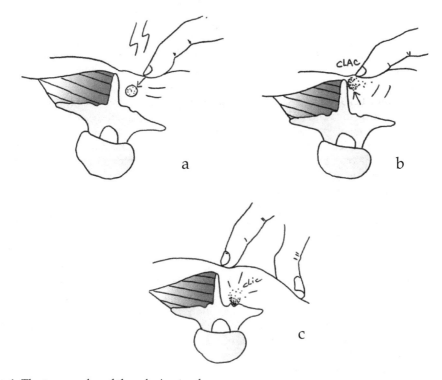

Fig. 1. The two modes of the *relaxing touch*

When they are close to a bone relief, the physiotherapist sharply pushes away the *tensive lesions* against this bone (Fig 1, a). He crushed them on the bone and makes them crack (Fig 1, b). If there is no close bone relief around, the therapist strongly squeezes them between thumb and index, as if they were a guitar string. This gesture is to be made two or three times at a go.

The second gesture consists in making the treated soft structures bulge while vibrating. It looks like the "roll and lift" method, but it is longitudinal instead of being transversal (Fig 1, c). It aims to make the tissues become detached, and to allow them to slide on each other again.

4. Control and normotensive postural corrections

4.1 The functions of the postural system

The sensorimotor control of our postures and movements, is subject to fluctuations in the course of our existence. Unfortunately, it turns out not to be very effective for most people, whether they are ill or not. Should this control be disturbed on a long term basis, some signs might appear such as: tiredness, pain, tendonitis, degenerative arthralgia, discal hernia. Four sensorial entries are mainly to blame: internal ear, podal afference, vision, jaw.

Very soon in life, from the age of 35, the postural extensive muscles weaken, which leads to some difficulties for the rachis to adapt to verticality. Besides, when an elderly has a bad fall, his balance can be definitely disturbed (clinical picture of "post fall" and dysexecutive syndrome).

In the Parkinson's disease, where sensorial afferences are highly disturbed, especially the graviceptive somesthetic information, it is essential that the balance be taken therapeutically into account. The habits in the use of the body are progressively disturbed. If the patient is elderly, myogene or neurogene atrophy can occur and lead to a muscular unbalance, whatever the gravity of the illness.

The human motor behavior is organized in reference to a biological vertical line, which is built by the brain from visual and graviceptive informations (otolithic and somesthetic). Evocating the notion of position in an environment implies a system of reference. The system of reference based on the gravity vertical line, is mainly informed by the vestibular system, whereas the one which is based on landmarks in the space is mainly informed by the vision. As for the one which is peculiar to the individual, it is based on information coming from the somesthetic system (one of the base of the NT treatment).

The search for balance is the decisive factor of the postural control. Some cerebral injuries can alter the ability to keep a certain position, or to change it, in the three fundamental postures: reclining, sitting and vertical position. Sometimes, serious abnormalities of the sense of verticality can occur from a tactile, visual, or postural perception of the vertical line. In neuronal (or vestibular) pathology, the abnormalities of the subjective vertical line consist in the existence of a slantwise direction, and/or an uncertainty about the verticality. Any cerebral injury concerning a zone which is involved in the graviceptive vestibular or somesthetic perception can lead to a disturbance in the construction of the subjective vertical line. An injury of the vestibular tracts affecting the graviceptive somesthetic tracts will give an angle to the subjective vertical line concerning the postural perception of the vertical line. The posterolateral thalamus is not only an intermediary for the vestibular tracts, but it could be a fundamental structure for the control of the upright position as well. In the patients suffering from Parkinson's, the postural mode of the subjective vertical line is disturbed.

The vestibular, somesthetic, and visceral graviceptors, contribute to the actualization of this subjective vertical line (21).

However, if the contribution of the visual and somesthetic information to the control of the biped posture is well determined, the one regarding the vestibular informations remains a controversial issue. A study mention sensitivity thresholds of the upper semicircular canal, to the quickening of the classic postural fluctuations observed in an undisturbed upright static position (22).

Our tactile sensitivity is conveyed by different mechanoreceptors (Meissner, Pacini and Ruffini corpuscules, Merckel discs...). They provide informations about the outer world to the central nervous system, mainly thanks to the hands and the feet. That is why the NT is seriously taking them into consideration. The tactile receptors of the plantar sole are quite important, but the other cutaneous informations should not be overlooked. From feet to head, the continuity of the sensorial information which allows our balance, relies on numerous muscles and joints which are associated in chains. The plantar arches give informations about the variety of supports, eyes give information about the position into the space. There is a direct link between jaw and neck, and between eyes and neck muscles. The stability of the head relies on the balance between the jaw joints (23). Some scientific studies suggest, on the one hand, that the central and peripheral visions play a complimentary role in the control of the biped posture, and, on the other hand, that the relative contribution of each of these visions depends on the information given by the other sensorial systems, especially the somatosensorial informations coming from the foot-ankle segment (24, 25). If the sensorial captors are situated in different parts of the body, the information they provide converge to common cortical or subcortical structures, which control the postural system through different reflexes. The vestibulo-ocular reflex allows the stabilization of the eyes, the vestibulo-spinal and vestibulo-oculo-cervical reflexes allow the global control and the maintenance of the posture by their action upon the myostatic reflex.

In the patient suffering from Parkinson's, the visual stimulation is usually shown as being supportive to the reconstruction of the motor activity. Nothing is less certain. The whole day long, the patient is aware of the risks due to his pathology, and the result is not conclusive. The movements with the eyes open are inefficient and ill adapted to the real needs of the patient, who is under constant stress while performing his daily routine. During the NT session, the vision is sometimes occulted in order to reinforce the patient's confidence in his other senses, as he often perceives the environment as hostile and full of potential and insurmountable difficulties. It is not possible for the patient to control everything: balance, postural correction, lengthening of the step. If the eyes are closed, and the therapist around, the patient can relax and focus on the reinforcement of his other senses, which later on will allow him to adapt better to the variations of his environment. In his everyday life, the extrinsic factors which are factors of falls such as: faulty lighting, carpets or furniture, will be more easily grasped, the vision becoming an asset adding to the other reinforced senses, instead of just being a substitute.

4.2 Posturo-normo-regulator examination

It is inspired by the medical clinical examination, and by the anamnesis. It is important to appreciate the comorbidity which could alter the conclusions of the examination: medical history of cardiovascular accident, heart failure, myocardial infarction, infectious illness, hypoglycemia if diabetic patient. The posturo-normo-regulator examination involves many maneuvers, which cannot all be mentioned in this paper which does not aim to be exhaustive.

The patient is examined when in underwear. The examination should not be more than 5/10 minutes long, as the patient will rapidly adopt wrong corrective postures which will alter the conclusions. It is important to look for faulty postures and maladjusted movements which might pose problems.

The examination regarding the balance control consists in checking the patient's ability to stay in a stable position when sitting, then standing, with the eyes wide open, then closed. The static and dynamic bipodal then unipodal phases are assessed (there is an abnormality if the patient cannot stand more than 5 seconds on his favorite foot, with his eyes wide open (26). The *Get-up-and-go test* consists in asking the patient, sitting on a chair which is 3 meters from a wall, to stand up, stay immobile for a few seconds, walk up to the wall, turn round and go back to the chair and sit again in no particular hurry. Between the age of 65 and 85, it normally takes the patient about 12 seconds to perform the exercise. If the exercise takes him more than 30 seconds, the patient is said to be highly dependent. The inability to stand on one foot for less than 5 seconds is said to be pathologic (27).

4.2.1 Postural bearing test

It aims to detect the degree of global corporal instability. This test is to be carried out both at the beginning and at the end of the physiotherapy session. The end of session test is expected to be better than the one carried out at the beginning of the session. In case it is not so, the following session must be optimized by either changing the time of the session, or by reinforcing the balance control exercises. All these sessions will be interrupted with NT normalization of the tissue maneuvers.

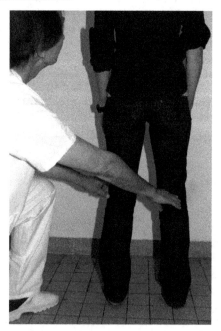

Fig. 2. Postural bearing test

The patient is standing up, eyes closed. Without any warning, the therapist is exerting a thrust in the popliteal space. The therapist can check the reaction of the different body segments, and then evaluate the restoration of the balance component, and the arms swing (Fig 2).

4.2.2 Test in the trunk diagonal with focus on the fluctuating effect

It is about the closing chain of the locomotion muscular chains, and it tests the mobility of the scapular and pelvic belt with each other.

This examination is to be carried out on both sides, as a comparison test. The therapist lays one hand on the patient's shoulder, and the other one on the opposite hip. Then he exerts a sudden thrust with his two hands, in order to test the articular mobility. For instance a thrust on the shoulder may harmoniously drag down the lateral hemithorax, whereas the opposite hip remains blocked in the high position, which evokes a flaw in the lombo-pelvic cinematic (Fig 3).

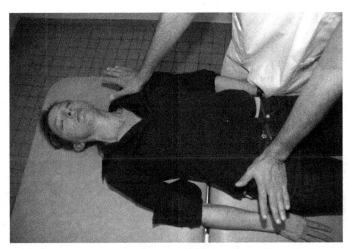

Fig. 3. Test in the trunk diagonal with focus on the fluctuating effect

5. Rehabilitation

In the patient suffering from Parkinson's, the poor speed and amplitude of the movements are to be seriously taken into consideration before any other parameter. The NT treatment is a combination of different balance control exercises on a Klein balloon and when wearing an elastic bandage, and also normotensive correction of the tissues carried out either before or during or even after the exercises. The sessions must be quite short in duration, interrupted with phases of rest. It is indeed important to hold the patient's attention during the session and even to make sure he enjoys it.

5.1 About the obstacle of dystonia

Dystonia is movements in profusion which is difficult to control. When walking, the patient takes long strides and swerves, and might easily fall. However disturbing they might be, this dystonia should not prevent the rehabilitation session to be carried out in a satisfactory way, even if they are painful or if they disturb the patient's balance because of their impact on the joints, or on any other body segment.

If the exercise in process is definitely disturbed, it is then necessary to carry on the session with other active or passive maneuvers, and to come back later on to the previously planned exercise, at a more convenient time.

5.2 The walking ability

We know that some factors predispose to falls, such as : being over 80, being a woman, depressed, suffering from a loss of strength or a bad coordination of movements, or from feet abnormality or ill-fitting shoes. In the patient suffering from Parkinson's, the main problem with the walking ability is that not only is the walking faulty, but it moreover lacks stimulation. Over the years, walking becomes slower, with a shortened step, a lengthening of the time when the two feet are supportive, a loss in the arms swing, and a tendency to stand with the trunk leaning backwards (28).

5.3 Improvement in walking by foot stimulation by TENS (Transcutaneous electro-neuro-stimulation)

Most of the patients suffering from Parkinson's are suffering from their feet. As a consequence the neuro-informational podal component, which is essential to the balance control, is disturbed. This leads to falls in the patients. However it is possible to improve the postural vertical component, thanks to a low frequency ambulatory transcutaneous neurostimulation. This stimulation improves the foot somesthetic perception. It stimulates the walking. The power reinforces the foot afferences, giving the patient a better perception of the support.

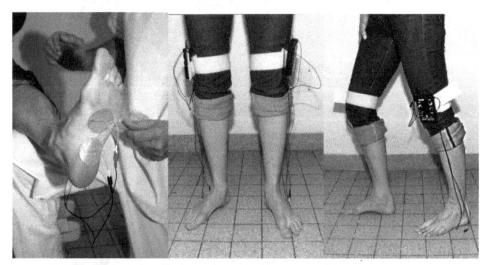

Fig. 4. The electrodes are installed in medioplantar. The stimulation must not be excitomotor. The power must be of a low intensity, just enough to be perceptible, and no algogenic. If one of the feet is less responsive, we must increase the stimulation on the less responsive side. It is possible to vary the treatment, for instance in stimulating only one of the feet, or in modifying the electrodes position, in order to get a better motor reaction.

5.4 Exercices and walking with an elastic bandage

It has been proved that wearing elastic adhesive bandages on different body parts, or Velcro bandages, could increase the intensity of tactile informations (29, 30). Taking this information as a starting point, I had the idea to initiate the occasional wearing of an elastic bandage (60mm wide coarsely woven flat elastic band, 10 m long roll), to be worn directly on the clothes. It is especially recommended in case of: weakness of a lower limb, osteoporosis, arthritis, backache, very old age, Alzheimer, hemiplegia, Parkinson's. This extensor system allows the patient to better apprehend his body from every angle. It helps him to feel the joints interaction, forces him to stretch his body, encourages the proprioception, and re-educates the vertebral erectors in restoring the balance of the chains of movements. In the Parkinson's case, the equinism of the ankle pushes the patient back even more. The elastic bandage partly makes up for that. It must be on while exercising, and even for a few hours a day if necessary. It is not to be kept on too long, nor when sleeping, sitting, or lying down.

Place the elastic bandage in the middle of the foot, and then pull it up to the shoulders, folding it tightly and firmly across the body. (Figures 5, 6, 7 and 8)

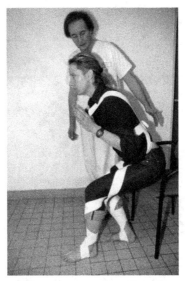

Fig. 5. Standing up after sitting. To restore the gravity line forward (its tendency being backward), the patient pull on his "suspenders".

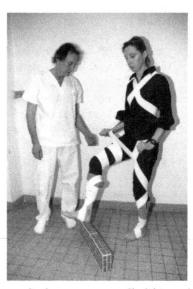

Fig. 6. Putting forward an upper limb or exaggeratedly lifting a lower limb, in making sure the movement doesn't push the patient backward, might be enough to initiate the step. The patient is asked to pull on the elastic bandage as he would do with suspenders (that he should wear later on, for the same use). When stepping over an obstacle, it is first the therapist who pulls on the bandage to help the patient move, and then it should be the patient himself who does it, as soon as he/she is able to.

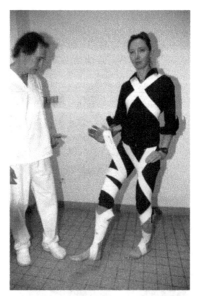

Fig. 7. Half a turn, initiated by the therapist (then by the patient), in waddling alternately to the left and to the right, in order to alight the body weight so that the foot can move forward

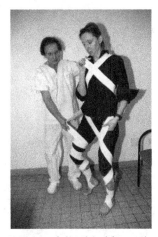

Fig. 8. Harmonization of the movements of the shoulder and pelvic girdle, during the moving

5.5 Specific exercises on the Klein balloon

"An active sitting position should be encouraged whereas a passive position should be avoided !"

Generally speaking, we should all sit on a balloon instead of using a chair, as a passive sitting position is very aggressive for our back, alter our balance, and doesn't make sense on the postural point of view.

A posture which is too long maintained is always harmful, especially when regarding elderly people or people who seldom move. It is the same problem with the patients suffering from Parkinson's. The elderly women who spend more than 9 hours a day sitting have one and a half more risks of suffering from a broken hip than the women who sit less

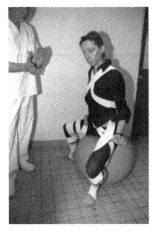

Fig. 9. Exercise of transfer of the body weight from one foot to the other one, a phase which is essential for the initialization of the step. The therapist can give a rhythm to the exercise. For example he claps his hands to help the patient change his support, and the exercise can be carried out more or less rapidly

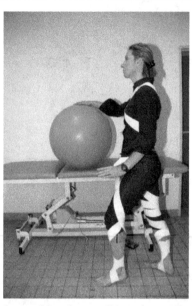

Fig. 10. Make a ball roll on a long table when walking alongside it. At the end of the table, change hands and go back to the starting point. Accelerate the pace progressively

than 6 hours a day (31). Unfortunately elderly people are most of the time made sitting in a chair the whole day long, especially in old people's homes. Because of that, the motor deprogramming is quick which makes the rehabilitation even more difficult. It would be much better to encourage the elderly, if their health condition allows it, to sit on the Klein balloon in order to reinforce their balance.

In the case of the patients suffering from Parkinson's, the balance of the head, as well as the setting of the body weight forward, should be thoroughly checked, as the akinesia leads to the gestures being scarce, to the body coiling itself up, and to retractions. The exercises while sitting on the balloon, backed up with manual maneuvers, try to make up for these problems.

6. Normotensive normalization of the tissues

The patient is checked according to the pattern of the above-mentioned posturo-normo-regulator examination. And then early corrective manual maneuvers are carried out for quite a short time (about ten minutes). Next, the patient performs some exercises on an oscillating board, with the eyes closed, for the same duration. Eventually, following a new normo-postural examination, ultimate corrections are made.

6.1 Example of manual treatment

The Normotensive Therapy is quite rich in different maneuvers and the therapist can pick up any of them , according to the specific need of the patient.

Here are some of them:

In this example, the patient shows up with a fixed facies. The walk is awkward: bent shoulders, accentuated cervical lordosis, accentuated and stiff kyphosis which lead to cervical and scapular bilateral pain. Furthermore the right ankle is scarcely mobile which causes the support to be faulty. The thoracic expansion is limited, and the respiratory amplitude affected. The patient can easily fall. In the Parkinson's stiffness very usually predominates on the flexors, when in flexion.

6.2 Myofascial Normotensive treatment
6.2.1 Treatment of the facies
There are close links between cervical biomechanics and manducator function. Only if the jaw joints are well balanced can the head remains stable. If the patient shows a fixed facies and a poor facial expression, it is necessary to treat him in order to soften the expression. The manducator function is quite important for the general balance of the body. The very specific NT massage increases the biting force and allows the peripheral muscles of the neck to relax, while they usually make the patient adopt a very poor posture in the severe phase of the illness. It has been proved that vibrating friction massage could improve the biting force (32).

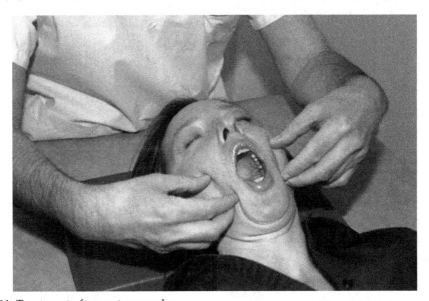

Fig. 11. Treatment of masseter muscles

This treatment mainly applies to the masseter and lateral pterygoid muscles, very much involved in the dysfunctions of temporo-mandibular joints.
The patient is asked to firmly and quickly close his mouth, whereas the therapist tries to prevent the movement with the tip of his fingers (Fig 11). Next the therapist carries out a *triggering touch* without the patient's participation, with thumb and forefinger first joined together, then, moving apart from each other, several times at a go. Maneuver to be carried out on both sides.
Then, the patient is asked to move his chin sideways, in opposition to the treated muscle while the therapist prevent the movement, and then carries out a *triggering touch* in separating thumb and forefinger on this muscle(Fig 12). Maneuver to be carried out on both sides.

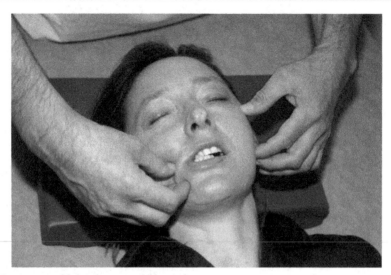

Fig. 12. Treatment of lateral pterygoid muscles

6.2.2 The Twist maneuver
It is a global NT maneuver which aims to the softening of the vertebral column.

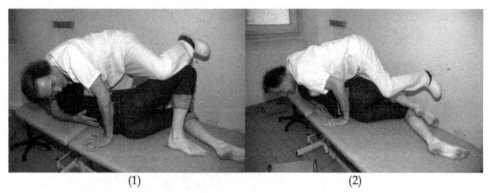

(1)   (2)

Fig. 13. The *twist maneuver*

The patient puts his shoulder forward and raises his knee in a rotary outward movement, whereas the therapist resists it (Fig 13 -1). Next the patient relaxes and follows the therapist who triggers a spiral movement while firmly holding the pelvis which must remain immobile (Fig 13 - 2). Maneuver to be carried out on both sides. If it is only a thoracic amplitude gain which is to be obtained, the hand which holds the pelvic should be placed slightly higher.

6.3 Cervical treatment
The cervicothoracic treatment always comes before the treatment of the shoulder as it relies on it. The balance of the head is to be thoroughly monitored. The cervical rachis should be softened, functional, and harmoniously following the eyes, as the vestibulo-ocular and

vestibulo-oculo-cervical reflexes have an important role in the preservation of a correct posture.

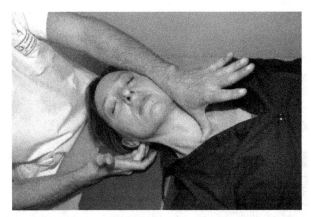

Fig. 14. *Dynamic triggering touch* on sternocleidomastoid muscle

The patient is in decubitus. The therapist resists to a contraction (isometric movement) of the muscle in rotation of head and neck, of the opposite side of the contraction (sternal head), and then in homolateral inclination (clavicular head). Next, he pulls on the extended muscle by a soft occipital traction, while gently rotating the head to and fro (Fig 14).

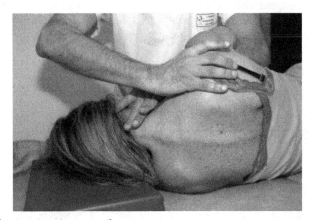

Fig. 15. Cervical maneuver in *nutcracker*

The patient is in lateral decubitus (Fig 15). He is asked to raise the shoulder three or four times, slightly backward, in opposition to a manual resistance (isometric movement). Next, the therapist makes the superior trapezius muscle stretch with hands apart, while simultaneously carrying out a static triggering touch with both hands. And then he carries out the same *static triggering touch*, then *relaxing touch* on the scapular insertion of the levator scapulae muscle, after the shoulder blade has been raised in the opposite direction. A regional *relaxing touch* is then carried out if needed, especially if there are *tensive lesions* left, the therapist's hands being placed the same way.

6.4 Thoracic treatment

Although deformations appear quite late, emphasis must be put on their prevention. Moreover, there is quite frequently a feeling of thoracic oppression occurring during the periods of *block*. Spinal or scapular pain often occur at the same time.

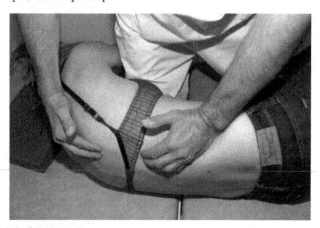

Fig. 16. Vertebral thoracic treatment

The patient is in lateral decubitus, with his back bent (Fig 16). While he is breathing out, the therapist's hands, moving apart from each other, exert *triggering touch traction* along the paravertebral thoracic muscles, on the side which doesn't lean on the table. At the same time, his knee placed in the thoracic zone exerts a pressure so that the treated zone is stretched. A relaxing maneuver is to be carried out if *tensive lesions* are detected. To be repeated in the opposite lateral decubitus.

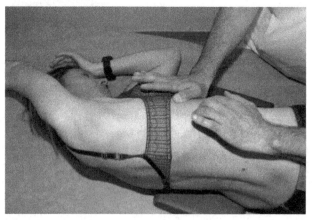

Fig. 17. Costal treatment

The therapist puts his fingers successively in each intercostal space, insisting on the area where the thoracic expansion is limited (Fig 17). The patient is asked to "breathe inside his ribs". The therapist carries out small stretching movements in *triggering touch*, with the hands moving apart while the patient breathes out.

Then, relaxing treatment, if necessary, mainly in the posterior thoracic zone, near the vertebras.

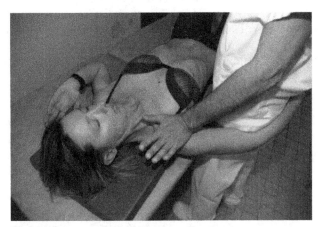

Fig. 18. Shoulder treatment

The patient being in dorsal decubitus, the therapist keeps stretching the upper limb of the patient along his back, while he gently pulls the head of humerus in decoaptation with his thigh (Fig 18). He uses the heel of the hand to push backward and downward the head of humerus with a *triggering touch*. This maneuver which is never painful, is to be repeated for two or three minutes at a go.

6.5 Lumbar treatment: Specific treatment of Iliopsoas muscle
The Iliopsoas muscle is often to blame in any lumbar mechanical pathology, even sometimes the only one to blame. It is necessary to check it or correct it, if necessary.
The patient finds it difficult to straighten up. His muscles are stiff and hypertonic, partly because of his posterior muscles "in flessum".

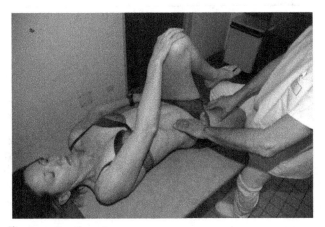

Fig. 19. Lumbar Iliopsoas treatment

The patient is in decubitus at the end of the table, with the thigh folded on the abdomen (Fig 19). The therapist tests the elastic resistance of the two Iliopsoas through a palpation of the abdomen (inferolateral part of the abdomen, rectus abdominis excluded) with the patient's hip bent in opposition (isometric movement), his hand being below the groin fold. And then he treats the lesional Iliopsoas: the patient bends his hip against resistance, the other being tucked up on the abdomen, and the therapist carries out a *triggering touch*, with both hands vibrating at the same time.

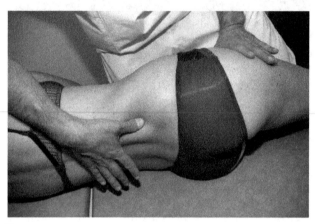

Fig. 20. Lumbar Iliopsoas treatment

Immediately after the maneuver before, the patient positions himself in laterocubitus, with the trunk in rotation (Fig 20). On the side which is to be treated, the thigh is kept in extension. The patient bends his hip (isometric) with opposition from the therapist, and then the therapist carries out a *relaxing touch* on the patient's lumbar rachis while pushing his shoulder back to the table.

6.6 Tibiofibular treatment
Treatment of the tibiofibular syndesmosis when blocked, in order to ease the flexion-extension movement of the ankle and to restore the support.

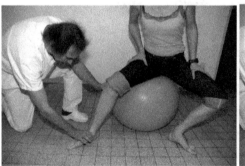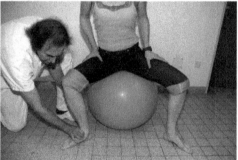

Fig. 21. and 22. Tibiofibular treatment

The patient is sitting on the Klein balloon (Fig 21, 22). He makes it roll from right to left (so that the ankle is mobile, which is the dynamic element of the maneuver) while the therapist carries out a *triggering touch* on the tibiofibular syndesmosis, followed by a *relaxing touch* if needed. It must lead to a mobility gain in the flexion-extension of the ankle. Otherwise, the maneuver must be repeated.

6.7 Minor joints

The different rehabilitation maneuvers often overlook the minor joints. However, the illness seriously alters the way they work, which can handicap the patient in all his daily activities, so he ends up forgetting to use them. Thanks to the NT, he realizes how important it is to reintegrate them in his body scheme, being aware that taking care of them will give him back a freedom of movement.

The tactile foot captors give very valuable information on the body oscillations in relation to the vertical line. However the skin sensitivity decreases over the course of years, and it can alter the balance, especially in the case of Parkinson's disease whereas it is important to keep a good support.

The graviceptive somesthetic tactile information brought by the *triggering touch* on the plantar soles, improves the patient's postural stability. Each session should include a *triggering touch* on the plantar soles just before the equilibration exercises on the oscillating board. When the skin receptors are stimulated by vibrations, the control of the biped posture is improved.

The patient is sitting on the balloon. He bents the hallux against slight resistance, then the therapist exerts a traction in line in *triggering touch*. Again the patient is asked to bend the hallux against resistance (Fig 23). Then, he can relax whereas the therapist keep the hallux bent while he carries out a *triggering touch* on the upper side of the joint. The maneuver is to be repeated between the proximal and the distal phalanges.

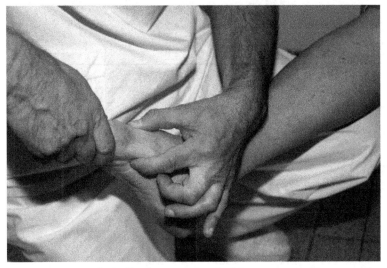

Fig. 23. *Triggering touch* on the hallux between head of first metatarsal bone and base of proximal phalange, on a Klein balloon

The patient suffering from Parkinson's tends to lose his sensitivity and his foot mobility. Nevertheless the plantar sole is an important sensorial entry for the body balance.

One hand is grabbing the calcaneus, the other one is picking the metatarsal bones, with the patient being asked to bend his foot (Fig 24). A *triggering touch* is being carried out on the plantar sole, in longitudinal stretching, with hands moving apart from each other.

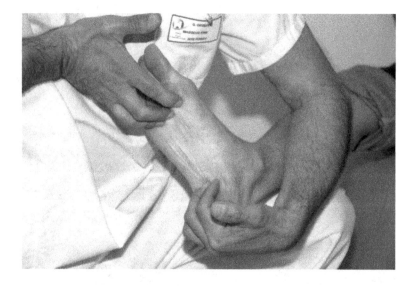

Fig. 24. Maneuver on the plantar sole

7. Late phase

When in the late phase of the illness, the NT maneuvers can still improve the patient's comfort, by easing the pain and improving the vertebral (spiral maneuvers) and thoracic mobility (thoracic amplitude and cardio respiratory capacity). Besides, the *normo-triggering touch* (which is antalgic) will allow the muscles to relax. (Figure 25)

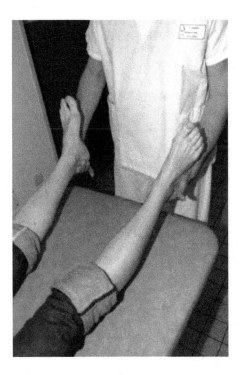

Fig. 25. Gentle shaking of the legs in order to make the muscles relax, and to ease the blood circulation. Shaking of the lower then upper limbs

8. Conclusion

The Normotensive Therapy doesn't stand in the way of other traditional rehabilitative methods. It just adds its personal touch, its *triggering and relaxing touches*. The NT not only treats the symptoms but also the patient in his complexity, without forgetting the comorbidities. Dystonia and diskinesia, unpredictable, often very disturbing in rehabilitation, are attenuated and less frequent, thanks to the gentle and adaptable side of the NT, which can adjust if necessary, if the patient's health is changing, so that his confidence is restored without any added stress.

The central neurology patient is usually a little deprived of physical contact. Consequently his loss of body marks gets worse, and he is even more depressed. It is important to assess his postural problems regularly, by using well chosen therapeutic tools, in order to avoid being overwhelmed by difficulties. The therapist must be ready to adapt quickly. His finger must be at the right place, at the right moment, where and when it hurts. It must be a *vibrating finger,* a *relaxing finger,* a *gentle finger* and a *stroking finger…* A finger which "recognizes the needs of the body", a neuro-informational finger. That is the point of the Normotensive Therapy, which consists in stimulating the patient's balance, his walk and consequently his autonomy, by closely associating manual therapy and original exercises with an elastic bandage and also the Klein balloon during the same session.

9. Acknowledgement

Special thanks to Roselyne De Waele my translator (rosydenys@yahoo.fr), and to Patrice Jones my photograph.

10. References

[1] Amarenco G, Césaro P, Chevrie-Muller C,Cornu Ph, Damier Ph, Destée A, Fabre N, Fénelon G, Laumonnier A, Mahieux F, Marion M-H, Rascol O, Roubeau B, Senard J-M, Tison F. Parkinson's Disease. Acanthe, Masson Smithkline Beecham, Paris, 1998. PP 41-43; 108-110.

[2] Bannwarth B, Bertin P, Trèves R, Dehais J. Affections articulaires induites par les médicaments. Le Concours Médical. 04. 12. 99. 121-39. P 3066-3070.

[3] Jego M et Viallet F. Maladie de Parkinson du sujet âgé. Prise en charge thérapeutique : médicaments à prescrire et médicaments à éviter. La Revue de Gériatrie. 2009.1; 34(1). A8-A11.

[4] Stacy M, Bowron A, Guttman M, Hauser MD, Hughes K, Petter J, Larsen MD, Lewitt P, Oertel W, Niall Quinn, Kapil Sethi, Stocchi F. Identification of motor and nonmotor wearing-off in Parkinson's disease : comparison of a patient questionnary versus clinician assessment. Mov disorders. 2005 ; 20(6) : 726-33.

[5] Bleton JP. Maladie de Parkinson et qualité de vie - 1ère et 2ème parties. Kinésithérapie Scientifique. 1999 ; 387: 56-388.55.

[6] Neiger H, Gilhodes JC, Roll JP. Méthode de rééducation motrice par assistance proprioceptive vibratoire. Kinésithérapie Scientifique.1986; 252: 6-21.

[7] Burke D, Hagbarth K. E. & Lofstedt L. & Wallin,B.G The responses of human muscle spindle endings to vibration during isometric contraction. J Physiol. 261, 695-711.

[8] Lackner J.R and Levine M.S. Changes in apparent body orientation and sensory localization induced by vibration of postural muscles: vibratory myesthetic illusions. Aviat Space Environ Med.1979. 50(4) : 346-54.

[9] Roll JP, Vedel JP, Ribot E. Alteration of propioceptive messages induced by tendon vibration in man : a microneurographic study. Exp Brain Res. 1986. 76 :203-222.

[10] Eklund G. Further studies of vibration-induced effects on balance. J Med Sci. 78. (1973) : 65-72.

[11] Bove M, Nardone A, Schieppatin M. Effects of leg muscle tendons vibration on group Ia and group II reflex responses to stance perturbation in humans. J Physiol Lond. 550. 2003. 617-630.

[12] Smetanin BN, Popov KE, Kozhina GV. Human postural responses to vibratory stimulation of calf muscles under conditions of visual inversion. Human Physiol 28. 2002. 554-558.

[13] Lekhel. H, Popov. K, Anastasopoulos D, Bronstein A, Bhatia K, Marsden CD, Gresty M. Postural responses to vibratin of neck muscles in patients with idiopathic torticolis. Brain. 1997; 120 : 583-91.

[14] Ivanenko YP, Talis VL and Kazennikov OV. Support stability influences postural responses to muscle vibration in humans. Eur J Neurosci. 1999 ; 11 (2) : 647-654.

[15] Ivanenko YP, Grasso R and Lacquantini F. Neck muscle vibratin makes walking humans accelerate in the direction of gaze. J Physiol. 2000 ; 525: 803-814.

[16] Kavounoudias A, Gilhodes JC, Roll R, Roll JP. From Balance regulation to body orientation : two goals for muscle propioceptive information processing ? Exp Brain Res. 1999. 124 : 80-88.

[17] Kavanoudias A, Roll R , Roll JP. Specific whole-body shifts induced byfrequency-modulated vibrations of human plantar soles. Neurosci Lett. 2000. 281 : 99- 102.

[18] Bloem B.R, Allum J.H, Carpenter M.G, Honegger F. Is lower leg propioception essential for triggering human automatic postural responses ? Experimental Brain Research. 2002. 130(3): 375-391.

[19] Polak J. Contractures persistantes: l'hypothèse d'une boucle beta. Kinésithérapie Scientifique. N°360. Octobre 1996. P 9.

[20] Orgeret G, Viel E. Thérapie manuelle du système myofascial. Coll. Bois Larris. Masson, Paris, 2000. P 57.

[21] Perennou D. Postural disorders and spatial neglect in stroke patients ; a strong association. Restor Neurol Neurosci. 2006. 24: 319-334.

[22] Fitzpatrick and MacCloskey. Propioceptive, visual and vestibular thresholds for the perception of sway during standing in humans. J Physiol. 1994, 478, 1, 173-186.

[23] Bogumila Sobczak. Influence de la kinésithérapie sur l'état fonctionnel des articulations temporo-mandibulaires, de la colonne vertébrale et des membres ; Kinésithérapie Scientifique. N° 328. Novembre 1993. P11-25.

[24] Amblard B. Les descripteurs du contrôle postural. Ann Réadaptation Méd. Phys. 1998, 41, 225-237.

[25] Uchiyama M, Demuras S. Low visual acuity is associated with the decrease in postural sway. Tohoku J Exp Med. 2008 nov ; 216 (3) : 277-85.

[26] Naudin-Rousselle P. Les chutes répétées des personnes âgées. Le Généraliste. Septembre 2009. N° 2495. P21.

[27] Podsiadlo D, Richardson S. The timed up and go: a test of basic functional mobility for frail elderly persons. J Am Geriat Soc 1991 ; 39 : 142-148.

[28] Kemoun G, Defevre L, Watelain E et al. Maladie de Parkinson comme modèle de vieillissement: analyse prospective des troubles de la marche. Revue Neurologique 2003; 159; 1028-37.

[29] Vaillant J, Barthalais N, Vuillerme N. Ankle strapping and postural control : Effetc of underwrap. Science & Sports. 23. 2008. 78-82.

[30] Menz HB, lord SR, Fitzpatrick R. A tactile stimulus applied to the leg improves postural stability in young, old and neuropathic subjects. Neuroscience Letters. Volume 406, Issues 1-2, 2 octobre 2006. P 23-26.

[31] Zouch M, Alexander Ch, Vico L. L'activité physique dans l'ostéoporose, avec modération. Impact Medecine. Exercice. N°215. 18 Octobre 2007. P 28.

[32] Iwatsuki h, Ikuta y, Shinoda K, Deep friction massage on the masticatory muscles, in stroke patients increases biting force. J Phy; Ther Sci; 2001; 1: 17-20.

6

Potentials of Telehealth Devices for Speech Therapy in Parkinson's Disease

Lilian Beijer[1] and Toni Rietveld[1,2]
[1]Sint Maartenskliniek Nijmegen, Section Research, Development & Education
[2]Radboud University Nijmegen, Faculty of Arts, Department of Linguistics
The Netherlands

1. Introduction

Rapidly evolving technological developments have been influencing our daily lives for a few decades now. In particular information and communication technologies enable more sophisticated and faster ways of communication than ever before. These developments have far reaching consequences for professional, domestic and leisure activities. Use of computers, whether or not with an internet connection, has become very common also in the field of education and health care. The primary benefits in these areas are believed to lie in cost reduction and enhanced efficiency.

In this chapter we will focus on the possibilities of technological developments in health care, particularly for patients with Parkinson's disease. This patient group is believed to benefit considerably from innovative applications of information and communication technologies since the number of parkinsonian patients is dramatically growing due to demographic developments. Moreover, Parkinson's disease pre-eminently concerns a chronic and progressive illness, increasingly disabling these patients in almost all domains of their lives. In this chapter we will explore how telehealth technology and speech technology relates to the maintenance of their communicative competence.

2. General aspects of speech disorders associated with Parkinson's disease

2.1 General motor functions and oral motor control

Parkinson's disease is caused by the progressive impairment of neurons in an area of the brain known as substantia nigra. This is due to an imbalance in two brain chemicals (i.e. dopamine and acetylcholine) which are responsible for the transmission of nerve messages from the brain to the motor nerves in the spinal cord which control muscle movement. As a result, the communication between the substantia nigra and the corpus striatum, required for coordinating smooth and balanced muscle movement, is distorted.

The diminished functioning and coordination of respiratory, laryngeal and supralaryngeal muscles obviously affects speech, swallowing and saliva control in parkinsonian patients (Ziegler, 2003). As a consequence, the quality of speech in patients with Parkinson's disease tends to be deteriorated to some degree. As it is, dysarthria is a common manifestation of Parkinson's disease (PD) which increases in frequency and intensity with the progress of the disease (Streifler, 1984). Hypokinetic dysarthria is mainly associated with PD; mixed dysarthria tends to occur in atypical parkinsonism.

General motor symptoms such as rigidity, bradykinesia (reduced speed of muscles), tremors or trembling are reflected in typical speech symptoms of hypokinetic dysarthria. Bradykinesia associated with Parkinson's disease causes difficulty in the initiation of voluntary speech. This can result in delay in starting to talk as well as very slow speech. According to Duffy (1995), there may be freezing of movement during speech. Rigidity can also occur. Additionally, parkinsonian patients have reduced loudness, imprecise consonant production, reduced pitch variability and festinating speech. The latter can result in extremely fast speech together with short rushes of speech (Ferrand and Bloom, 1997). Perceptual features of parkinsonian speech associated with hypokinetic dysarthria, are a weak, breathy (hoarse) voice, monotone and monoloud speech, low volume, articulatory imprecision and rate disturbances (Darly et al., 1969). The syndrome of parkinsonian dysarthria is by no means homogeneous with respect to speech rate. This might be due to different consecutive stages in the development of parkinsonian dysarthria or to different degrees of impairment (Ackermann & Ziegler, 1991). In general, more pronounced phonatory than articulatory disturbances tend to occur as far as clinical-perceptual ratings are observed.

2.2 Speech intelligibility

As a consequence of distorted oral motor functions and coordination, speech intelligibility in patients with PD obviously tends to be reduced. Prevalence studies point out that about 70% of patients living at home with Parkinson's disease have speech complaints (Kalf et al., 2008a), which are mainly associated with hypokinetic dysarthria. Diminished communication skills, in addition to the fact that these patients are increasingly disabled in their physical condition and motor abilities in the course of their disease, frequently lead to patients experiencing a deteriorating quality of life (Slawek et al., 2005). Improving or at least maintaining speech quality as long as possible is essential to enable optimal social participation and to maintain relationships. As a consequence, patients with PD are often eager to practice and improve their speech quality.

Although the majority of patients with PD are dysarthric speakers, only a minority of this group with diminished speech quality receives speech therapy (20-30%). The small percentage of PD patients under 'speech therapeutical control' might be partially due to the fact that a majority of speech language therapists consider themselves not capable to adequately treat dysarthric speakers with PD. Another reason might be the fact that speech therapy often is provided to patients that have only recently been diagnosed with PD. Therapists lose sight of their patients once face-to-face therapy sessions have been completed. Thus, dysarthric patients tend to be deprived of speech therapy in the chronic and deteriorating course of their disease. As it is, this tendency of 'undertreatment' of dysarthric patients with PD is likely to continue in the course of the coming years. That is, the incidence and prevalence of PD will increase due to our aging population. It is estimated that in 2030 about 30% of our population will be 65 years of age or older.

2.3 Guidelines for diagnostic and treatment procedures

Apart from the observed 'undertreatment' of patients with PD, large variability exists in therapeutical approaches of this patients group. In the Netherlands, evidence based guidelines for diagnostic and treatment procedures for patients with PD were developed in order to provide speech-language therapists with recommendations for their clinical practice (Kalf et al., 2008b). It should be noted that methodological quality of comparative studies is often insufficient to meet the conditions of highest level of evidence (Deane et al., 2001). Therefore, evidence is mainly based on comparative studies of less methodological quality, noncomparative studies or experts' opinions. Five key points for treating dysarthric speech in patients with PD were formulated in the evidence based guidelines (Kalf et al., 2008b):

1. Patients with PD have basically normal motor skills, requiring to be elicited in an adequate way.
2. Hypokinesia increases when duration and complexity of motor acts increase. Therefore, complex acts should be divided into more simple acts.
3. Separate acts should therefore compensate for failing automatic motor acts
4. External cues could support initiation and continuation of motor acts.
5. Simultaneous execution of motor and cognitive tasks should be avoided, since execution of motor tasks already puts considerable demands on cognitive functions.

For diagnosis and treatment of dysarthria in patients with PD, two procedures are strongly recommended. 1) As far as diagnostic procedures are concerned, the initial situation should be assessed by documenting spontaneous speech and establishing to what extent speech can be stimulated by means of maximum performance tests. 2) For treatment, the Lee Silverman Voice Treatment (LSVT) (Ramig et al., 2001) and the Pitch Limiting Voice Treatment (PLVT) (de Swart et al., 2003) are strongly recommended. The LSVT focuses on tasks to maximize respiratory and phonatory functions in order to improve respiratory drive, vocal fold adduction, laryngeal muscle activity and synergy, laryngeal and supralaryngeal articulatory movements, and vocal tract configuration. The PLVT also aims at increasing loudness but at the same time sets vocal pitch at an adequate level. The LSVT and the PLVT produce the same increase in loudness but PLVT limits an increase in vocal pitch and claims to prevent a strained or stressed voicing (de Swart et al., 2003). Both therapy programs concern intensive training periods of four sessions weekly during a training period of four weeks. Intensive speech therapy is preferred if diagnostic results allow highly intensive and frequent training. That is, voice quality, intrinsic motivation, physical condition and cognitive abilities are vital conditions for intensive training of newly acquired speech techniques. In case a patient's condition does not allow intensive training, augmentative and alternative procedures or devices could provide a solution to the communication problems experienced by dysarthric speakers with PD.

In the next sections, we will go into more detail with respect to current trends in speech therapy for patients with PD. These result from rapidly evolving developments in information-, communication- and speech technology. Not only will these developments provide patients with new therapy facilities; they are also expected to bring about some crucial changes for health care providers (i.e. speech therapists) and influence health care processes.

3. Current trends in the therapy of speech disorders related to Parkinson's disease

3.1 Increased need for speech training

A considerable percentage of PD patients experience oral motor disorders, causing problems with swallowing, speech and saliva control. With 70% of PD patients being dysarthric, it is obvious that therapeutical interventions are required. That is, the speech of PD patients with predominantly hypokinetic dysarthria, needs treatment in order to improve speech intelligibility. Since communication skills are vital for adequate social participation, improvement of these abilities can significantly contribute to quality of life.

A number of current trends seem to influence the developments in speech therapy for parkinsonian patients. Firstly, there is an increased attention for dysarthria and its treatment. This is partially due to the results of scientific research in the field of PD, enhancing care givers' awareness of the relevance for long lasting communication skills in parkinsonian patients. Secondly, recent social and demographic developments have caused patients to be more aware of possibilities for treatment and to be more assertive in their call for adequate information. Patient centred health care has even gained considerable importance for reimbursement companies that find themselves increasingly confronted with clients searching for the best quality of care. Apart from this, the economic instability in this decade urges the health care community to treat the growing number of elderly patients with neurological diseases with less financial means. It is obviously a challenge to maintain a sound balance between the need (and call) for speech training on the one hand, and the availability of professionals and financial means for speech training on the other hand. Particularly with current speech training programs for PD such as the LSVT (Ramig et al., 2001) and the Dutch PLVT (de Swart et al., 2003), involving intensive speech training for several weeks to enhance speech intelligibility, it becomes clear that traditional speech therapy does no longer meet the actual needs of our current society.

3.2 Telehealth in the field of speech-language pathology
Telehealth applications, resulting from recently developed information and communication technologies in health care, could provide solutions to overcome barriers of access to therapy services caused by factors such as decreasing financial resources, shortage of professionals and increasing number of clients. The terms 'telemedicine' and 'telehealth' are sometimes used interchangeably. Telemedicine is considered a subset of telehealth. Telemedicine uses communication networks for delivery of healthcare services and medical education from one geographical location to another, primarily to address challenges like uneven distribution and shortage of infrastructural and human resources (Sood et al., 2007). 'Telehealth' is a broader term and does not necessarily involve clinical services. It can be defined as the use of telecommunication technologies both to provide health care services and to enable access to medical information for training and educating health care professionals and consumers. As such, telehealth concerns all applications of information and communication technologies, enabling the retrieval, recording, management and transmission of information to support health care. In this chapter, we refer to this latter definition when discussing telehealth.

Mashima and Doarn's (2008) overview of telehealth activities in the field of speech-language pathology provide a strong foundation for broader applications of telehealth technologies in this area. Also telehealth applications for treatment of patients with neurogenic communication disorders have been reported. Theodoros et al. (2006) report an online speech training for PD patients which turned out to be effective. Ten patients with PD followed the LSVT online using video conferencing, during a four-week program of intensive training, involving 16 therapy sessions. Comparison of sound pressure level, pitch measurements and perceptual ratings from audio recordings pre- and posttreatment, containing participants' reading and conversational monologue, showed significant improvements, comparable to previously reported outcomes for the LSVT when delivered face-to-face. This example shows that remote diagnosis and treatment of speech in parkinsonian patients has vital benefits, in particular for patients who are less mobile and easily fatigued due to their deteriorated physical condition. Ziegler and Zierdt (2008) report an online version of a computer-based intelligibility assessment tool: the Munich Intelligibility Profile. The web based MVP-version is reported to have potentials for dysarthric speech of patients with PD and other underlying neurological diseases such as stroke.

3.3 E-learning based Speech Therapy (EST)
Quite recently, in the Netherlands a web based speech training device 'E-learning based Speech Therapy' (EST) has been developed (Beijer et al., 2010a). EST primarily aims at patients with dysarthric speech resulting from acquired neurological impairment such as stroke and Parkinson's disease. According to our clinical experience, these patients suffer from their deteriorating quality of speech. Particularly in the chronic phase of their disease, once therapy sessions have been completed, the lack of practice results in diminished speech intelligibility. With verbal communication being a vital condition for adequate social participation, diminished abilities in this field can be considerably invalidating. A vital benefit of EST is the possibility to follow a tailor-made speech training program in the patients' home environment. That is, time, energy and costs normally involved with speech training can be reduced for these patients who tend to be less mobile and easily fatigued due to their physical condition. In addition, the possibility to practice speech in the home environment at any moment, allows intensive speech training, which is known to be effective in patients with acquired neurological diseases (Kwakkel et al., 1999). Repetitive training in chronic phases also has been proven to have positive effects on speech intelligibility (Rijntjes et al., 2009).

Since telehealth applications tend to differ in many respects, Tulu et al., (2007) made an effort to provide insight into the large number of innovative web based devices that are available. They introduced a taxonomy of telehealth applications along five dimensions: communication infrastructure, delivery options, application purpose, application area and environmental setting. According to this classification, EST concerns a store-and-forward web application for treatment (i.e. training) purposes in the area of speech pathology that is commonly used in the home environment.

The keystone of the EST infrastructure is formed by a central server. The server hosts two types of audio files: target speech files in MP3 format and recorded speech files uploaded by patients in wav format (Figure 1). A desktop computer or a laptop with internet connection provides users with access to the server. Using their EST therapist account, therapists are able to, at a distance, provide their patients with a tailor-made speech training program, which is compiled from audio examples of target speech, stored at a central server.

Patients have access to this program using their client account. In the EST training procedure patients listen to audio examples of target speech which is downloaded from the server. Subsequently they imitate the audio example, in order to approach the target speech. The target and the own speech are then aurally compared. Finally the patients' speech is uploaded and stored at the server (Figure 2).

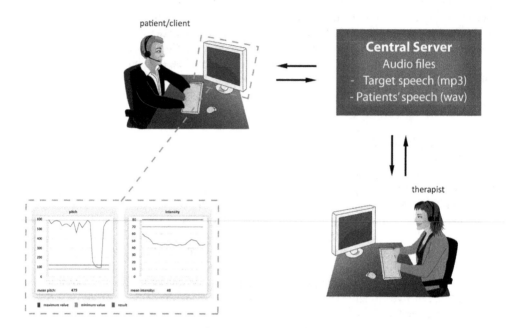

Fig. 1. Infrastructure of E-learning based Speech Therapy (EST). (Reproduced with credit of the Telemedicine and eHealth journal)

Obviously, this training procedure puts considerable demands on patients' auditory speech discrimination skills. However, indications have been reported that patients with PD experience problems with estimating the own speech volume (Ho et al., 2000) and with auditory speech discrimination (Beijer, Rietveld & van Stiphout, in press). Although this diminished auditory discrimination might be caused by cognitive problems and hearing loss, these patients would benefit from additional visual feedback on their own speech realization. That is, visualization of speech might support them in the auditory discrimination task of the EST training procedure. Although this visualization is already implemented in EST, the abstract graphs (Figure 1) and the delayed, post hoc display of visual feedback did not appear suitable for all patients (Beijer et al., 2010b). Therefore, the development of an intuitive visualisation of loudness and pitch is currently underway in order to apply to patients with various backgrounds (i.e. educational levels, age, gender). Not only should the graphic form of the visual feedback apply to the patients, indicating into what direction a new speech attempt should be adjusted to approach the target. It should also be assessed to what extent different visualisations contribute to the improvement of speech intelligibility. In section 4.4. we will go into some detail with respect to visual feedback on pitch and intensity (loudness).

Therapists are allowed to download audio files of their patient's speech from the server. Thus, they are able to listen to their patient's speech at different points across time. In addition they may analyze the acoustic speech signal for objective measures of speech dimensions that are relevant for an individual patient.

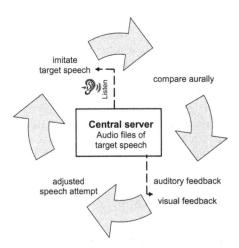

Fig. 2. EST training procedure. (Reproduced with credit of Telemedicine and eHealth)

Despite the improvements to be made, a case study conducted with a male patient with PD suggested that EST is a suitable web based speech training device with potential efficacy for patients with PD (Beijer et al., 2010b). The patient had completed face-to-face sessions of PLVT practice, and was able to conduct the training program that he was already familiar with, independently at home. He followed an intensive, protocolized four-week program, involving the PLVT (de Swart et al., 2003) by means of EST. His speech intelligibility had significantly improved immediately after the EST training period. Speech intelligibility was measured by the percentage correctly (orthographically) transcribed words in semantically unpredictable sentences (SUS). After several weeks without practice, the patient's speech intelligibility declined. Apparently, practice of speech maintained speech quality. As mentioned in section 1.3, the PLVT primarily aims at improving speech intensity (the acoustical correlate of perceived loudness) with, for vocal hygiene reasons, limited vocal pitch raise and laryngeal tension. It appeared that the participant appreciated weekly contact via telephone with his speech therapist. Apparently there was a need for additional therapeutical suggestions and a therapeutical relationship. Nevertheless, the results of this case study are hopeful. Currently, the efficacy and the user satisfaction of the web application EST are subject of investigation.

3.4 Research issues for EST

It will be clear that innovative web based applications for diagnostic and treatment purposes should be evaluated from several perspectives. First of all, the technological feasibility should be proven. Secondly, patients as well as therapists should be able to operate the web based devices. Hence, user satisfaction should be evaluated since this is obviously vital for successful implementation. The term 'user satisfaction' needs to be accurately defined to ensure comparison of user satisfaction across time and across different web based devices. This brings us to the need to establish minimum user requirements regarding physical condition, motor coordination skills and auditory or cognitive abilities. Assessing these conditions for successful use of web based devices is vital for parkinsonian patients who tend to experience constraints in more domains than communication or speech alone. Thirdly the efficacy and the effectiveness of EST should be evaluated. This brings us to the vital issue of reliable outcome measures for treatment outcomes. In the case of parkinsonian speech, these treatment outcomes primarily concern speech intelligibility. Most of these outcome measures concern subjective, perceptual measures of speech quality (FDA, rate scaling, etc.). Along with health care reimbursers' call for objective outcome measures however, current trends point into the direction of objective acoustical measures of speech quality as a vital outcome measure for speech intelligibility in addition to traditional perceptual measures.

Employment of web based applications for diagnosis and treatment tend to go perfectly along with the need for speech technological developments. That is, speech data can be easily collected, thus generating an automatic data base of pathological speech. We will elaborate on this in section 4.5.

4. The role of speech technology in speech therapy

4.1 Introduction

For more than 25 years phoneticians, speech technologists and speech therapists have systematically investigated the phonetic correlates of speech disorders. These investigations were carried out with a number of explicit or implicit objectives: a) to corroborate subjective judgements of speech therapists, b) to find objective evidence for progress as a result of therapy, c) to facilitate the distinction of subgroups of pathologies, and d) to find evidence for theories on the nature of pathologies, which could not be obtained on the basis of subjective measurements. As has been the case in phonetics sciences, the progress of computer and information technology made available a number of additional applications, which form the core of the current chapter:

a.   Gathering objective evidence based on acoustic and/or physiological data,
b.   The development of systems which can be used by patients to obtain direct or indirect feedback on their realizations in a training program,
c.   The implementation of feedback systems in telehealth applications in order to facilitate intensive training at home.

In the following we will focus on a number of applications of speech technology to be used in the assessment and treatment of dysarthria in general and that of dysarthria associated with Parkinson's disease in particular. We should be aware of the fact that phonetics and the associated speech technology are language bound, that is to say that phenomena which are relevant in one language, may be irrelevant in another.

Kent et al. (1999) published a seminal overview of acoustic correlates of quite a number of phenomena associated with dysarthria. The overview distinguishes the conventional phonetic components of the speech production process: Initiation, Phonation, Articulation, Velopharyngeal functioning and Prosody. As is the case with most acoustic correlates of speech disorders, stochastic relations between perceptually distinctive disorders on one side and acoustic correlates on the other are more evident than inferential procedures which boil down to statements like: the F1 and F2 (first and second formants) of segment X are higher/lower than 'normal', so we can be sure that this segment was not realized in a canonical way. The fact that trade-off relations exist between speech production and speech perception is the nuisance factor. Trade-off relations in phonetics occur when an effect in one domain – say segment duration – can compensate for the absence of a feature in another domain, say voicing. In English, for instance, a relatively long pre-consonantal vowel can perceptually compensate for an obstruent which is incorrectly realized as voiceless.

The presence of this kind of trade-off relations is an obstacle in finding clear and unambiguous acoustic correlates of the perception of speech and speech disorders. This fact is not a direct problem in group studies, which aim at finding tendencies in signal characteristics between pathological groups and a control group. In set-ups in which the aim is to provide stable and robust feedback to a patient, the presence of trade-offs can be disturbing.

Providing instrumental feedback to speakers has quite a long history. As a matter of fact, there are two parallel developments. One development focuses on learning a foreign language ("L2"), and the other on correcting speech disorders. It is quite obvious why these developments are parallel: the dimensions on which deviations of target speech can be projected are – most of the time – equal or similar: prosodic dimensions, dimensions of segmental quality, phonatory dimensions and dimensions of velopharyngeal functioning. Like in speech pathology, it is hardly ever the case that all dimensions are equally relevant. For French as L2, nasality is more important than for English or Dutch. Intonation and tone is extremely important for languages like Chinese, and much less important for English, French or Dutch. These facts have directed research both in systems which provide feedback in L2 learning and in speech therapy. Until now, it has proven not to be worth the effort in this context to assess all characteristics of speech which are imitations of target speech. It is better to direct efforts to specific segments which are known to be vulnerable and/or relevant in L2 learning and speech pathology. This brings us to two different lines in feedback:

a.   Direct, quasi real time feedback on the realization of global parameters like intensity, tempo and intonation and parameters associated with segmental quality, and

b.   Indirect, post-hoc feedback on the realization of speech parameters.

Direct feedback is meant to help the patient in non-face-to-face training sessions; indirect, post-hoc feedback is often only needed when the therapist has to have access to assessment scores; it is only available after quite a number of speech materials have been collected.

There might be a misunderstanding when it is decided to provide web based speech therapy, in the sense that it is often assumed that a computer system which provides feedback is immediately applicable in an e-health application. That is not true. Supervised training/learning often cannot be directly applied in an environment in which direct assistance is absent. Supervised learning is much more robust than its non-supervised counterpart. An example is provided by Carmichael (2007). In his study, which aimed at the development of objective acoustic measures for the Frenchay Dysarthria Assessment Procedure (Enderby, 1980), the calibration of the 'loudness' measurements might be somewhat complicated to be performed at home. It involves the use of a Sound meter at a standard distance. In his set-up the test administrator performs the calibration procedure. In order to avoid this kind of calibration at home, we opted in our telehealth application for the production of a long nasal consonant [*mmmm*]. As the production of this consonant does not involve any mouth opening and variable jaw movements, the radiated sound can be assumed to be quite constant, and to function as a reliable calibration.

Speech technology in the context of speech pathology can be divided in a number of approaches, which also depend on the objectives to be achieved. In this chapter we restrict our review to applications in assessment, therapy and training. We distinguish five dimensions on which the approaches can vary:

Dimension I: Either the parameters focus on global parameters like intensity, tempo and pitch, or on characteristics which reflect segmental quality.

Dimension II: There are two types of results to be obtained, viz. global assessment, or direct feedback.

Dimension III: Types of speech: the assessment of free speech, or the assessment of read, known speech.

Dimension IV: The inclusion of physiological parameters, like reflexes and respiration.

Dimension V: The inclusion of facial expressions as parameter(s).

A more general dimension is the user-interface. Of course, the interface for the therapist requires less attention, but the one for the patient asks for robustness and psychological validity.

Dimension I: In specific therapies, like the PLVT (de Swart et al., 2003), global parameters are of great importance. As explained in section 1.3 of this chapter, it involves two therapy goals: "speaking loud" while not increasing pitch at the same time. The rationale is that speaking loud generally leads to an increase of articulatory precision, while increasing pitch above habitual level may harm the vocal cords.

Dimension II: Global assessment – not to be confused with global parameters – involves the assessment of speech on a long-term scale. That is, direct feedback is not provided, only feedback after some amount of speech materials has been realized, recorded and analyzed. In an application for direct feedback, the user is provided with quasi real time feedback on the quality of the speech parameters at issue: global parameters like intensity and F0, or feedback on specific segments, like vowels or consonants.

Dimension III: Very often, known and consequently read speech will be used in assessment and therapy sessions. The automatic recognition of speech and the detection of deviations from it, are enormously facilitated by the use of this kind of texts (it implies what is called forced recognition). The drawback is that the use of read speech may decrease the ecological validity of the measures and indices thus obtained.

Dimension IV: As is well-known, the initiation phase in speech, which refers mainly to respiration, is crucial for the generation of speech. There are, to our knowledge, no applications available yet which provide assessment and feedback on initiation (respiration) parameters.

Dimension V: In a number of speech pathologies the assessment of facial expressions is a relevant issue. This is also the case with dysarthria. The recognition and assessment of facial expression demand dedicated software, which is quite difficult to tune to the demands of the patient and/or therapist.

4.2 Realization of assessment and feedback systems

For the realization of feedback and assessment on global parameters (F0, Intensity), relatively simple algorithms are needed, often implemented in current software packages for signal analysis, like PRAAT (Boersma & Weenink, 2011). The problem there is not the analysis of the parameters itself, but the display of the results and the feedback on deviations from the goal values. No significant changes in the detection of the global speech parameters are to be expected, but work has to be done in order to provide displays which facilitate insight in possible errors and stimulate improvements.

For the realization of feedback and assessment of segmental quality, speech technology comes to play. There are a number of approaches, depending again, on the objectives of the application: direct/indirect feedback on the realization of each target speech sound (phoneme), direct/indirect feedback on the realization of single words, direct/indirect feedback on the realization of a short text, direct/indirect feedback on fixed or free texts, and feedback on the overall intelligibility of words and texts. The two main technical approaches are: the analysis of speech based on Automatic Speech Recognition (ASR) and ASR-free analysis of speech (Middag et al., 2010). If ASR is used, the Hidden Markov Model (HMM) is the main tool. HMMs constitute the default tool for automatic speech recognition, although other approaches are also possible (Middag et al., 2010). Hidden Markov Models are based on probabilities of states of speech segments and transitions from one state to another, or to the same state. In light of the popularity of HMMs we present a short account of this approach below. To illustrate HMMs we give a fictitious example of the use of an HMM for the recognition of the vowel /i/. The acoustic parameter used is the second formant (F2) only. In that respect the example is already fictitious: HMMs hardly ever use formants as acoustic parameters, let alone just one formant. The default parameters used to reflect the spectra of the sound segments are Mel-Frequency-Cepstral Coefficients (MFCCs), which also take into account human perception (Davis & Mermelstein, 1980).

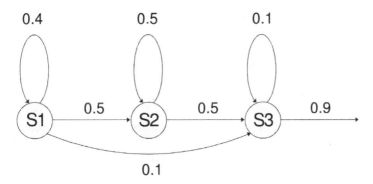

Fig. 3. A hypothetical Hidden Markov Model of the vowel /i/. (Reproduced from Rietveld & van Heuven, 2009, with permission).

In the above figure we display a model of the second formant (F2) of the vowel /i/. We see an inner loop from state 2 to state 2, which occurs with a probability of 0.5; this means that the model has a relatively high probability of staying in state 2, which boils down to the realization of a long vowel. The probability of going from state 1 (initial state) to the final state (S3) is small, only 0.1. The probabilities of obtaining discrete values of F2 for state 2 (low, rather low, rather high and high: E1, E2, E3, E4) are 0.05, 0.10, 0.15 and 0.70 respectively. Thus the probability of finding a high value of F2 in the middle of the vowel /i/ is rather high.

In reality we observe small speech frames, with – in our restricted and hypothetical example – only values of F2. The sequence of values of the F2, for instance E2, E4, E4, E4, E3 (each frame covering 20 ms), has to be compared with the probabilities implied by the model. The model which has the largest probability of having generated the observed sequence of states, will be labelled as the 'realized segment'. Of course, there will be differences in confidence that a sequence X should be labelled as segment $/x/$.

A confidence index is a possible measure of the quality of the realized segment. This procedure is used in an ASR application for the detection of errors in L2 (Cucchiarini et al., 2009). There is a complication. In most speech recognition algorithms, a so-called 'language model' plays a role. That language model contains transitional probabilities of going from one word to another. In Dutch, for instance, the probability of finding a word with the neutral gender – like '*house*' – is extremely low after the non-neutral determiner 'de' ('the'). In some ASR approaches language models even pertain to phoneme sequences. In Dutch, for instance, the sequence $/l\ r/$ is very low, whereas the probability of observing a sequence $/s\ t/$ is relatively high. Of course, this language knowledge should be used in speech recognition, but not in a system that aims at assessing the quality of speech segments. Knowledge of the language model is a well-known obstacle to the subjective assessment of speech. We all know that in '*the cat p...*' '*p*' will be followed with a high probability by '*urrs*'. That is why subjective measurement has an intrinsic problem: the expectation of the listener.

HMMs are used in a number of formats, depending on:

- the number of states used in modelling speech segments,
- the amount of training material needed,
- the dimensionality of the statistical distributions of the parameters used.

A word-based account of errors is often not informative, even if the language model in the HMM is "switched off". The reason is that segment mispronunciations have to be weighted in order to obtain a valid error score for an utterance (Preston, Ramsdell, Oller, Edwards & Tobin, 2011). That is why most systems developed for providing feedback on the adequacy of pronunciation are segment based. Before a robust ASR system can be set up to provide feedback on speech performance, it has to be established to which extent target speech segments meet the following criteria, which, as a matter of fact, are quite similar to the criteria used in systems for error detection in second language acquisition (see Cucchiarini et al. 2009).

a. The influence of an incorrect realization has an impact on intelligibility and communication; this implies that for every language different segments and features are important. Tonal movements are less important for languages like English or German, but crucial in Chinese.

b. The errors are perceptually salient;

c. The errors are frequent;

d. The errors occur in the speech of relatively many speakers;

e. The errors are persistent;

f. Robust automatic error detection is possible;

g. Unambiguous feedback is available.

4.3 Speech materials to be used

An often neglected subject is the nature of the speech materials to be used. Of course, the materials should contain language samples which are prone to be incorrectly realized – see above -, but there are also other aspects which should be considered. There are a multitude of factors which affect the realization of speech segments and global parameters of speech. We mention: the prosodic position: in the English word *rhododendron,* for example, *'den'* carries word stress. Word stress affects duration, intensity and spectral characteristics, the length of the utterance: the longer an utterance is, the shorter the speech segments which make it up are (the *'i'* in *'stride'* is shorter than in *'side'*, the distinction between function words and content words (for instance *'in'* vs. *'bin'*) is influential in speech tempo, intensity and spectral characteristics. If speech materials are to be used in subsequent assessment procedures, it is worthwhile to have the speech segments realized in balanced conditions.

4.4 Technical requirements

The American Telemedicine Association published a valuable list of "Core Standards for Telemedicine Operations" (2007). For speech applications an additional number of technical requirements have to be met, as a function of the goals of the application. Most of them are self-evident. We mention a number of requirements, and will give some more information on requirements which are less self-evident:

1. *The presence of a reliable and robust server,* with personnel that can answer technical questions at well-defined time intervals and can update the system as required by IT-developments (firewalls, browsers etc.);
2. *A cross-platform browser-based application* which delivers uncompromised viewing of applications;
3. *A clear distribution of roles* with an associated system for authorizations: user, therapist and administrator;
4. *Quick uploading* of target utterances;
5. *A psychologically valid and quick presentation of feedback with sufficient screen resolution.*
   The configuration of visual feedback for speech is not self-evident, and needs some scrutiny in order to adapt it to the user population. In this domain, speech technologists should be supplemented with experts in the integration of auditory and visual perception (Sadakata et al., 2008). For patients with neurogenic communication disorders such as PD, who are likely to suffer from other disorders than distorted speech alone, visual or cognitive distortions might be a serious constraint in the perception of visual displays that aim at providing feedback on different speech dimensions, such as pitch and intensity (loudness). This is particularly the case when two or more speech dimensions of a dysarthric speaker are displayed, such as pitch and intensity in the case of the PLVT for parkinsonian speakers. Rather than abstract graphs, which are difficult to interpret for a large number of predominantly elderly speakers, visualization should be simple and intuitive. That is, the form of visual feedback should apply to patients and give cues for approaching and adequate realization of speech.
   An example: how should one display the time course of pitch and intensity, as a simple graph (see Figure 4a), or as a picture which might intuitively be more appealing (Figure 4b)? The solution might obviously lie in an integrated, multidimensional picture of more speech dimensions.
   Currently, in the Netherlands, web based experiments are set up in order to evaluate what graphic form appeals to healthy controls. In addition, it will be evaluated whether or not preferences for visual forms in healthy controls also goes for neurological patients such as speakers with PD or after stroke.

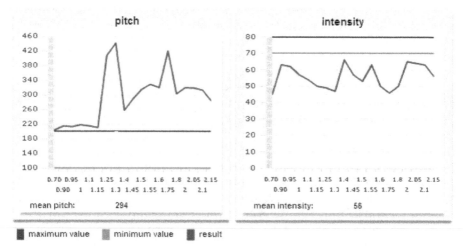

mean pitch: 294   mean intensity: 56

■ maximum value   ▨ minimum value   ▪ result

Fig. 4a. Separate displays of the time course of pitch and intensity (female speaker)

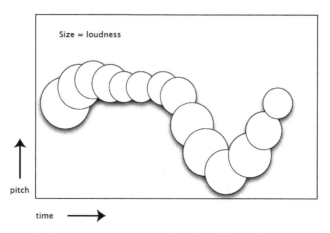

Fig. 4b. Integrated display of the time course of pitch and intensity

6. *Easy use of the PC/laptop;*
7. *Adjustable text fonts;*
8. Possibility to *personalize* protocols for exercises;
9. *Privacy guarantees;*
10. *Adequate format of speech files.*

If (subsets of) realized utterances are stored for subsequent assessment by a speech therapist or an automated computer procedure, the format of the speech files should be suited for those procedures. The main element of the format is the sampling frequency (22.05 kHz or 44.1 kHz). Preferably no signal coding should be used to reduce the amount of data. MP3 coding and the associated data reduction (with bit rates of 128 or 192) does not have any effects on perception, but may lead to some effects on the spectral representation. WAV-files have an advantage: they are files without any data-coding. Important factors in the decision on the sampling frequency and the possible data reduction are the characteristics of the parameters to be extracted from the signal. The upper bound of the frequency range relevant for the acoustic description of vowel-like sounds is around 3 kHz. For the analysis of fricatives – for instance speech sounds like /s/ and /ʃ/ - we need a wider frequency range, with an upper bound of at least 6 kHz (Olive et al., 1993).

11. *Robust and well-defined recording conditions.*

The basic principle underlying eHealth applications is that patients can use the application at home. Conditions at home vary to a great extent. Some people will use the application in a quiet office, others in a kitchen with neon tubes, or in a garden with traffic noise in the background. In the following figure we show the waveform of an utterance with an added 50 Hz-signal; the latter is not a pure sinus wave. The sinusoidal signal might hinder subjective judgement, and create biases in the spectral representation of the realized utterances, see panel (b) in Figure 5, where a strong 50 Hz component and the associated harmonics are displayed. The presence of the harmonics is due to the fact that the sinus wave was not 'pure'.

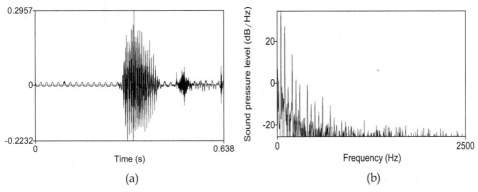

(a)   (b)

Fig. 5. (a) Waveform of a fragment of the Dutch word 'buitenboord' ([bœytəb...]:'English: 'outboard') with an added 50 Hz signal generated by an external source and (b) spectrum of the (intended silent) initial part of the waveform.

In many approaches to the (semi-automatic) assessment of the segmental quality of speech segments, the silent interval associated with the closing phase of stop consonants like /p, t, k/ is relevant. If this interval is filled with some 'humming' it may be an indication that the speaker was not able to firmly close his/her lips for the stop consonant (Kent et al., 1999).

4.5 Secondary outcomes of telehealth applications for speech technology

Apart from therapeutical aims, which mainly focus on the benefits for clients and therapists, telehealth applications such as EST provide a vital source of data for researchers in the field of speech pathology and speech technology. That is, uploading patients' speech by means of web based systems, automatically generates a data base of pathological speech (Figure 6). This data base is vital for clinical outcome research in the field of speech pathology. That is, a data base allows perceptual and acoustical measurements of speech across time in order to evaluate therapy outcomes. This will increasingly gain importance in the context of decreasing financial resources for health care, where evidence based treatments finally will prevail. Although guidelines for diagnosis and treatment have been formulated (section 2.3), these are not based on the highest level of evidence. Objective outcome measures on the basis of a central data base of pathological speech are likely to enhance evidence based guidelines. Government policies and hence requirements of health care reimbursers will be based on objective therapy results, to be derived from data sources as generated by web based applications such as EST. For therapists the objective speech data over time of an individual patient is expected to provide useful information to evaluate therapy results and to adjust therapy focus if necessary.

In addition to its relevance for clinical outcome research, a data base of pathological speech contains vital information for speech technological and language technological research. In general, speech and language technology has considerably gained importance in health care during the last few decades. Particularly for patients with communicative problems this research area is of vital importance. These problems can be due to cognitive disorders (e.g. aphasia or dyslexia), sensory disorders (blindness or hearing loss) or voice and speech disorders (e.g. dysarthria, stuttering, dysphonia). Speech and language technology also applies to the needs of patients with communication problems in a broader sense. That is, constraints in the interaction with their environment as a result of motor system disorders such as Repetitive Strain Injury (RSI) or movement disorders such as paralysis after stroke or distorted arm movement coordination due to PD. Only recently, a report on needs and future possibilities for speech and language technologies for patients with communicative problems appeared (Ruiter et al., 2010).

Applications of speech and language technology are expected to contribute to more efficient and more effective health care. Patients can stay longer in their home environment without putting demands on health care givers and, hence, on financial resources. For example, patients with PD could benefit from speech synthesis applications for text-to-speech conversions, facilitating patients with severely diminished speech intelligibility in their verbal communication. Automatic error detection could provide parkinsonian patients who are eager to practice their speech in their home environment using web applications such as EST, with automatic feedback on segmental speech quality (i.e. articulation of speech sounds). An ASR application in dysarthric speech for example would lie in the field of domotica. PD patients with severe motor constraints could gain considerable independence from remotely (i.e. speech) controlled domestic equipment.

In general, speech synthesis, as applied in text-to speech conversions, is usually relatively simple and is not dependent on features of pathological speech. Automatic speech recognition (ASR) and automatic error detection of pathological speech however, are complex issues in the field of speech technology. This is primarily due to the large variability within and between pathological speakers, in particular in the case of neurogenic speech disorders such as dysarthria. Hence, large amounts of data are required for the development of ASR and automatic error detection in pathological (i.e. dysarthric speech). Applications of automatic error detections concern for instance feedback on segmental speech quality in EST, in addition to feedback on loudness and overall pitch. This would enhance patients' independent web based speech training.

Obviously, apart from research in the field of speech technology, an automatically generated data base of pathological speech, is an essential source for additional fundamental research into acoustical features of parkinsonian dysarthria for instance. Outcomes of acoustical studies might even lead to adjustments of speech training programs for patients with PD.

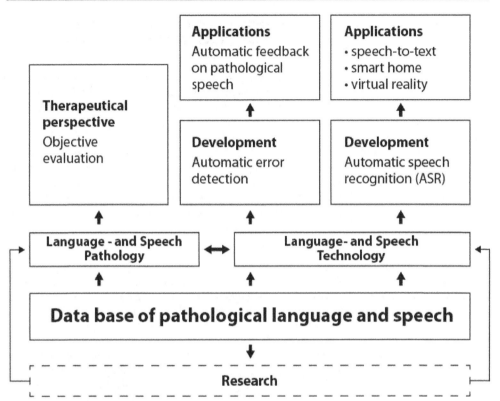

Fig. 6. A data base of pathological speech as a vital source for clinical outcome research and speech and language technological research.

A data base of pathological speech should contain speech at various linguistic levels. Audio recordings stored at the data base should be adequately annotated. That is, identification of standardized speech tasks, orthographic and phonetic annotation and linguistic level should be well documented. In addition, anonymous speaker identification should be ensured. An adequately structured data base should facilitate researchers' search for audio files of pathological speech. In Belgium, the Corpus of Pathological and Normal Speech (COPAS) (Middag et al., 2010) has been collected. Researchers employ the COPAS data base for the development of an automated intelligibility assessment, based on phonological features. These phonological features refer to articulatory dimensions. This information should reveal underlying articulation problems in dysarthric speakers. The Nemours Data Base of Dysarthric Speech is another example of a corpus of pathological speech (Menendez-Pidal et al., 1996). It should be noticed however that the COPAS and the Nemours data bases were not generated by a web based system, whereas a data base generated by means of EST involves upload and storage of audio files by means of a telehealth application. Vital conditions must be met to ensure audio recordings with adequate quality for perceptual and acoustical assessment. Obviously, a data base of pathological speech is language specific. Cross-language comparisons however should be enabled by similar structures of speech data bases for different languages.

5. Research areas with respect to the development, implementation and evaluation of telehealth applications for speech training of patients with Parkinson's disease

Telerehabilitation has a potential in a large number of fields. We are still in the first phase of a development which may revolutionize medical care and cure. The heterogeneous applications – be they in psychiatry, asthma or diabetes care, speech and language therapy – share a number of factors which have to be fulfilled in order to warrant success, but which are not always met yet. A dangerous aspect of the phase we are in now is that we focus on technology and just admire its realized or promised possibilities. Thus we might overlook the key human factors for telerehabilitation applications in general as reviewed by Brennan and Barker (2008). In this section we give an overview of the four research areas formulated by the American Telemedicine Association (Krupinsky et al., 2007), and will zoom in on those aspects which are relevant for telehealth applications for people with Parkinson's disease.

a) Attention should be paid to definition of infrastructure and integration of various infrastructural components of web based devices

Of course, the definition of infrastructure and the integration of various infrastructural components of web based devices is a prerequisite for the application and evaluation of results obtained with web based devices (see section 3.3), but the central component of the applications in our field remains the availability of robust speech recognition and/or error detection systems, if at least providing automatic feedback on realized utterances in speech training is (one of) the goal(s) of the web-application. Both speech and language pathology and speech and language technology are language bound. That is, they share underlying principles (HMMs, for instance, are used for very diverse languages like Chinese, English or Russian), and pathological reduction of vowels, consonants and pitch excursions occur in all languages, but the details of the technologies have to be developed for every specific language and the phenomena associated with speech pathology of specific languages have to be studied. In this context much attention has to be paid to the form of feedback, as was already pointed out in section 4.4.

Speech disorders and the associated symptoms may show considerable variability between and within speakers. While intensive training may help some patients to partially recover and improve their speech skills, other patients will show no improvement or perhaps even deterioration. Therefore, novel speech recognition and natural language processing techniques will have be developed that can cope with the dynamics of the speech disorder.

b) Clinical utility of telehealth should be established

The establishment of the clinical utility of a telehealth application for speech therapy of patients with PD is not a simple one. The first prerequisite is the presence of a robust infrastructure and a robust feedback system. While students using a feedback system on the quality of their pronunciation of a second language may be "robust" themselves, we cannot assume the same extent of robustness in patients with PD. That is why a very small number of studies have been conducted on the clinical utility of eHealth applications in our field. In order to test the clinical utility in phase III or phase IV studies, quite a number of conditions have to be fulfilled:

- A clear definition of the effect one wants to attain with the application. There are different possible and/or positive effects: (1) after a pre-specified time interval the speech quality of the telehealth group has improved more than that of the control group, (2) after the time interval the speech quality of the telehealth group was more stable than that of the control group, (3) in the long run, maintenance of achieved results is made possible by the telehealth application. Each of these possible outcomes has to be crossed with outcomes regarding the cost-effectiveness of the treatment (see under d) and user satisfaction.

- Relatively large numbers of patients are needed in order to ensure sufficient power to detect possible differences between a treatment and a control group. In light of the heterogeneity of the patients with respect to a large number of relevant background variables (age, SES, cognitive and motor skills, hearing and vision, computer skills, mobility, home situation), matching on these variables is a crucial issue in the effect studies to be carried out. As it is not very simple to include large numbers of patients, it is difficult to obtain a complete overview of the importance of these variables (see under c).

- An important aspect of effect studies is a clear definition of the outcome variables to be used. For telehealth applications for patients with Parkinson's disease we mention five variables which are directly related to speech dimensions:
  - Articulatory precision
  - Intelligibility
  - Naturalness of speech
  - Speech effort
  - Listening comfort

Much research is needed to find generally accepted operationalizations of the above-mentioned variables. Reviewing the relevant international journals in this domain makes clear that research is still going on, and that final results are not in view. This is in contrast to related questions on the intelligibility and naturalness of synthesized speech, where researchers agreed on a number of well-documented protocols to assess these aspects of computer speech (see the Blizzard Challenge, a yearly competition among speech synthesis systems based on corpora, see http://www.cs.cmu.edu/~awb/). For a review of problems encountered in subjective methods to assess intelligibility we refer to Beijer, Clapham & Rietveld (submitted) and Hustad (2006).

Even if the correct operationalizations are available, a number of other questions have to be answered before ecologically valid effectiveness studies can be carried out. Here are two examples of the questions still to be answered: (1) Articulatory precision can be achieved at the cost of naturalness ("speak loud", the message of the Lee-Silverman therapy): what is more important: articulatory precision or naturalness? (2) Intelligibility is obviulsy related to articulatory precision, but to what extent can outcomes of current intelligibility tests and tests of articulatory precision be generalized to daily life?

c) Human and ergonomic factors should be taken into account in research activities.

At first sight the condition under c) is stating the obvious; however, enthusiasm for technology might obscure the importance of these factors. It is well known that diseases like PD may come with other problems: comorbidity is not uncommon (Lowit et al., 2005). The problems may be such that a telehealth application is not suitable for a patient, neither in daily practice, nor in a research setting. For a research setting which aims at finding evidence for the effectiveness of an application itself – out of the social/psychological context - the problem may be that some of the participants are not suited to fully appreciate the application. There are a multitude of possible reasons for this; we mention impaired auditory processing and impaired vision as possible and obvious obstacles to the use of a telehealth application. In section 3.3 we describe an Auditory Discrimination Test on a number of speech dimensions (Beijer, Rietveld, & van Stiphout, in press) to assess participants' suitability to use auditory feedback.

There are also less obvious factors which should be taken into account, and which are often also region-determined. In densely populated areas like the Netherlands, with short distances, a patient has the choice to opt for face-to-face sessions or to stay at home with an eHealth application. A number of aspects may influence the choice: (1) finances – in the Dutch context hardly ever a factor for a patient, as even taxi expenses will often be reimbursed, (2) the wish to see other people at a regular basis; this opportunity is provided by face-to-face sessions and not by a telehealth application, (3) mobility; some people are home-bound, while others may be mobile, (4) the need to be intelligible for people others than direct partners.

d) Economic analysis should point out whether the balance of costs and benefits is beneficial to the actual economic and social situation.

This research area becomes an important one against the background of an ageing population and limited financial resources. A prerequisite for cost-effectiveness studies is the availability of effectiveness measures accepted by the community of speech and language pathologists and therapists. The question how to decide whether a number of beneficial units of web based speech therapy (less effort for a listener, less repetitions needed to achieve complete understanding, less absence from home, less transport, better maintenance of communication etc.) are in a positive trade-off relation with additional costs (implementation and maintenance of infrastructure, availability of a help-desk etc.) is a matter of politics and society.

6. Conclusion

Employment of telehealth devices for dysarthric patients with PD seems promising with respect to their possibilities to practice their speech independently. As such, they might provide a solution for the foreseen imbalance between the need (and call) for speech training on the one hand, and the reduced availability of therapeutical resources on the other hand. Although technological feasibility of various web based training devices has been established, user requirements for parkinsonian patients with frequently observed deficits in cognitive and motor functioning demand further adjustments. Apart from therapeutical goals, web based training devices such as EST provide the possibility of generating a data base of pathological speech. This data base not only provides required information for clinical outcome research. It is also of vital importance for the development of automatic speech recognition and automatic error detection of pathological (i.e. parkinsonian) speech.

7. Acknowledgement

The authors wish to thank Dike Ottoy for her corrections of the English text and Gaetano Ambrosino for his assistance with the illustrations.

8. References

Ackermann, H. & Ziegler, W. (1991). Articulatory deficits in parkinsonian dysarthria: an acoustic analysis. *Journal of Neurology, Neurosurgery & Neuropsychiatry*, 54 (12), pp. 1093-1098, ISSN 00223050.

American Telemedicine Association. http://atmeda.org/news/definition.html. Last accessed 20.2.2011.

Beijer, L.J., Clapham, R.P., & Rietveld, A.C.M. 'Evaluating the suitability of orthographic transcription and intelligibility scale rating of semantically unpredictable sentences (SUS) for speech training efficacy research in dysarthric speakers with Parkinson's disease.' *Journal of Medical Speech-Language Pathology* (Accepted for publication, November 2011).

Beijer, L., Rietveld, T., van Beers, M, Slangen, R., van den Heuvel, H., de Swart, B. & Geurts, S. (2010a). E-learning based Speech Therapy (EST) as a web application for speech training. *Telemedicine and e-Health*, 16(2), pp. 177-180, ISSN 1530-5627.

Beijer, L., Rietveld, T., Hoskam, V., Geurts, A. & de Swart, B. (2010b). Evaluating the feasibility and the potential efficacy of e-Learning-Based Speech Therapy for speech training in dysarthric patients with Parkinson's disease: a case study. *Telemedicine and e-Health*, 16(6), pp. 732-738, ISSN 1530-5627.

Beijer. L., Rietveld, A. & van Stiphout, A. (in press). Auditory discrimination for E-learning based Speech Therapy: a proposal for an Auditory Discrimination Test (ADT) for adult dysarthric speakers. *Journal of Communication Disorders*, ISSN 0021-9924.

Blizzard Challenge: http://www.cs.cmu.edu/~awb/).

Boersma, P. & Weenink, D. (2011). *Praat: Doing Phonetics by Computer*. www.praat.org. Downloaded 8.3.2011.

Brennan, D.M. & Barker, L.M. (2008). Human factors in de the development and implementation of telerehabilitation systems. *Journal of Telemedicine and Telecare*,14, pp. 55-58, ISSN 1758-1109.

Carmichael, J.N. (2007) *Introducing Objective Acoustic Metrics for the Frenchay Dysarthria Assessment Procedure*, Unpublished PhD-thesis, University of Sheffield.

Cucchiarini, C., Neri, A., Strik, H. (2009). Oral Proficiency Training in Dutch L2: the Contribution of ASR-based Corrective Feedback. *Speech Communication*, 51(10), pp. 853-863, ISSN 0167-6393.

Davis, S. & Mermelstein, P. (1980). Comparison of parametric representations for monosyllabic word recognition in continuously spoken sentences. *IEEE Transactions on Acoustics, Speech, and Signal Processing*, 28, pp. 357-366, ISSN 0096-3518.

Darly, F.L., Aronson, A.E., & Brown, J.R. (1969). Differential diagnostic patterns of dysarthria. *Journal of Speech and Hearing Research*, 12, pp. 246-269, ISSN 1092-4388.

Deane, K.H.O., Whurr, R., Playford, E.D., Ben-Shlomo, Y., Clarke, C.E. (2001). Speech and language therapy versus placebo or no intervention for dysarthria in Parkinson's disease. Cochrane *Database of Systematic Reviews*, Issue 2. Art. No.: CD002814, ISSN 1469-493x.

Duffy, J.R. (1995). *Motor Speech Disorders: Substrates, Differential Diagnosis and Management*. Mosby-Year Book, ISBN 0801669448, St. Louis.

Enderby, P. (1980). Frenchay Dysarthria Assessment, *British Journal of Disorders of Communication*, 21, pp.165-173, ISSN 0007-098x.

Ferrand, C. & Bloom, R. (1997). *Introduction to Organic and Neurogenic Disorders of Communication*. Allyn and Bacon, ISBN10: 0205168671, Needham Heights, MA.

Ho, A.K., Bradshaw, J.L. & Iansek, R. (2000).Volume perception in parkinsonian speech. *Movement Disorders* 15 (6), pp. 1125-1131, ISSN 1531-8257.

Hustad, K.C. (2006). Estimating the intelligibility of speakers with dysarthria. *Folia Phoniatrica et Loopaedica*, 58, pp. 217-228, ISSN 1021-7762.

Kalf, J.G., de Swart, B.J.M., Zwarts, M.J., Munneke, M., Bloem, B.R. (2008a). Frequency of oral motor impairments in Parkinson's disease and implications for referral to speech therapists. *Movement Disorders*; 23:S328, ISSN 1531-8257.

Kalf, J.G., de Swart, B.J.M., Bloem, B.R., Munneke, M. Guidelines for speech-language therapy in Parkinson's disease (2008b). *Movement Disorders*; 23:S328, ISSN 1531-8257.

Kent, R.D., Weismer, G., Kent, J.F., Vorperian, H.K. & Duffy, J.R. (1999). Acoustic studies of dysarthric speech: methods, progress, and potential. *Journal of Communication Disorders*, 32, pp. 141-186, ISSN 0021-9924.

Krupinsky, E, Dimmick, S., Grigsby, J., Mogel, G., Puskin, D., Speedie, S., Stamm, B., Wakefield, B., Whited, J., Whitten, P., Yellowlees, P. Research recommendations for the American Telemedicine Association. *Telemedicine and e-Health*, 12(5), pp. 579-589, ISSN 1530-5627.

Kwakkel, G., Wagenaar, R.C., Twisk, J.W.R., Lankhorst G.J., Koetsier, J.C. (1999). Intensity of leg- and arm-training after primary middle-cerebral- artery stroke. Lancet, 354 (9174), pp.191-196, ISSN 0140-6736.

Lowit, A., Howell, P. & Brendel, B. (2005). Cognitive impairment in Parkinson's disease. Is it a unfied phenomenon? *Journal of Brain Impairment*, 6 (3), pp. 191-204, ISSN 1443-9646.

Mashima, P. & Doarn, C. (2008). Overview of telehealth activities in speech-language pathology. *Telemedicine and e-Health*, 14, pp. 1101-1109, ISSN 1530-5627.

Menéndez-Pidal, X., Polikoff, J.B., Peters, S.M., Leonzio, J.E. & Bunnell, H.T. (1996). The Nemours Database of Dysarthric Speech. *Proceedings of the Fourth International Conference on Spoken Language Processing*. Philadelphia, PA, USA.

Middag, C., Saeys, Y. & Maryens, J-P. (2010). Towards an ASR-free objective analysis of pathological speech. *Proceedings Interspeech 2010, Makuhari, Japan*, pp. 294-297 ISSN 1990-9772.

Neri, A., Cucchiarini, C. & Strik, H. (2006). Selecting segmental errors in L2 Dutch for optimal pronunciation training. *International Review of Applied Linguistics in Language Teaching*, 44, pp.357-404, ISSN 1613-4141.

Olive, J.P., Greenwood, A. & Coleman, J. (1993). *Acoustics of American English Speech: A Dynamic Approach*. Springer Verlag, ISBN 0-387-97984, New York.

Preston, J.L., Ramsdell, H.L., Oller, D.K, Edwards, M.L. & Tobin, S.J. (2011). Developing a Weighted Measure of Speech Sound Accuracy. *Journal of Speech, Language, and Hearing Research*, 54, pp.1-18, ISSN 1558-9102.

Ramig, L.O., Sapir, S. Countryman, S., Pawlas, A.A., O'Brien, C., Hoehn, M. & Thompson, L.L. (2001). Intensive voice treatment (LSVT) for patients with Parkinson's disease:

a 2 year follow up. *Journal of Neurology Neurosurgery and Psychiatry*, 71, pp. 493-498, ISSN 00223050.

Rietveld, T. & Stoltenberg, I. (2005). *Taal- en spraaktechnologie en communicatieve beperkingen*. ('Language and speech technology for people with communication disorders', in Dutch). Dutch Language Union, ISBN-13: 9789070593063, The Hague.

Rietveld, T. & van Heuven, V.J. (2009). *Algemene Fonetiek ('General Phonetics', in Dutch)*, 3rd edition. Coutinho, ISBN 978 90 469 0163 2, Bussum.

Rijntjes M, Haevernick K, Barzel A, van den Bussche H, Ketels G, Weiller C.(2009). Repeat therapy for chronic motor stroke: a pilot study for feasibility and efficacy. *Neurorehabilitation & Neural Repair*. 23(3), pp. 275-80, ISSN 0888-4390.

Ruiter, M.B., Rietveld, Toni C.M., Cucchiarini, C., Krahmer, E.J. & Strik, H. (2010). Human Language Technology and Communicative Disabilities: Requirements and Possibilities for the Future in Dutch. *Proceedings Seventh International Conference of Language Resources and Evaluation* (LREC), pp. 2839-2846, ELRA: ISBN 2-9517408-6-7, Malta.

Sadakata, M., Hoppe, D., Brandmeyer, A., Timmers, R. & Desain, P. (2008). Real-Time Visual Feedback for Learning to Perform Short Rhytms with Variations in Timing and Loudness. *Journal of New Music Research*, 37, pp. 207-220, ISSN 1744-5027.

Sanders, E., Ruiter, M., Beijer, L. & Strik, H. (2002). Automatic recognition of Dutch dysarthric speech: A pilot study. *Proceedings of ICSLP-2002*, Denver, USA, pp. 661-664.

Slawek, J., Derejko, M., Lass, P. (2005). Factors affecting the quality of life of patients with idiopathic Parkinson's disease – a cross-sectional study in an outpatient clinic attendees. *Parkinsonism & Related Disorders*, 11 (7), pp. 465-468, ISSN 1353-8020.

Sood, S., Mbarika V., Jugoo, S., Dookhy, R., Doarn, C.R., Prakash, N., Merrell, R.C. (2007). What is telemedicine? A collection 104 peer-reviewed perspectives and theoretical underpinnings. *Telemedicine and e-Health*,13 (5), pp. 573-590, ISSN 1530-5627.

Strik, H., Truong, K., de Wet, F., Cucchiarini, C. (2009). Comparing different approaches for automatic pronunciation error detection. *Speech Communication*, Volume 51, Issue 10, October 2009, pp. 845-852, ISSN 0167-6393.

Swart, B.J.M. de, Willemse, S.C., Maassen, B.A.M. & Horstink, M.W.I.M.   (2003). Improvement of voicing in patients with Parkinson's disease by speech therapy. *Neurology*, 60, pp. 498-500, ISSN 0028-3878.

Streifler, M. & Hofman, S. (1984). Disorders of verbal expression in parkinsonism. *Advances in Neurology*, 40, pp. 385, ISSN 0091-3952.

Teasell, R.W. & Kalra, L. (2004). Advances in stroke 2003. What's new in stroke rehabilitation? *Stroke*, February, pp. 383-385, ISSN 1524-4628.

Von Campenhausen, S., Bornschein, B., Wick, R., Botzel, K., Sampaio, C., Poewe, C., et al. (2005). Prevalence and incidence of Parkinson's disease in Europe. *European Neuropsychopharmacology*, 15(4), pp. 473-490, ISSN 0924-977x.

Theodoros, D.G., Constantinescu, G., Russell, T.G., Ward, E.C., Wilson, S.J.& Wootton, R.(2006). Treatin the speech disorder in Parkinson's disease online. *Journal of Telemedicine and Telecare*, 12: S3, pp. 99-91, ISSN 1758-1109.

Tulu, B. Chatterjee, S. and Maheshwari, M. (2007). Telemedicine Taxonomy: a classification
    tool. *Telemedicine and e-Health*, 13 (3), pp.349-358, ISSN 1530-5627.
Ziegler, W. (2003). Speech motor control is task-specific: Evidence from dysarthria and
    apraxia of speech. *Aphasiology*, 17 (1), pp. 3-36, ISSN 1464-5041.
Ziegler, W. & Zierdt , A. (2008). Telediagnostic assessment of intelligibility in dysarthria: A
    Pilot investigation of MVP-online. *Journal of Communication Disorders*, 41(6), pp. 553-
    577, ISSN 0021-9924.

7

Rehabilitation Versus no Intervention – Only a Continued Intensive Program Conducted Statistically Significant Improvements Motor Skills in Parkinson's Disease Patients

Jesús Seco Calvo and Inés Gago Fernández
University of León,
Spain

1. Introduction

Parkinson's disease (PD) is a degenerative disease characterised by movement disorder, which consists of bradykinesia (movement slowness), hypokinesia (reduced movement), tremor, rigidity and alterations in gait and posture; mood changes also constitute a main component of PD (Marsden, 1994), which is also related to postural instability and often to cognitive deficits (Carne, et al., 2005). Working memory —which is defined as the capacity to maintain, supervise and use inner information for behavioural self-control— is an essential cognitive skill which works as base for other more complex and executive functions affected by PD (Baddeley, 1992). Since 1987, the Parkinson Study Group has undertaken a series of random controlled tests. In these studies, researchers used standardized clinical scales to examine the impact of pharmaceutical interventions on the progression of PD symptoms (Carne, et al., 2005). Other authors (Hiroyuki, et al. 2003) have studied modifications in balance, demonstrating that balance exercises lead to improvement in the function of static balance and that gait exercises improve dynamic balance and wandering functions in fragile or dependent elderly patients(Hiroyuki, et al. 2003). Quantitative reduction of muscular strength in the back, hips, ankles, with damage in propioception —visual sense and the lowest support base— are the main cause of instability in patients with Parkinson's disease. Motor complications caused by the disease have an important effect on physical and functional capacity.

Regarding gait, Herman et al., (Herman, et al. 2007), have evaluated the effects of 6 weeks of treadmill exercises, which allow rhythmic training of gait, functional mobility and quality of life in PD patients; the results obtained show the exercises' potential to improve gait rhythmically in PD patients and suggest that a progressive and intensive training program in treadmill may be used to reduce gait alterations and falling risk, and increase the quality of life of such patients[5]. In this sense, some authors (Brichelto, et al. 2006) showed potential short-term effectiveness of gait-slowness training in PD patients. Positive results were documented by clinic position scales and gait objective evaluation. Quick loss of clinical advantage suggests that further researches are necessary for a more precise definition of optimum frequency and treatment duration (Brichelto, et al. 2006). In order to reduce bradykinesia, the combination of motor imagery and real practice of motor movement might turn out to be efficient in PD treatment. Putting into practice such treatment regime allows improving quality of life involving non-significant risks and low cost (Tamir & Huberman, 2007). Several standard guidelines as well as interdisciplinary measures have been established with the purpose of achieving overall improvement of personal wellbeing, such as physical exercise, occupational and speech therapies, and psychological, food and social guidance, obtaining encouraging results (Quality Standars Subcommitte, American Academy of Neurology, 1993; Köler, et al., 1994). According to observations, occupational and behavioural therapies based on psychological and motivational aspects might induce improvements in movement initiation and quality (Muller, et al., 1997). Treatment by functional recovery or physiotherapy has already shown its effectiveness in PD patients (Comella, et al., 1994; Formisano, et al., 1992; Franklyn, et al., 1981; Gibberd, et al., 1981; Pederson, et al., 1990), although such evidence is questioned in several reports (Ellgring, et al., 1990). Physical therapy generally works as reinforcement for the motor program, but such kind of intervention generally lacks of motivational and emotional spheres which might explain why physiotherapy traditionally achieves little influence on mood condition and is not easily incorporated into the patient's way of life (Ellgring, et al., 1990). On the other hand, it is also well-known that psychosocial variables such as emotional or psychosocial tension have a strong influence on gait and postural anomalies, as well as on other motor functions (Carne, et al., 2005; O'Shea, et al., 2002). '

In order to quantify improvement in patient's motor condition and be able to show variations in his/her quality of life, the use of the Unified Parkinson's Disease Rating Scale (UPDRS) has prevailed (Movement Disorder Society Task Force on Ratio Scales for Parkinson's Disease, 2003). Pellecchia et al. (Pellecchia, et al., 2004) observed that —after a physiotherapy protocol— a significant improvement of UPDRS scoring took place in the section of daily-life activities and the motor section, but also in the Self-rating Scale for PD Incapacity, the 10-metre walking test and Zung Self-rating Depression Scale; after three months such clinic improvements were maintained to a great extent (Pellecchia, et al., 2004). In the same way, Ellis et al. (Ellis, et al., 2005) found out that total scoring within the mental and motor sections was not much different among different groups and that significant differences were only found three months after treatment in the UPDRS section devoted to daily-life activities and its total scoring (Ellis, et al., 2005), observing that PD patients obtain short-term benefits from physiotherapeutic group treatment and long-term advantages in UPDRS total scoring, although significant variations were found among different groups(Ellis, et al., 2005). Therefore, it seems to be evident that sustained improvement in motor skills can be achieved in PD patients through a physiotherapy program within a reasonable long term time-period (Pellecchia, et al., 2004; Ellis, et al., 2005).

Therefore, the aim of the present study is to demonstrate the effectiveness of a physiotherapy protocol in PD patients, quantified in terms of improvement in UPDRS scoring within its motor subscale.

2. Material and methods

2.1 Sample

27 PD patients (12 females and 15 males), members of the PD Patient Association from Astorga and its Region (Spain), of 69.50± 10.34 years of age —ranging from 55 to 80 years of age— and with an average number of disease evolution years of 11.39±1.614, ranging from 10 to 15 evolution years.

All subjects met the following inclusion criteria: Stable reaction to anti-Parkinson medication; Hoehn and Yahr stage I, II or III; At least one mobility-related activity limitation within the core areas of physiotherapy practice in PD (gait, balance and posture); No severe cognitive impairment, defined by Mini-Mental State Examination, score ≥24; No other severe neurologic, cardiopulmonary, or orthopedic disorders and not having participated in a physical therapy or rehabilitation program in the previous 4 month.

We divided our patient into two groups: control group (n=9, received only medication therapy) and experimental group (n=18, received physical therapy and medication therapy).

2.2 Kind of study

Descriptive study which consists of analysis —within the particular context of a PD association— of the relation between physiotherapeutic treatment and scoring obtained through motor examination in UPDRS scale; and Transversal study, since two measurements are carried out within two particular time periods (beginning and end of physiotherapeutic treatment).

2.3 Method

Qualitative: carried out on a reduced population (n=27), analysing physiotherapeutic strategy; and Quantitative: analysis of data obtained through motor examination in UPDRS scale.

2.4 Data collection process

We interview each patient and one of his/her relatives, who were provided with a complete description of the project. Through the following weeks we undertook data collection of the study variables composing the section of motor examination in the UPDRS scale (O´Shea, et al., 2002; Movement Disorder Society Task Force On Ratio Scales For Parkinson´s Disease, 2003) with each patient in both on and off phases. The physical therapist involved in conducting UPDRS was not involved in performing the intervention. All subjects were required to take their medications at the same time of day for all assesment sessions. All subjects usage: L-dopa, dopamine –agonist and amantadine. It should be pointed out that — during study development— we decided to carry out greater incidence on physical work focused on the variables of neck rigidity, posture, postural stability and gait in each patient; as a consequence of such approach, we analyse —apart from results of global scoring in motor examination in UPDRS scale— the results of these four variables.

2.5 Intervention protocol

For the application of the study, we undertook a program of physiotherapeutic treatment according to protocol (Ellis, et al., 2005; Keus, et al., 2007; Morris, 2000; Scandalis, et al., 2001), in which all patients in the sample received physiotherapy group sessions.

The group sessions took 90 minutes. All treatment sessions occurred at the same time of the day throughout the study. The physiotherapist involved in performing the intervention was not involved in conducting UPDRS scale.

The treatment consisted of cardiovascular warm-up activities (5min), stretching exercises (15min), strengthening exercises in a functional context (15min), functional training (15min), gait training overground and on a treadmill with external auditory cueing (15min), balance training and recreational games (15min), and relaxation exercise (10min).

According to the frequency of attendance to such sessions, we divided our experimental group (n=18) into four different subgroups: Subgroup 1 (from 1 to 3 monthly sessions), Subgroup 2 (from 4 to 6 monthly sessions), Subgroup 3 (from 7 to 9 monthly sessions) and Subgroup 4 (from 10 to 12 monthly sessions); each group will obtain different scores in motor examination, as it will be demonstrated in the section corresponding to result analysis.

We also undertook program revision after 32 weeks, in that the physical therapist entrusted to gather to the beginning of the study the punctuations in the subscale engine of the scale UPDRS with every subject of the study so much in the stadium on as (like) in the off, returns to gather the corresponding punctuation in identical conditions to those of the beginning of the study (at the same hour in two interviews). All the subjects finished the study, so much those of the group control as those of the experimental group.

2.6 Statistical analysis

These study design was a Prospective, Randomized, Placebo-Controlled, Double-Blinded Study. For data analysis we use statistical software SPSS® in its 16.0 version.

We calculate measures for central trend (mean, median, mode, standard deviation, minimum and maximum value); we use Student's t-test to analyse the existing relation among the four study variables. Significance level was fixed with $p<0.05$ and $p<0.01$, with a confidence interval of 95% and 99%, respectively.

3. Results

3.1 Experimental group

Regarding measures of central trend of global scoring obtained in the section of motor examination in the UPDRS scale achieved in pre- and post-intervention stages, it is obtained in the on phase that the value of the mean comes from 64.22 ±16.383 before physiotherapeutic intervention to 50.89±19.499 after intervention; in the off phase the value of such mean comes from 85.78±12.549 to 75.78±17.745.

If one compares data obtained in the pre- and post-intervention stages, apart from the decrease in global average scoring, it is also obtained a decrease in the values of the means of the central trend in variables of neck rigidity, posture, postural stability and gait (Table1).

In the neck-stiffness variable, it is where greatest difference among mean values of pre- and post-intervention are obtained, for both on (from 3.33 to 2.11) and off (from 3.72 to 2.94) phases.

The Table2 shows study-variable changes in the different modalities in on phase; by comparing data (expressed in percentages) obtained in pre- and post-intervention stages, it can be pointed out: a decrease in normal-posture modality from 0% to 11.1%;an increase postural stability (recovered without help) from 11.1% to 50% and a decrease in severe-gait-condition modality from 38% to 22.2%.

Table 3 shows study-variable changes in different modalities in off phase; by comparing data (expressed in percentages) obtained in pre- and post-intervention stages, it can be pointed out: a decrease of severe-rigidity modality from 72.2 % to 27.8 %; a variation in slight-rigidity modality or only in neck activity from 0% to 11.1% after physiotherapeutic intervention; a decrease in postural stability (unable to stand) from 38.9% to 22.2% and a decrease in severe-gait-condition modality from 55.6% to 16.7%.

	Valid N	Missing N	Mean	Median	Mode	Standard deviation	Min.	Max.
PHASE ON								
Pre-intervention								
Neck rigidity	18	0	3,33	3,00	3	,594	2	4
Posture	18	0	2,33	2,50	3	,907	1	4
Postural stabillity	18	0	2,33	2,00	2	,686	1	3
Gait	18	0	2,33	2,00	2	,840	1	4
Post-intervention								
Neck rigidity	18	0	2,11	2,00	2	,900	1	4
Posture	18	0	1,89	2,00	2	1,231	0	4
Postural stabillity	18	0	1,50	1,00	1	,985	0	3
Gait	18	0	1,94	2,00	2	,938	0	3
PHASE OFF								
Pre-intervention								
Neck rigidity	18	0	3,72	4,00	4	,461	3	4
Posture	18	0	3,11	3,00	3	,676	2	4
Postural stabillity	18	0	3,22	3,00	3	,732	2	4
Gait	18	0	3,11	3,00	3	,676	2	4
Post-intervention								
Neck rigidity	18	0	2,94	3,00	3	,938	1	4
Posture	18	0	2,72	2,00	3	,958	1	4
Postural stabillity	18	0	2,56	3,00	2	,984	1	4
Gait	18	0	2,78	3,00	4	1,166	1	4

Table 1. Experimental group, measures of central trend in on and off stages in pre- and post-intervention stages.

			Fq	%	Valid %	Cumulative %
Neck rigidity pre-intervention.	Valid	mild/moderate.	1	5,6	5,6	5,6
		marked, but full range of motion easily achieved.	10	55,6	55,6	61,1
		severe.	7	38,9	38,9	100,0
		Total	18	100,0	100,0	

			Fq	%	Valid %	Cumulative %
Neck rigidity post-intervention.	Valid	slight or only with activation.	4	22,2	22,2	22,2
		mild/moderate.	7	38,9	38,9	61,1
		marked, but full range of motion easily achieved.	4	22,2	22,2	83,3
		severe.	3	16,7	16,7	100,0
		Total	18	100,0	100,0	
Posture pre-intervention.	Valid	slightly stooped posture.	4	22,2	22,2	22,2
		moderately stooped posture.	5	27,8	27,8	50,0
		severely stooped posture with kyphosis.	8	44,4	44,4	94,4
		marked flexion with extreme abnormality of posture.	1	5,6	5,6	100,0
		Total	18	100,0	100,0	
Posture post-intervention.	Valid	normal erect.	2	11,1	11,1	11,1
		slightly stooped posture.	5	27,8	27,8	38,9
		moderately stooped posture.	8	44,4	44,4	83,3
		severely stooped posture with kyphosis.	2	11,1	11,1	94,4
		marked flexion with extreme abnormality of posture.	1	5,6	5,6	100,0
		Total	18	100,0	100,0	
Postural stability pre-intervention.	Valid	recovers unaided.	2	11,1	11,1	11,1
		would fall if not caught by examiner.	8	44,4	44,4	55,6
		falls spontaneously.	8	44,4	44,4	100,0
		Total	18	100,0	100,0	
Postural stability post-intervention.	Valid	normal.	1	5,6	5,6	5,6
		recovers unaided.	9	50,0	50,0	55,6
		would fall if not caught by examiner.	4	22,2	22,2	77,8
		falls spontaneously.	2	11,1	11,1	88,9
		unable to stand.	2	11,1	11,1	100,0
		Total	18	100,0	100,0	
Gait pre-intervention.	Valid	walks slowly.	3	16,7	16,7	16,7
		walks with difficulty, but requires little or no assistance.	7	38,9	38,9	55,6
		severe disturbance of gait, requiring assistance.	7	38,9	38,9	94,4
		cannot walk.	1	5,6	5,6	100,0
		Total	18	100,0	100,0	
Gait post-intervention.	Valid	normal .	2	11,1	11,1	11,1
		walks slowly.	6	33,3	33,3	44,4
		walks with difficulty, but requires little or no assistance.	5	27,8	27,8	72,2
		severe disturbance of gait, requiring assistance.	4	22,2	22,2	94,4
		cannot walk.	1	5,6	5,6	100,0
		Total	**18**	**100,0**	**100,0**	

Table 2. Experimental group, modifications in scores of variables neck rigidity, posture, postural stability and gait in the *on* phase of the pre- and post-intervention stage.

			Fq	%	Valid %	Cumulative %
Neck rigidity pre-intervention	Valid	marked, but full range of motion easily achieved.	5	27,8	27,8	61,1
		severe.	13	72,2	72,2	100,0
		Total	18	100,0	100,0	
Neck rigidity post-intervention	Valid	slight or only with activation.	2	11,1	11,1	11,1
		mild/moderate.	2	11,1	11,1	22,2
		marked, but full range of motion easily achieved.	9	50	50	72,2
		severe.	5	27,8	27,8	100,0
		Total	18	100,0	100,0	
Posture pre-intervention	Valid	moderately stooped posture.	3	16,7	16,7	16,7
		severely stooped posture with kyphosis.	10	55,6	55,6	72,2
		marked flexion with extreme abnormality of posture.	5	27,8	27,8	100,0
		Total	18	100,0	100,0	
Posture post-intervention	Valid	slightly stooped posture.	2	11,1	11,1	11,1
		moderately stooped posture.	5	27,8	27,8	38,9
		severely stooped posture with kyphosis.	7	38,9	38,9	77,8
		marked flexion with extreme abnormality of posture.	4	22,2	22,2	100,0
		Total	18	100,0	100,0	
Postural stability pre-intervention	Valid	would fall if not caught by examiner.	3	16,7	16,7	11,1
		falls spontaneously.	8	44,4	44,4	61,1
		unable to stand.	7	38,9	38,9	100,0
		Total	18	100,0	100,0	
Postural stability post-intervention	Valid	recovers unaided.	2	11,1	11,1	11,1
		would fall if not caught by examiner.	9	44,4	44,4	55,6
		falls spontaneously.	4	22,2	22,2	77,8
		unable to stand.	2	22,2	22,2	100,0
		Total	18	100,0	100,0	
Gait pre-intervention	Valid	walks with difficulty, but requires little or no assistance.	3	16,7	16,7	16,7
		severe disturbance of gait, requiring assistance.	7	55,6	55,6	72,2
		cannot walk.	7	27,8	27,8	100,0
		Total	18	100,0	100,0	
Gait post-intervention	Valid	walks slowly.	3	16,7	16,7	16,7
		walks with difficulty, but requires little or no assistance.	5	27,8	27,8	44,4
		severe disturbance of gait, requiring assistance.	3	16,7	16,7	61,1
		cannot walk.	7	38,9	38,9	100
		total	18	100,0	100,0	

Table 3. Experimental group, modifications in scores of variables neck rigidity, posture, postural stability and gait in the *on* phase of the pre- and post-intervention stage.

Thus, as it can be observed in Tables 2 and 3, better results were obtained in on phases than in off phases after physiotherapeutic intervention.

According to attendance to group sessions, different results were obtained for the four study-variables:

The results obtained by applying Student's t-test with a $p<0.05$ significance level were: Subgroup 1: the difference among the four variables — in on phase and pre- and post-intervention stages— is not statistically significant ($p>0.05$) and t-test could not be calculated in the off phase since the standard error of the difference equals zero; Subgroup 2: the difference among the four variables in both on and off phases of the pre- and post-intervention stages is not statistically significant; Subgroup 3: in the on stage, the difference between stiffness in pre- and post-intervention stages is statistically significant ($p<0.05$), as well as the difference in posture between pre- and post-intervention stages. However, the difference regarding balance in pre- and post-intervention stages could not be calculated, since the standard error of the difference equals zero; regarding posture and gait in pre- and

	Mean	Standar desviation	Standard error of mean	95% confidence interval		t-value	Degrees of freedom	Critical level
				Min	Max			
PHASE ON								
Neck rigidity pre-intervention_ neck rigidity post-intervention.	1,875	,354	,125	1,579	2,171	15,000	7	,000
Posture pre-intervention_ posture post-intervention.	1,250	,463	,164	,863	1,637	7,638	7	,000
Retropulsion test pre-intervention_ retropulsion test post-intervention.	1,375	,518	,183	,942	1,808	7,514	7	,000
Gait pre-intervention_ gait post-intervention.	,875	,354	,125	,579	1,171	7,000	7	,000
PHASE OFF								
Neck rigidity pre-intervention_ neck rigidity post-intervention.	1,375	,744	,263	,753	1,997	5,227	7	,001
Posture pre-intervention_ posture post-intervention.	1,000	,535	,189	,553	1,447	5,292	7	,001
Retropulsion test pre-intervention_ retropulsion test post-intervention	1,500	,535	,189	1,053	1,947	7,937	7	,000
Gait pre-intervention_ gait post-intervention.	1,000	,535	,189	,553	1,447	5,292	7	,001

Table 4. Experimental group: Student's t-test fro Subgroup 4 in on and off phase between pre- and post-intervention stages with a 95 % confidence interval.

post-intervention stages, statistical difference is not significant. T-test could not be calculated for stiffness in the on phase since standard error of the difference equals zero; differences were not either significant in the other three variables; and Subgroup 4: the difference among the four variables in the on and off phases in pre- and post-intervention stages is statistically significant (Table 4).

The results obtained by applying Student's t-test with a p<0.01 significance level, were: Subgroups 1, 2 and 3: No statistically significant difference was obtained among the four study variables in on or off phases (p>0.01) and Subgroup 4: the difference among the four variables in on and off phases in pre- and post-intervention stages is statistically significant (Table 5 and Figure 2).

	Mean	Standar desviation	Standard error of mean	99% confidence interval		t-value	Degrees of freedom	Critical level
				Min.	Max.			
PHASE ON								
Neck rigidity pre-intervention_ neck rigidity post-intervention.	-,556	,527	,176	-1,145	,034	-3,162	8	,000
Posture pre-intervention_ posture post-intervention.	-,556	,726	,242	-1,368	,257	-2,294	8	,000
Retropulsion test pre-intervention_ retropulsion test post-intervention.	-,444	,726	,242	-1,257	,368	-1,835	8	,000
Gait pre-intervention_ gait post-intervention.	-,556	,527	,176	-1,145	,034	-3,162	8	,000
PHASE OFF								
Neck rigidity pre-intervention_ neck rigidity post-intervention.	-,556	,726	,242	-1,368	,257	-2,294	8	,001
Posture pre-intervention_ posture post-intervention.	-,444	,726	,242	-1,257	,368	-1,835	8	,001
Retropulsion test pre-intervention_ retropulsion test post-intervention	-,333	,707	,236	-1,124	,458	-1,414	8	,000
Gait pre-intervention_ gait post-intervention.	**-,444**	**,726**	**,242**	**-1,257**	**,368**	**-1,835**	**8**	**,001**

Table 5. Experimental group: Student's t-test fro Subgroup 4 in on and off phase between pre- and post-intervention stages with a 99 % confidence interval.

3.2 Control group

The results obtained by applying Student's t-test with a p<0.05 significance level were: the difference among the four variables —in on and off phases and pre- and post-intervention stages— is not statistically significant. The results obtained by applying Student's t-test with a p<0.01 significance level were: the difference among the four variables —in on and off phases and pre- and post-intervention stages— is not statistically significant (Table 6).

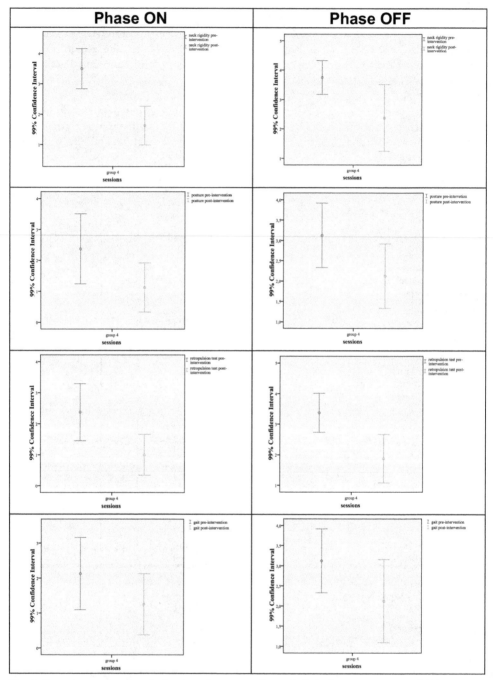

Fig. 1. Experimental group, Subgroup 4: mean values of clinical measurements (99% confidence Interval).

	Mean	Standar desviation	Standard error of mean	99% confidence interval		t-value	Degrees of freedom	Critical level
				Min.	Max.			
PHASE ON								
Neck rigidity pre-intervention_ neck rigidity post-intervention.	-,556	,527	,176	-,961	-,150	-3,162	8	**,013**
Posture pre-intervention_ posture post-intervention.	-,556	,726	,242	-1,114	,003	-2,294	8	**,051**
Retropulsion test pre-intervention_ retropulsion test post-intervention.	-,444	,726	,242	-1,003	,114	-1,835	8	**,104**
Gait pre-intervention_ gait post-intervention.	-,556	,527	,176	-,961	-,150	-3,162	8	**,013**
PHASE OFF								
Neck rigidity pre-intervention_ neck rigidity post-intervention.	-,556	,726	,242	-1,114	,003	-2,294	8	**,051**
Posture pre-intervention_ posture post-intervention.	-,444	,726	,242	-1,003	,114	-1,835	8	**,104**
Retropulsion test pre-intervention_ retropulsion test post-intervention	-,333	,707	,236	-,877	,210	-1,414	8	**,195**
Gait pre-intervention_ gait post-intervention.	**-,444**	**,726**	**,242**	**-1,257**	**,368**	**-1,835**	8	**,104**

Table 6. Student´s t-test fro control group in on and off phase between pre- and post-intervention stages with a 95% confidence interval

4. Discussion

As Morris et al. (Morris, 2000) state, there is a need to devise and evaluate locomotor training programs for both the on an off phases of the levodopa cycle. The effects of PD medications on movement and functional capacity should not be overlooked.

Following Jacobs et al. (Jacobs & Horak, 2006), greater validity and sensibility is achieved in balance valuation in PD patients by supplementing the retropulsion test of the UPDRS scale with the test on postural stability developed. Our work achieves global improvement in motor capacity in PD patients, as it is demonstrated by the decrease of average scores in motor examination and by significant modifications regarding the variables of neck rigidity, posture, postural stability and gait. Regarding the effectiveness of physiotherapy programs, we agree with De Goede et al. (De Goede, et al., 2001) and Ellis et al. (Ellis, et al., 2005), who demonstrate the benefits of a physiotherapy program supplementary to medical treatment; however, we have observed a significant increase in the improvement of the four variables studied in patients belonging to the Subgroup 4 of the present study.

It has been studied (Lun, et al., 2005) the effect of a self-supervised home exercise program and a therapist-supervised exercise program on motor symptoms in PD; Lun et al., (Lun, et al., 2005), −through an evaluator-blinded clinical trial− observed that (confidence intervals at 95 % were calculated for change in secondary results measures with an 8-week duration) a statistically significant decrease took place in the motor-examination section of UPDRS during those scarce 8 weeks in both treatment groups; no difference was found in the confidence interval at 95 % of secondary results measures (Lun, et al., 2005). Although patients in our work have followed the protocol under strict professional guidance (undertaken by the physiotherapist in charge of their treatment), it can be found in the bibliographical references that the validity of a self-supervised home exercise program is similar to that of a physiotherapist-supervised program regarding improvement of motor symptoms in PD patients (Lun, et al., 2005). Such finding is important for advising PD patients with regard to co-adjuvant treatment through exercise (movement) of DP motor symptoms.

Apart from traditional treatments, a series of supplementary methods are also applied, such as Qigong. Studies in such line by Schmitz-Hübsch et al., (Schmitz-Hübsch, et al., 2006) demonstrated −after 3, 6 and 12 months− that there were more patients whose symptoms improved in the Qigong group than in control group within a 3 and 6-month period (P = 0.0080 for 3 months and P = 0.0503 for 6 months; using the Fisher's exact test); depression scores diminished in both groups, while the incidence of non-motor symptoms only diminished in the treatment group (Schmitz-Hübsch, et al., 2006). Nallegowda et al. (Nallegowda, et al., 2004), showed that medication improves muscular strength, gait-speed and ankle optimization when gaiting, and did not observe worsening of the propioceptive sense. However, it was observed a correlation among muscle strength, static and dynamic balance, and gait in both on and off phases (Nallegowda, et al., 2004).

5. Conclusions

In short, quantitative reduction of muscle strength in back, hip and ankle −with damage to propioception and visual sense, and lower supporting base− are the main causes for postural instability in PD patients. We have observed in the present study that when increasing the number of sessions up to 7-12 (subgroups 3 and 4), scoring in motor subscale is higher, which indicates that neck rigidity, posture, postural stability and gait improve, and that such improvement is longer lasting; such fact is demonstrated establishing significance level at $p < 0.01$, for which subgroup 4 is the only group obtaining statistically significant improvements.

Definitively, since Jöbges et al., (Jöbges, et al., 2007) demonstrated the clinical relevance of rehabilitation programs for patients of PD is estimated to be sufficient if the following seven criteria are met: effectiveness, everyday life relevance, long-term effect, therapy frequency+setting, duration of therapy units, quality of live, timing of assessment+medication; for it, we conclude that the relevant of our work is to have demonstrated the long-term efficiency of a physiotherapy protocol in PD.

6. Acknowledgements

The authors would like to thank the members of the Association of PD Patients from Astorga and its Region (Spain) for their interest and collaboration, and of the physicians and physical therapists who participated in the study.

No sources of funding were used to assist in the preparation of this text. The authors have no conflicts of interest, that are directly relevant to the content of this text.

7. References

Baddeley, A. (1992). Working memory: the interface between memory and cognition. *Journal of Cognitive Neuroscience*, Vol.4, No.3, (Summer 1992), pp. 281–288, ISSN 898-929

Brichetto,G; Pelosin, E.; Marchese, R.& Abbruzzese, G. (2006). Evaluation of physical therapy in parkinsonian patients with freezing of gait: a pilot study. *Clinical Rehabilitation*, Vol.20, No.1, (January 2006), pp. 31–35, ISSN 02692155

Carne, W.; Cifu, DX.; Marcinko, P.; Baron, M; Pickett, T.; Qutubuddin, A.; Calabrese, V.; Roberge, P.; Holloway, K. & Mutchler, B.(2005) Efficacy of multidisciplinary treatment program on long-term outcomes of individuals with Parkinson's disease. *Journal of Rehabilitation Research and Development*, Vol.42, No.6, (November-December 2005), pp. 779–86, ISSN 0748-7711

Comella, JC.; Stebbins, GT.; Brown-Tomas, N. & Goetz, CG.(1994) Physical therapy and Parkinson's disease: a controlled clinical trial. *Neurology*, Vol.44, No.3, (March 1994), pp. 376–78, ISSN 0028-3878

De Goede, CJ.; Zeus, S.; Kwakkel, G. & Wagenaar, R. (2001). The effects of physical therapy in Parkinson's disease: a research synthesis. *Archives of Physical Medicine and Rehabilitation*, Vol.82, No.4, (April 2001), pp.509–15, ISSN 0003-9993

Ellgring, H.; Seiler, S.; Nagel, U.; Perleth, B.; Gassr, T. & Oertel, WH. (1990). Psychosocial problems of Parkinson patients: approaches to assessment and treatment. *Advances in Neurology*, Vol.53, (June 1990), pp. 349–353, ISSN 0091-3952

Ellis, T.; de Goede, CJ.; Feldman, RG.; Wolters, EC.; Kwakkel, G. & Wagenaar, RC. (2005). Efficacy of a physical therapy program in patients with Parkinson's disease: a randomized controlled trial. *Archives of Physical Medicine and Rehabilitation*, Vol.86, No.4, (April 2005), 2005, pp.626-632, ISSN 0003-9993

Formisano, R.; Pratesi, L.; Modarelli, F.; Bonifanti, V. & Meco, G. (1992). Rehabilitation and Parkinson's disease. *Scandinavian Journal of Rehabilitation Medicine*, Vol.24, No.3, (September 1992), pp. 157–160, ISSN 0036-5505

Franklyn, S.; Kohout, IJ.; Stern, GM. & Dunning, M. (1981). Physiotherapy in Parkinson's disease, In: *Research progress in Parkinson's disease*, Rose, FC. & Capildeo, R. (Ed.), pp. 397-400, Pitman Medical, ISBN 9780272796016, Kent, UK

Gibberd, FB.; Page, GR. & Spencer, KM. (1981). A controlled trial in physiotherapyfor Parkinson's disease, In: *Research progress in Parkinson's disease*, Rose, FC. & Capildeo, R. (Ed.), pp. 401-403, Pitman Medical, ISBN 9780272796016, Kent, UK

Goetz, CG.; Fahn, S.; Martínez-Martín, P.; Poewe, W.; Sampaio, C.; Stebbins, GT.; Stern, MB.; Tilley, BC.; Dodel, R.; Dubois, B.; Holloway, R.; Jankovic, J.; Kulisevsky, J.; Lang, AE.; Lees, A.; Leurgans, S.; Lewitt, PA.; Nyenhuis, D.; Olanow, CW.; Rascol, O.; Schrag, A.; Teresi, JA.; Van Hilten, JJ. & LaPelle, N. (2007). Movement Disorder Society-sponsored revision of the Unified Parkinson's Disease Rating Scale (MDS-UPDRS): Process, format, and clinimetric testing plan. *Movement Disorders*, Vol.22, No.1, (January 2007), pp. 41-47, ISSN 0885-3185

Herman, T.; Giladi, N.; Gruendlinger, L. & Hausdorff, JM. (2007). Six weeks of intensive treadmill training improves gait and quality of life in patients with Parkinson's disease: a pilot study. *Archives of Physical Medicine and Rehabilitation*, Vol. 88, No.9, (September 2007), pp. 1154-1158, ISSN 0003-9993

Hiroyuki, S.; Uchiyama, Y. & Kakurai, S. (2003). Specific effects of balance and gait exercises on physical function among the frail elderly. *Clinical Rehabilitation*, Vol.17, No.5. (August 2003), pp. 472–479, ISSN: 02692155

Jacobs, JV. & Horak, FB. (2006). An alternative clinical postural stability test for patients with Parkinson's disease. *Journal of Neurology*, Vol.253, No.11, (November 2006), pp. 1404-1413, ISSN: 0340-5354

Jöbges, E.; Spittler-Schneiders, H.; Renner, C. & Hummelsheim, H. (2007). Clinical relevance of rehabilitation programs for patients with idiopathic Parkinson syndrome. II: symptom-specific therapeutic approaches. *Parkinsonism & Related Disorders*, Vol.13, No.4, (May 2007), pp. 203-213, ISSN 1353-8020

Keus, S.; Bloem, BR.; Hendriks, E.; Bredero-Cohen, A. & Munneke, M. on behalf of the Practice Recommendations Development Group. (2007). Evidence-based analysis of physical therapy in Parkinson's disease with recommendations for practice and research. *Movement Disorders*, Vol.22, No.4, (March 2007), pp. 451-460, ISSN 0885-3185

Köller, WC.; Silver, DE. & Lieberman, A. (1994). An algorithm for the management of Parkinson's disease. *Neurology*, Vol.44, No.12 Suppl 10 (December 1994), pp. 51-52, ISSN 0028-3878

Lun, V.; Pullan, N.; Labelle, N.; Adams, C. & Suchowersky, O. (2005). Comparison of the effects of a self-supervised home exercise program with a physiotherapist-

Rehabilitation Versus no Intervention – Only a Continued Intensive Program Conducted Statistically
Significant Improvements Motor Skills in Parkinson's Disease Patients
163

supervised exercise program on the motor symptoms of Parkinson's disease. *Movement Disorders*, Vol.20, No.8,(August 2005) pp. 971-75, ISSN 0885-3185

Marsden, CD. (1994). Parkinson's disease. *Journal of Neurology, Neurosurgery & Psychiatry*, Vol.57, No.6 (June 1994), pp. 672-681, ISSN 00223050

Morris, ME. (2000) Movement disorders in people with Parkinson's disease: a model for physical therapy. *Physical Therapy*, Vol.80, No.6, (June 2000), pp. 578-597, ISSN 2079-9209

Movement Disorder Society Task Force on Ratio Scales for Parkinson's Disease. (2003). The Unified Parkinson's Disease Rating Scale (UPDRS): status and recommendations. *Movement Disorders*, Vol.18, No.7, (July 2003), pp. 738-750, ISSN 0885-3185

Muller, V.; Mohr, B.; Rosin, R.; Pulvermuller, F.; Muller, F. & Birbaumer, N. (1997). Short-term effects of behavioral treatment on movement initiation and postural control in Parkinson's disease: a controlled clinical study. *Movement Disorders*, Vol.12, No.3, (May 1997), pp. 306-314, ISSN 0885-3185

Nallegowda, M.; Singh, U.; Handa, G.; Khana, M.; Wadhwa, S.; Yadav, SL.; Kumar, G. & Behari, M.(2004). Role of sensory input and muscle strength in maintenance of balance, gait and posture in Parkinson's disease: a pilot study. *American Journal of Physical Medicine & Rehabilitation*, Vol.83, No.12, (December 2004), pp. 898-908, ISSN 0894-9115

O'Shea, S.; Morris, ME. & Iansek, R. (2002). Dual task interference during gait in people with Parkinson disease: effects of motor versus cognitive secondary tasks. *Physical Therapy*, Vol.82, No.9, (September 2002), pp. 888-897, ISSN 2079-9209

Pederson, SW.; Oberg, B.; Insulander, A. & Vretman A. (1990). Group training in Parkinsonism: quantitative measurements of treatment. *Scandinavian Journal of Rehabilitation Medicine*, Vol.22, No.4, (October 1990), pp. 207-211, ISSN 0036-5505

Pellecchia, MT.; Grasso, A.; Biancardi, LG.; Squillante, M.; Bonavita, V. & Barone, P. (2004). Physical therapy in Parkinson's disease: an open long-term rehabilitation trial. *Journal of Neurology*, Vol.251, No.5, (May 2004), pp. 595-598, ISSN 0340-5354

Quality Standards Subcommittee, American Academy of Neurology. (1993). Practice parameters: initial therapy of Parkinson's disease. *Neurology*, Vol.43, No.7, (July 1993), pp. 1296-1297, ISSN 0028-3878

Scandalis, TA.; Bosak, A.; Berliner, JC.; Hellman, LL. & Wells, MR. (2001). Resistance training and gait function in patients with Parkinson's disease. American Journal of physical Medicine & Rehabilitation, Vol.80,No.1, (January 2001), pp. 38-46, ISSN 0894-9115

Schmitz-Hübsch, T.; Pyfer, D.; Kielwein, K.; Fimmers, R.; Klockgether, T. & Wüllner, U. (2006) Qigong exercise for the symptoms of Parkinson's disease: a randomized, controlled pilot study. *Movement Disorders*, Vol.21, No.4, (April 2006), pp. 543-548, ISSN 0885-3185

Tamir, R.; Dickstein, R. & Huberman, M. (2007). Integration of motor imagery and physical practice in group treatment applied to subjects with Parkinson's disease. *Neurorehabilitation and Neural Repair*, Vol.21, No.1, (January-February 2007), pp. 68-75, ISSN 1545-9683

8

Improving Transfer of Parkinson's Disease Patients – Sit-to-Stand Motion Assistance

Yoshiyuki Takahashi[1], Osamu Nitta[2] and Takashi Komeda[3]
[1]Toyo University,
[2]Tokyo Metropolitan University,
[3]Shibaura Institute of Technology,
Japan

1. Introduction

In many areas of the world, population aging is steadily increasing. Japan became an aged society in 1995 and the numbers of Japanese citizens aged 65 years and above (elderly) continues to increase. In 2010, the percentage of elderly people in Japan reached 23.1%. In such a "super-aged" society, health maintenance, along with the prevention and treatment of diseases, are important long-term social care issues affecting elderly people.

Because the incidence of Parkinson's disease (PD) onset increases among persons over 50 years of age, it can be considered an age-related ailment, and there were approximately 145,000 confirmed PD patients in Japan at the time of this research. PD is caused by the death of dopamine-containing cells in substantia nigra of the brain. Common symptoms of PD are tremors, muscle stiffness, slow movement and poor balance, as well as other movement-related problems. When walking and during sit-to-stand motions, persons afflicted with such symptoms face increased risks from falls and subsequent injuries.

Ensuring efficient and safe transfer motions helps ensure self-reliant lifestyles, especially among elderly and physically disabled people, including PD patients. Transfer motions are among the basic activities of daily life. To help such persons, there are a number of commercially available sit-to-stand assistance devices on the market today, most of which assist users in rising from chairs by means of a lift seat that reduces the load on their lower limbs. However, from the viewpoint of maintaining lower muscle strength, excessive assistance is undesirable. Because of this, we have developed an effective sit-to-stand assistance system that provides the minimum assistance necessary.

In this paper, an outline of our developed sit-to-stand assistance system is introduced and experiments with this system involving individuals diagnosed with PD are described. It was found that the proposed system effectively permitted individuals to rise from a seated position.

2. Research background

There are numerous different tools and devices designed to assist transfer maneuvers. Most commonly, handrails are provided for individuals who have problems standing up and walking. However, handrails are difficult to adjust once installed. This can pose difficulties in situations where an individual's physical abilities change over a short period of time due to age and/or disease, because such changes often require that the position of an installed handrail be modified.

Such modifications often require reconstruction of the facilities. The typical position of a handrail that meets industrial standards e.g. Japanese Industrial Standard (JIS) is not suitable for all people because of differences in body size and physical abilities. Accordingly, the primary purpose of this research was the development of a moveable handrail system that provides sit-to-stand assistance that can be personalized to individual users.

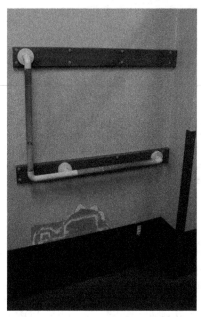

Fig. 1. Typical handrail installation

Previous handrail studies focused primarily on finding generalized heights and shapes, and no reports discussing active handrails for stand-up assistance were found. However, a number of active stand-up assistance devices have been developed. These include the Rehabilitation Robot Cell for Multimodal Stand-Up Motion Augmentation and the Stand-Up Motion Assistance System. Furthermore, the following devices are already available commercially: a seat lift chair, a lifting cushion, and a toilet seat lift. Such devices, which are not aimed at rehabilitation efforts, assist users in getting up from chairs by means of a lift seat that reduces the load on their lower limbs.

However, from the viewpoint of maintaining the lower muscle strength of a patient, excessive assistance is undesirable. Based on observations of the standing motions of large numbers of PD patients and elderly persons, it is clear that a significant percentage of such individuals would be able to stand up, despite poor motor function, if the transfer motion could be assisted in some ways. Therefore, we attempted to develop an effective sit-to-stand assistance system that provides the minimum degree of assistance necessary.

3. Sit-to-stand motion assistance system

Our prototype sit-to-stand assistance system was designed for elderly and disabled persons, including PD patients, who find it difficult to stand up from a sitting position. Figure 2 shows an overview of this sit-to-stand assistance system, which consists of two 650 mm stroke AC servo motor driven linear actuators combined in a square configuration and a handrail installed at the intersection of these actuators. When a user begins to stand from a seated position on a chair, the handrail moves to lead his or her motions. A personal computer was used to control the handrail movements, which was designed to move a 490 N load at a maximum velocity of 125 mm/s.

Figure 3 shows the system diagram. A six-axis force sensor (100M40A, JR3, Inc., California, USA) was attached to the base of the handrail. Figure 4 shows the six-axis force sensor coordinate system. The control program of the system calculates the trajectory of the handrail, and the force exerted on the handrail can be used to actuate the handrail movement. The direction and the actuating speed can be set on the control panel.

In our experiment, two force detection plates were positioned under the feet of the users, as shown in Figure 5. Each plate was 400 mm in length and 300 mm wide. The plates were designed to detect the floor reaction force exerted as the subject was standing up. A maximum force of 1500 N could be measured at a resolution lower than 2.5 N.

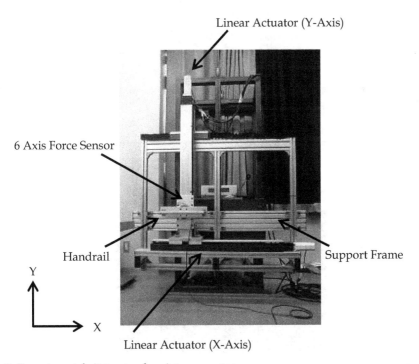

Fig. 2. Experimental sit-to-stand assistance system

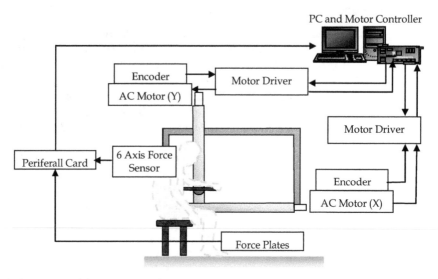

Fig. 3. Overview of the sit-to-stand motion assistance system

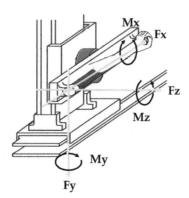

Fig. 4. 6 Axis force sensor coordinate system

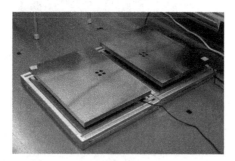

Fig. 5. Force detection plates for measuring feet pressure

4. Handrail motion

4.1 Concept of the sit-to-stand motion assistant strategy

People normally utilize two different strategies when executing a sit-to-stand maneuver. One is a sudden, rapid torso bend-and-straighten motion that generates and utilizes inertia to propel the person to a standing position. The other involves moving the person's center of gravity (CG) position slowly forward, balancing on the legs, and then straightening into the standing position. Normal healthy people can flex their torsos very rapidly, so they do not need to make excessive motions. In contrast, elderly people with low muscle strength are unable to make rapid torso motions. As a result, they normally move their torso forward to shift their CG, and then straighten up using the muscle strength of their legs.

In case of PD patients, it is often difficult for such persons to flex their torsos forward and back quickly enough to execute the first method and (due to increased muscle tone) they lack the knee joint extension power and flexibility needed to rise to the standing position, which is necessary for the second method. Furthermore, since their CG position does not move forward sufficiently, it is easy for such persons to fall backwards, as shown in Figure 6. Therefore, to assist such persons' sit-to-stand motions, the following method was considered to be effective. First, pulling their torso forward slowly until their CG positions moved onto their base of support and then leading their torsos upwards in a straight motion.

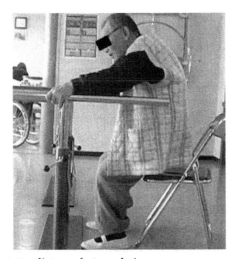

Fig. 6. Elderly PD patient standing up from a chair

4.2 Design of the individualized handrail trajectory system

In previous experiments, we examined three different handrail trajectories for PD patient sit-to-stand motion assistance. These included a horizontal motion, a diagonal motion and a curvature motion that was based on the shoulder motions of a normal healthy adult. Our examinations indicated that, in most cases, a trajectory based on the shoulder motion of a normal healthy individual in the process of standing up was effective for PD patient sit-to-stand motion assistance because it successfully assisted patients who were unable to stand using a fixed handrail. In these experiments, it was confirmed that the patient CG moved onto the base of support before the seat-lift and the handrail pulling force was decreased.

However, the curvature trajectory was not suitable for all PD patients. We then examined a fixed trajectory and determined that it would not be able to accommodate different user heights. Finally, we designed a new approach, which was to adjust the timing of the handrail motions using measurements of the force applied to the floor beneath the patient's feet in order to determine whether the CG had moved onto the base of support.

In this evolution, the handrail first moves slowly forward and downward to bend the patient's torso and shift his or her CG onto the base of support. Then, when the force under the patient's feet exceeds the preset threshold, the handrail begins moving upwards and slightly backwards to extend the patient's torso vertically. The original curvature trajectory was segmented and set to an approximate curve. Figure 7 shows a typical handrail trajectory and its formula.

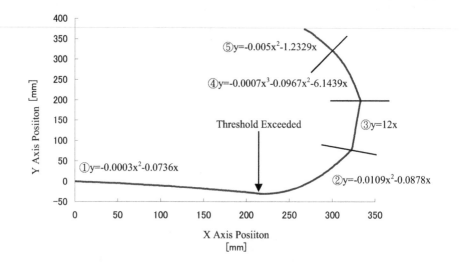

Fig. 7. Typical handrail trajectory

5. Materials and methods

The prototype sit-to-stand assistance system was designed and tested in conjunction with the handrail trajectory control program, and experiments were conducted to evaluate the sit-to-stand motion of PD patients as compared with normal healthy subjects.

5.1 Subjects

Two PD patients and two healthy adults (selected as the control subjects) participated as text subjects in this experiment. Both PD test subjects were diagnosed as Stage 4 patients based on the Hoehn and Yahr Scale. The mean age of the PD test subjects was 73.5 years (SD, 1.5 years). Their average weight was 48.5 kg (SD 5.5 kg); average height was 1.60 m (SD 0.03 m). Neither subject could stand up from a chair unassisted. The average weight of the control subjects was 70.5 kg (SD, 1.5 kg). The average height was 1.73 m (SD, 0.01 m). Informed consent was obtained from all test subjects.

5.2 Tasks and protocols

The initial posture of the subjects is shown in Figure 8. The X axis of the coordinate system is horizontal and the Y axis is vertical. Test subjects were positioned on a height-adjustable stool with an initial lower limb posture as follows: hips were flexed at 90° and knees were flexed at 80°. The height of the stool was set between approximately 370 and 390 mm. The height of the stool and the posture of the test subject were selected to simulate the position of a user on a toilet seat, as set in the Japanese Industrial Standard. The handrail was set to fit initial upper limb posture: the elbow position was 110°.

The PD test subjects were asked to perform sit-to-stand motions from a stool using the proposed sit-to-stand assistance system. Figure 7 shows an example of the handrail trajectories. Here, it can be seen that the handrail moves forward (X axis) and then curves upward (Y axis). In this experiment, the reaction force exerted on the floor under the feet of the test subjects was used to switch the handrail motion direction. Three different levels of reaction force, equal to 50%, 70% and 80% of the test subjects' body weight were used as thresholds. Each subject was asked to perform the sit-to-stand motion two times.

5.3 Measurements

A total of 11 optical markers were placed on key points of the subjects (the head of the 5th metatarsal bone, the lateral malleoluses, knee joints, hip joints, shoulders, top of the head, elbow, and wrist) and on the edge of the handrail. The locations of the optical markers are shown in Figure 5. A Vicon motion analysis system (Vicon 370, Oxford Metrics, Ltd. Oxford, UK) operating at a rate of 60 Hz was used to measure the various positions and calculate the posture of the subjects. Four floor-mounted force detection plates were used to measure the reaction force exerted on the chair and floor. The six-axis force sensor, operating at a rate of 30 Hz, measured the force exerted on the handrail and the two floor mounted force detection plates were used to determine when to switch the handrail motion direction. The marker positions, along with the pressures applied to the handrail and force detection plates, were all measured simultaneously. The corrected data was low-pass filtered using a 7 Hz Butterworth filter.

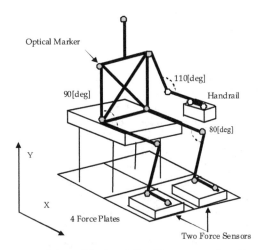

Fig. 8. Initial posture of the subject and the force sensor locations

The position of the test subject's CG was calculated by the positions of the 11 optical markers. A rigid link model, which consisted of the feet, lower legs, thighs, torso and head of the test subject, was used. The values used for the moment of inertia and the center of mass of body parts were taken from a database of body part characteristics for Japanese elderly people. The timing of the seat-off event was set at the point when Y-axis force on the floor mounted force plates became 0 N. Figure 9 shows a PD test subject participating in the experiment.

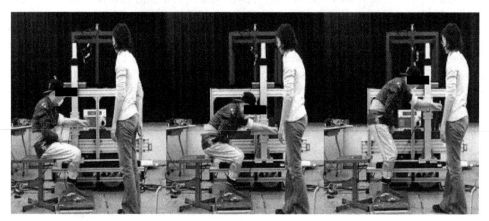

Fig. 9. PD test subject participating in the experiment

6. Results

6.1 CG position

Figure 10 shows examples of the handrail trajectories. The origin is set to the initial position of the handrail. Table 1 shows the average handrail positions that were moving direction switching position in X axis. The handrail trajectory was programmed to switch movement directions at certain points. Measurements equal to 50%, 70% and 80% of the test subject's body weight were set as thresholds. For the 80% threshold, the handrail was extended further forward than when the 50% and 70% threshold were set.

Figure 11 shows the CG trajectories. The X and Y axes positions were divided by the subject's body height and normalized. Table 2 shows the average CG positions when the seat-off point and maximum forward position occurred. The CG positions were then divided by the subject's foot length and normalized.

For healthy test subjects that did not use the handrail, the CGs were found to have moved forward and slightly down at first, following which, they moved upward in a curve. The seat-off position was designated at the point when the CG moved 10% of the test subject's foot length. At the 50% threshold, the maximum forward position of the CG was -18% of the test subject's foot length, at which point the PD test subjects were unable to stand. Therefore, it was considered likely that the CG had not moved onto the base of support. In the case of the 70% threshold, the subject could stand, however when the CG started to rise its movement distance was found to be less than that of a normal healthy test subject. At the 80% threshold, the test subject was able to stand smoothly and the CG trajectory was similar to that of a healthy test subject. The maximum recorded forward position of the CG was 54% of the test subject's foot length, which was roughly similar to that of a healthy test subject.

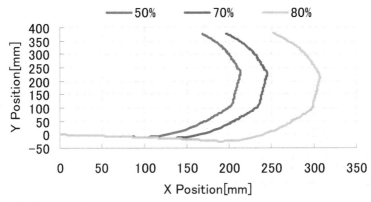

Fig. 10. Handrail trajectories

Threshold (% of body weight)	Handrail Position [mm]
50%	92
70%	232
80%	272

Table 1. Average handrail positions actuated by the handrail trajectory

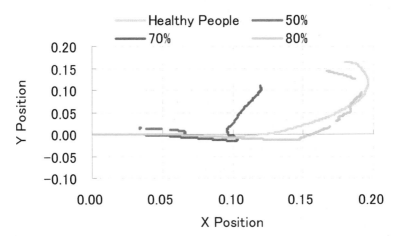

Fig. 11. CG trajectories

Threshold (% of body weight)	Seat-off Position [% of foot length]	Max. Forward Position [% of foot length]
Control (Healty Subject)	10	54
50%	–	−18
70%	16	37
80%	20	54

Table 2. Maximum forward CG position

6.2 Torso and thigh angle

Figure 12 shows the torso and thigh angles of the healthy test subjects. Figures 13 and 14 show the torso angle, thigh angle and X axis position of the handrail for the PD subjects at the 70% and 80% thresholds. The horizontal axis indicates the timeline, which was divided by the total time and normalized. The origin of the torso angle is set on the horizontal line that extends through the hip joints. The origin of thigh angle is set on the horizontal line that extends through the knee joint. The initial position of the handrail is set as the origin point.
For the healthy test subjects, thigh angles increased before seat-off occurred, after which the torso angles also increased. For the 70% and 80% thresholds, the torso angle increased after the handrail moved backward in the horizontal direction. In the case of the 80% threshold, the torso angle began increasing after seat-off occurred, at which time the handrail began moving backwards. This indicates that, in the case of 80% threshold, the test subject's body bent forward during the standing motion and the CG remained within the base of support. This motion assistance allowed the achievement of a stable sit-to-stand motion.

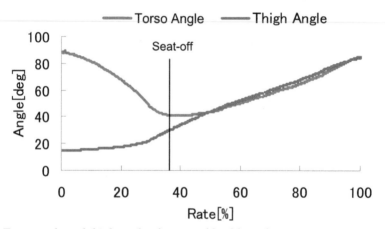

Fig. 12. Torso angle and thigh angle of a normal healthy subject

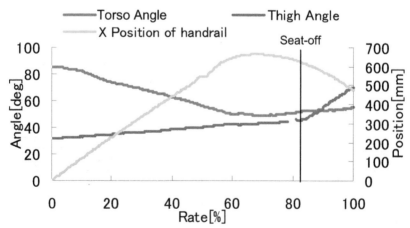

Fig. 13. Torso angle, thigh angle and handrail position of a PD subject at the 70% threshold

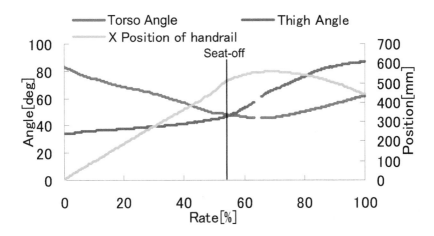

Fig. 14. Torso angle, thigh angle and handrail position of a PD subject at the 80% threshold

Threshold (% of body weight)	Minimum Trunk Angle [deg]
Control (Healthy Subject)	43
50%	58
70%	47
80%	43

Table 3. Minimum torso angle

6.3 Knee joint moment

Figure 15 shows the knee joint moment. Here, it can be seen that the flexion direction is positive and the extension direction has a negative value. This measurement was divided by the subject's height and normalized. The time for sit-to-stand motion was divided by the total time and normalized. Table 4 shows the maximum knee joint moment.

The variation of knee joint moment for healthy test subjects was larger than those measured for PD subjects in extension. At the 50% threshold, the subject could not achieve seat-off and the variation of the knee joint moment changed only fractionally. At the 70% and 80% thresholds, no significant difference was found in the maximum values. However, the timing of peak was different it caused by the different timing of seat-off.

Threshold (% of body weight)	Maximum Knee Joint Moment [Nm/kg]
Control (Healthy Subject)	−1.19
50%	−0.26
70%	−0.98
80%	−0.94

Table 4. Maximum knee joint moment

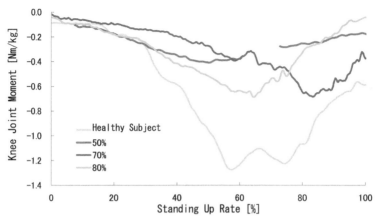

Fig. 15. Knee joint moment

6.4 Force exerted on the handrail

Figures 16 and 17 show the force exerted on the handrail on the X and Y axes. Here, the forward and down directions were positive (Figure 4). The X and Y axes of Table 5 and 6 show the maximum force exerted on the handrail.

There were no significant differences between the 50%, 70% and 80% thresholds on the X axis. However, in the case of the 80% threshold, the maximum force exerted on the handrail on the Y axis was less than the 50% and 70% thresholds.

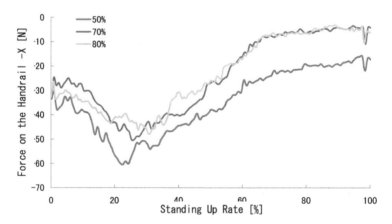

Fig. 16. Force exerted on the handrail as plotted on the X Axis

Threshold (% of body weight)	Max. Force on the Hnadrail −X [N]
50%	−60
70%	−65
80%	−61

Table 5. Maximum force exerted on the handrail as plotted on the X axis

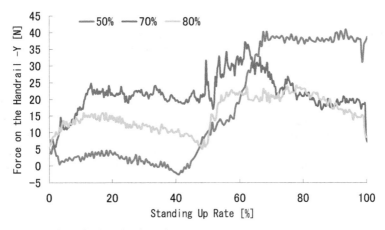

Fig. 17. Force exerted on the handrail on the Y Axis

Threshold (% of body weight)	Max. Force on the Hnadrail −Y [N]
50%	30
70%	32
80%	17

Table 6. Maximum force exerted on the handrail as plotted on the Y Axis

7. Discussion

The CG trajectory of a normal healthy test subject increased in a curve after seat-off. At that time, the torso was angled forward. After seat-off, the angle of the torso increased as the subject straightened into a standing posture. The CG was found to have shifted forward a maximum of 54% of the subjects' foot length, and the knee joint moment was measured at 1.19 Nm/kg in the extension direction.

The PD test subjects were unable to stand up at the 50% threshold assistance level. In that situation, the CG shift was -18% and the CG did not enter the base of support.

At the 70% threshold level, the PD test subject was able to stand, but the CG trajectory was different from that of a normal healthy subject, and the timing of the straightening motion was earlier than that for a normal healthy subject. When the handrail started to move backward, the subject's torso angle shifted to vertical. Additionally, it was found that the handrail had moved backward and torso angle had shifted to vertical before seat-off occurred. Thus, it was determined that the CG and posture transition sequence of PD subjects was different from that of normal healthy subjects, and that the PD subjects straightened their torsos before their CG had moved sufficiently forward. They also used stronger downward pushing pressure on the handrail than was exerted at the 80% threshold.

At the 80% threshold, PD subjects were able to stand successfully and the CG trajectory was similar to that of a normal healthy subject. It was also determined that PD subjects straightened their torsos after the CG had moved forward onto their base of support. When the subject seat-off occurred, the CG had moved forward approximately 20% of the subject's foot length and the maximum CG position was 54% of the foot length.

These results indicate that moving the handrail forward until the normal force under the feet exceeds 80% of total body weight, and then actuating the vertical rise of the handrail to perform seat-off could assist PD subjects in performing the sit-to-stand motion in a stable manner.

8. Conclusions

A sit-to-stand assistance system was developed and experiments with PD test subjects were performed. The results indicate that a moveable handrail with a forward trajectory (X axis) and upward curve motion (Y axis) could be used to assist individuals as they transition from a seated to a standing position. The motion direction was actuated by the reaction force exerted on the floor under the feet of the subject, and it was found that the 80% threshold was the most effective point for initiating assistance to their standing up motion.

9. Acknowledgment

I would like to acknowledge the generous support received from Mr. Tomuro, Dr. Takagi and students of the Tokyo Metropolitan University who joined the experiments conducted during this research.

10. References

Oshima T., Ito A., Endo Y. (2000). Research of a taste of "diameter and height" of handrail. *Proceedings of Architectural Institute of Japan,* pp. 1031-1032, ISSN 13414518

Takashima T., Nakanishi Y., Higaki H. (2005). Study of Design of Handrail, Proceedings of the Japan Society of Mechanical Engineers. *Proceedings of the Japan Society of Mechanical Engineers, Bioengineering Division,* 2005(18), pp. 315-316

Kamnik R., Bajd T., Williamson J., Murray-Smith R. (2005). Rehabilitation Robot Cell for Multimodal Standing-Up Motion Augmentation. *Proceedings of the 2005 IEEE International Conference on Robotics and Automation, ICRA 2005,* pp. 2277-2282, ISSN 0-7803-8914-X

Chugo D., Okada E., Kawabata K., Kaetsu H., Aasama H., Miyake N. (2005). Force Assistance System for Standing-Up Motion: 1st Report: Required Assistance Power for Standing-Up Motion: 1st Report: Required Assistance Power for Standing-Up. *The JSME Symposium on Welfare Engineering Vol.2005(20051207),* pp. 257-260

Hoehn M.M, Yarh D. M. (1967). Parkinsonism: onset, progression and mortality. *Neurology* 17, pp. 427-442

Ichirou H. (2001). *Living climate of welfare coordinator second class text,* The Tokyo Chamber of Commerce and Industry, ISBN 978-4924547476

Takahashi Y, Osamu N, Komeda T. (2008). Development of a Sit-to-Stand Assistance System. *Lecture Notes in Computer Science, 2008, Volume 5105/2008,* pp. 1277-1284, ISSN 0302-9743

Uplift Technologies Inc., 17.04.2011, Available from
        http:// www.up-lift.com/

TOTO LTD., 17.04.2011, Available from
        http:// www.toto.co.jp/

Part 2

Invasive Methods Examine in Patients with Parkinson's Disease

9

Human Central Nervous System Circuits Examined in Patients with Parkinson's Disease Using the Electrodes Implanted for Deep Brain Stimulation

Joao Costa[1,2], Francesc Valldeoriola[2] and Josep Valls-Sole[2]

[1]Institute of Molecular Medicine, Lisbon Faculty of Medicine
[2]Neurology Department, Hospital Clínic, Centro de Investigación Biomédica en Red sobre
Enfermedades Neurodegenerativas (CIBERNED) and Institut d'Investigacio Biomedica
August Pi i Sunyer (IDIBAPS), Facultad de Medicina, Universitat de Barcelona
[1]Portugal
[2]Spain

1. Introduction

Epidural or subdural electrodes are often used in humans in order to identify eloquent structures by stimulation or recording. Neurosurgeons are able to use the motor maps gathered more than 50 years ago by Penfield and Jasper (1954) for delineation of the functions of non-lesioned cortical tissue. These and other contributions have been made during surgical procedures in humans by either applying direct cortical stimulation (Woolsey et al., 1979; Burke and Hicks, 1998) or recording from the spinal cord tracts after cortical or peripheral nerve stimulation (Burke and Hicks, 1998; Di Lazzaro et al., 2006). Peroperatory neurophysiological monitoring offers also great opportunities for learning from using neurophysiological techniques, at the same time as helping the surgeon to reach a better outcome (Rainov et al., 1997; Horikoshi et al., 2000; Deletis and Sala, 2008).

These procedures have not only helped to improve the surgical procedure but they have allowed the use of neurophysiological tests to expand our knowledge on human central nervous system circuitry and functional connectivity. Nowadays, stereotactically placed electrodes with therapeutic aims such as deep brain stimulation (DBS), offer the possibility to reach structures that could not be otherwise targeted in humans and investigate further physiological aspects of brain circuits. For these purposes, authors have used the DBS electrodes inserted either in the nucleus ventralis intermedius of the thalamus (Vim), the globus pallidus internus (GPi), the subthalamic nucleus (STN), the pedunculopontine nucleus (PPN) or others in which the results of research are still scarce (Weinberger et al., 2008; Galati et al., 2008; Shimamoto et al., 2010; Alessandro et al., 2010). The information brought by these studies has already shed some light on the functioning of some central nervous system circuits. However, many questions remain to be answered and further research on the subject is required to 1) understand fully the physiological mechanisms underlying the beneficial effects of chronic repetitive high frequency DBS, and 2) strengthen our knowledge on human brain circuitry and connectivity.

In this chapter, we revise the contributions that have been made to various physiological questions by the use of the electrodes implanted for therapeutic purposes in patients with Parkinson disease (PD) or dystonia. We have not included works on clinical effects of deep brain stimulation or clinical correlations, unless they were considered relevant for understanding physiological processes. The reader interested on clinical aspects may look for recent reviews on the topic (Limousin and Martinez-Torres, 2008; Lozano and Schneider, 2008; Benabid et al., 2009; Foltynie et al., 2010).

2. Recording

2.1 Neuronal spikes and local field potentials
2.1.1 Localization of targets
During the surgical procedure, at the operating room, it is possible to perform direct microelectrode recording of neuronal activity along the structures crossed by the electrode to reach the target nucleus. This is part of routine practice in most centers to help in localizing the target basal ganglia (Hutchison et al., 1998; Benazzouz et al., 2002; Sterio et al., 2002a; Molinuevo et al., 2003; Mrakic-Sposta et al., 2008). An example of such recordings taken from a patient along the trajectory of the electrode to the STN is shown in Figure 1.

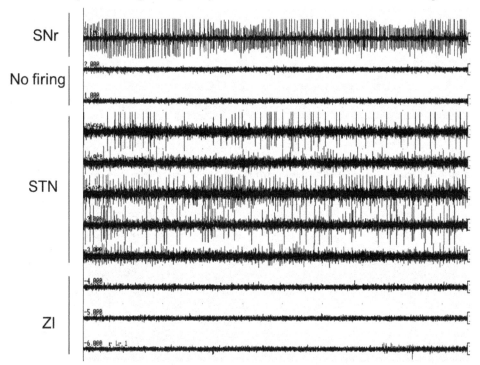

Fig. 1. Neurophysiological recording of various sites while inserting the electrode. From the bottom to the top: The electrode in the zona incerta (ZI) records almost no activity. When it enters the subthalamic nucleus (STN), the spikes become grouped in various bursts. Exiting the nucleus, there is a zone with no activity and then a continuous firing of spikes at a relatively high frequency, when the electrode enters the substantia nigra pars reticulata (SNr).

The possibility exists of recording from different nuclei in the circuitry. It is known, for instance, that the globus pallidus externus (GPe) shows a typical pauser neuronal firing, with activity in bursts. Sani et al. (2009) hypothesized that the characteristics of such firing might be different in patients with different disorders. They examined pause characteristics in 224 GPe units in patients with primary generalized dystonia, PD and secondary dystonia. The results showed that the characteristics of the pauses recorded in the GPe in awake humans distinguished primary dystonia from PD and secondary dystonia. Patients with primary dystonia had longer pause length, shorter interpause interval and higher mean pause frequency than PD patients. Interpause interval was also shorter in primary than in secondary dystonia. These results indicated an increased phasic input from striatal D2 receptor positive cells in primary dystonia.

A method to help localizing the border between the STN and the substantia nigra pars reticulata (SNr) has been shown by Lafreniere-Roula et al. (2009). These authors stimulated at low and high frequency through the electrode intended for the STN. When the electrode was at the border area between the STN and the SNr, they observed that high frequency stimulation caused a long lasting pause in the SNr firing but not in the STN. This is, therefore, an interesting technique to be used as a landmark for the STN electrode positioning. The same authors found inhibition in the GPi, similar to that induced in the SNr, although there were differences in threshold (Lafrenière-Roula et al., 2010), and suggested that such activity depression could contribute to the therapeutic effects of high frequency stimulation. A wavelet-based measure for quantitative assessment of neural background was used by Snellings et al. (2009) to show increase background levels within the STN that would help in identifying better the nucleus boundaries.

In our institution, we use the following criteria to consider electrode placement: For the GPi or the STN we consider signs of appropriate placement: 1) the observation of neuronal activity linked to limb movements, 2) a good therapeutic response such as improvement of bradykinesia, rigidity or tremor with intraoperatory high frequency stimulation, and 3) the absence of capsular, visual or ocular effects with the high frequency stimulation or its presence only when the stimulus intensity is increased above therapeutic threshold. For the Vim, we consider the finding of tremor cells within the boundaries of the nucleus and the disappearance of tremor when stimulating in the absence of motor or sensory side effects.

In 2002, various authors reported their observations on the preferred technical approach to reach the anatomical location for the electrodes to be implanted in the STN, GPi or Vim (Benazzouz et al., 2002; Lanotte et al., 2002; Starr et al., 2002; Saint-Cyr et al., 2002). However, good outcome measures of the surgical procedure should consider not only the precise localization of the appropriate target but, also, the lowest occurrence of residual symptoms and the lowest occurrence of side effects (Guehl et al., 2007).

Recognizing the target structure is a very important task at the time of electrode implantation. Knowing where the stimuli are actually applied or where they are more effective is another important piece of information for feedback. An attempt at knowing where the stimuli were actually applied through the STN electrode for the best clinical outcome was made by Maks et al. (2009). These authors used neuroimaging to measure the theoretical volume of tissue activated (VTA) by clinically defined best therapeutic stimulation parameters. They showed that therapeutic benefit was mainly achieved when the majority of VTA was in the area of the STN, mainly at its dorsal region, but outside the atlas defined boundaries of the nucleus. This, therefore, underlines the importance of the axons surrounding the STN for therapeutic efficacy. A similar observation was made by

Herzog et al. (2007) using electrodes implanted in the thalamus for the treatment of tremor. These authors observed a better effect on tremor using leads that were located closer to the STN rather than in the thalamus itself.

2.1.2 Assessment of activity and connectivity

Once in the target nucleus, the microelectrode can record both neuronal spikes and local field potentials (LFPs) originating in the same nucleus or in neighbouring neuronal groups. Such recordings have been used to characterize the physiological relationship between the target nuclei and its surroundings, as well as to provide evidence for disease-related neurophysiological abnormalities and their modulation by treatment (pharmacological and/or DBS).

Microelectrode recordings from within the STN show relatively rich background and spontaneously firing single neurons. Interestingly, however, if spikes are removed (obtaining a 'despiked' trace), the analysis of the STN signal still provides for the possibility to identify a pattern of activity typical of the STN (Danish et al., 2008). Various authors have reported high firing rates of neuronal spikes in PD patients in both, the STN (Rodríguez-Oroz et al., 2001; Sterio et al., 2002a), and the GPi (Hutchison et al., 1997; 2003), fitting well with the hypothesized hyperactivity of the indirect circuit of the basal ganglia in PD patients (Alexander and Crutcher, 1990; Wichmann and DeLong, 1996). An interesting finding has been recently reported by Novak et al. (2009) to provide a cue to understand why patients with unilateral STN DBS show bilateral benefit. These authors found that during high frequency STN DBS, there was an increase in multiunit spiking activity in the contralateral STN, an observation that provides also many questions to be answered in future studies. Apart from increased firing frequency, Levy et al. (2001; 2002) observed that neuronal spikes recorded from PD patients with tremor showed a prominent oscillatory pattern, which was substantially modified under dopaminergic activity. In the case of dystonia, however, the hypothesized low frequency firing rate of the GPi neurons has not always been found. While Vitek et al. (1999) reported firing rates lower than in PD in 3 patients with dystonia and one patient with hemiballismus, other authors have suggested that anesthesia played an important role in decreasing neuronal firing rate (Hutchison et al., 2003). The effect of anesthesia has not always been confirmed (Sanghera et al., 2003) and, according to Pralong et al. (2005), the lower firing rate of GPi neurons is independent of the type of anesthetic drug used.

Tremor is usually treated with thalamic high frequency stimulation both in PD and in essential tremor (ET). To see if there were differences between the two disorders in regard to the spontaneous neuronal firing in thalamic neurons, Chen et al., (2010) analyzed the recordings from the ventral oral posterior and the ventral intermediate nuclei. These authors concluded that there were significant differences between the two disorders, with decreased ventral oral posterior firing frequency in ET and increased neuronal firing rates in the ventral intermediate nucleus in patients with PD. The authors speculated on the possible pathophysiological implications of their findings.

Neuronal activity can be recorded also as LFPs, which have been confirmed to be time-locked to spikes generated in neighbouring neurones by recording spike-triggered LFP averages (Kuhn et al., 2005a) or examining coherence with multiunit recordings (Weinberger et al., 2006). The analysis of the LFPs may help confirming that the electrode is between the dorsal and ventral borders of the STN (Miyagi et al., 2009).

The LFPs can be recorded from the macroelectrode leads left externalized after surgery prior to connection to the impulse generator and, therefore, they can be analyzed while patients perform cognitive or motor tasks (Brown and Williams, 2005). Three prevailing frequency bands have been identified in the LFPs recorded from the basal ganglia: <8, 8-30 and >60 Hz. The band dominating the spectrum in the 'off' medication stage is the frequency in the alpha-beta range (8-25 Hz), while in the 'on' medication state baseline frequencies are higher (70-80 Hz). Brown et al. (2002) reported an increase in the amplitude of the frequency band of 25 Hz in the GPi of 2 PD patients that occurred prior to completion of a bimanual timing task. Because of a strong correlation between band amplitude changes and task duration, the authors suggested that modulation of this GPi frequency band could be involved in the prediction of movement timing. The band of 8-30 Hz predominates in the STN and GPi of PD patients withdrawn from their dopaminergic medication and is, therefore, considered antikinetic, likely contributing to the bradykinesia.

The high frequency LFP oscillations can only be recorded with normal levels of dopaminergic activity, while the band of 8-30 Hz is suppressed by dopaminergic treatments, behaviourally relevant stimuli and voluntary movement. Therefore, it seems that the subthalamo-pallidal-thalamo-cortical circuit undergo an opposite modulation by dopaminergic activity that may be a fundamental feature of the pathophysiological mechanisms of bradykinesia in PD (Brown, 2003). Actually, a correlation has been reported between the efficacy of the pair of leads used for chronic stimulation and the energy of the beta and gamma frequency band detected initially with LFP recordings during movements (Ince et al., 2010; Zaidel et al., 2010).

Foffani et al. (2003; 2005) described a distinct 300 Hz band in the STN that was more consistently seen during movement than at rest and more robust after apomorphine treatment. The authors suggested that such high frequency band represented a distinct mode of operation of the STN that could be a pathophysiological clue for PD. However the same group reported a similar high frequency band in the STN of two patients with diagnosis other than PD (one with dystonia and another with ET), hence suggesting that this finding may represent a broader feature of human STN function rather than being specific for PD (Danish et al., 2007).

Various loops are likely to run between the cortex and the basal ganglia that can be segregated by the amplitude of the frequency band. Williams et al. (2002) examined coherence between neuronal oscillatory activity recorded from electrodes inserted into the STN (8 patients) or the GPi (2 patients) and the EEG activity. They found significant coherence in three major frequency bands: 2-10 Hz, 10-30 Hz and 70-85 Hz, which differed in their cortical topography. Cortical activity led by around 20 ms the basal ganglia activity in frequencies <30 Hz, while it was the other way around with frequencies in the 70-85 Hz band.

An exaggerated synchronization in the band between 8 and 35 Hz (alpha/beta) might be implicated in the pathophysiology of Parkinson's disease. The power in this band decreased with dopamine treatment, as shown by several authors in the analysis of STN-LFP oscillations (Giannicola et al., 2010). The same effect has been obtained with STN DBS (Kuhn et al., 2008; Bronte-Stewart et al., 2009; Giannicola et al., 2010) although the intensity of the effect has not been the same in all reports. The abnormally enhanced beta band oscillations are encountered in certain sites of the STN and some authors have found a correlation between localization of the electrode in sites of the STN where there was a predominating beta band and the efficacy of STN DBS in alleviating the patient's symptoms (Ince et al.,

2010; Zaidel et al., 2010). Interestingly, the activity was transiently suppressed between 200 and 600 ms after transcranial magnetic stimuli (TMS), regardless of it being applied to the motor cortex or to the supplementary motor area (Gaynor et al., 2008). The effect was seen even with subthreshold intensity for elicitation of a motor evoked potential and, therefore, the authors dismissed the possibility for peripheral reafferentation as the cause of the transient interruption. This observation could underline the beneficial effects of repetitive TMS (rTMS) in patients with PD but the differences between L-Dopa, STN DBS and rTMS point out to the existence of other contributory mechanisms.

The high frequency oscillatory activity (gamma band) is more prominently recorded in patients treated with L-Dopa, suggesting that this may be an important correlate of dopaminergic activity. Although initially considered to be related to the L-Dopa induced dyskinesias, an increase power in the gamma band was actually seen at movement onset in patients in the OFF medication state, to increase significantly in the 'on' medication state (Androulidakis et al., 2007). Therefore, there is evidence that the L-Dopa related increase in gamma band power is a sign of restoration of physiological pattern of oscillatory activity in Parkinson's disease. An abnormally low ratio between beta and gamma activity has been found in the STN during tremor (Weinberger et al., 2009), suggesting that the balance between these two oscillatory frequency bands may be associated with the clinical manifestation of tremor.

Kuhn et al. (2006a) examined event-related desynchronization (ERD) by recording LFPs from the STN region in 8 PD patients 'off' dopaminergic medication. Patients were instructed to either extend the wrist or to imagine performing the same task without any overt movement. They found that imagining a motor action was accompanied by ERD of oscillatory beta activity in the region of the STN that was similar in frequency, time course and degree to the ERD occurring during real execution of movement. The event-related synchronization (ERS) occurring after completion of movement was significantly smaller in movement imagination than in movement execution. According to these observations, neuronal activity in an area around the STN might have a role in trial-to-trial motor learning and in the re-establishment of postural set after movement.

In dystonia, Chu Chen et al. (2006), using a multielectrode that combined 4 platinum-tungsten fibers in a glass insulation with 4 circular contacts, reported the finding of a high power 3-12 Hz band in the analysis of LFP from the GPi, which has been considered relevant in the pathophysiology of dystonia (Silberstein et al., 2003; Liu et al., 2006). Again, computed spike-triggered averages demonstrated that the oscillations were actually generated by GPi neuronal spikes. Consistent with the expected basal ganglia functional activity, a significantly lower firing rate was found in the GPi neurons in dystonic patients than in PD patients (Tang et al., 2007). When recording from the STN of dystonic patients, Schrock et al. (2009) found a frequency of firing of 26.3 Hz (SD 13.6), which was lower than that in the PD patients (35.6 Hz, SD 15.2), but higher than published values for subjects without basal ganglia dysfunction. In Tourette's syndrome, Marceglia et al. (2010) reported the observation of bursting neuronal activity in the ventralis oralis (VO) complex of the thalamus, known to improve tics in patients with Tourette's syndrome. These bursts occurred at low frequencies (2-7 Hz) and in the alpha-band (8-13 Hz), while there was virtually absent beta band activity. Microelectrode recording was performed in the GPi by Zhuang et al. (2009) to explore the relationship between basal ganglia output and electromyographic activity during tics and demonstrate that the basal ganglia motor circuit is involved in tic movements. In 232 neurons, these authors found 45% of them that were related to either a burst of activity or a pause in ongoing tonic activity.

The correlation between LFP oscillatory changes and movements has been reported by many authors, supporting the hypothesis that the GPi and the STN are somehow involved in movement preparation in humans. An increase in high frequency activity (>60 Hz) has been found to occur before voluntary movement (Cassidy et al., 2002). Alegre et al. (2005) reported bilateral changes in the neuronal oscillatory activity of the STN during voluntary unilateral hand movements, suggesting that movement-related activity in the STN has a bilateral representation and probably reflects cortical input. Alegre et al. (2010) also reported, during movement observation, a bilateral beta reduction in subthalamic power, similar to that observed in the EEG, , and decreased cortico-STN coherence, suggesting that the basal ganglia might be engaged by the activity of the human mirror system. Likely, there are multiple circuits linking the motor cortex with the basal ganglia that are segregated by not only topography but also frequency (Lalo et al., 2008).

Interestingly, Paradiso et al. (2003) reported the finding of pre-movement potentials recorded from the STN similar to those recorded from the scalp. These authors found a bilateral slow rising negative pre-motor potential beginning at a latency of more than 2 seconds before onset of self-paced wrist extension movements. Further support for the implication of the cortico-basal ganglia-thalamocortical circuit in movement preparation has been brought recently by the same group. Purzner et al. (2007) reported a phase reversal of the pre-movement potential when simultaneously recorded the activity preceding self-paced or externally cued movements with scalp electrodes and STN electrodes. The possibility that rhythms of neuronal oscillatory activity determine the participation of the basal ganglia on movement preparation, movement execution and post-movement recovery was pointed out by Foffani et al. (2005), while Marceglia et al. (2006) suggested that the key factor could be the interaction between rhythms generated in different neuronal circuits.

There is some evidence for the human STN area to be involved in the processing or transmission of emotional information: Kuhn et al. (2005b) recorded LFPs through the STN electrode in 10 PD patients while viewing pleasant and unpleasant emotionally arousing and neutral pictures. They found a significant, unspecific, ERD in the alpha power (8 to 12 Hz), starting at about 0.5 seconds after stimulus presentation, and a later ERD (at about 1 to 2 seconds post-stimulus), that was larger in trials containing pleasant or unpleasant images than in those with neutral stimuli. These findings suggest some kind of link between the STN and limbic structures that could be a clue for understanding the pathophysiology underlying the mood changes observed in patients with PD and high frequency STN stimulation. The basal ganglia may be involved in the evaluation of changes in the environment and their significance, which could explain the behavioural impairment that can follow basal ganglia lesions or dysfunctions (Sauleau et al., 2009).

2.1.3 Responses of nearby neuronal groups

In search for an explanation of the effects of high frequency stimulation, investigators have used microelectrode recording of neuronal spikes and LFPs in response to local stimuli. Technical development has brought up the possibility of recording from one contact while stimulating by another at a few hundred microns distance only, allowing for the construct of a functional stereotactic mapping around the microelectrode. Dostrovsky et al. (2000) reported inhibition of the GPi neurons by high frequency stimulation through another electrode inserted in the same nucleus, between 250 and 600 microns apart. This was re-examined in 2007 by Pralong et al., who reported opposite effects of high frequency stimulation (100 Hz) over neurones located in different parts of the GPi nucleus, with a pattern of local inhibition and distant excitation. A similar study was done in STN neurons by Filali et al. (2004), who reported an inhibitory effect of stimulation applied through another electrode located in the same nucleus at a distance of about 600 microns. Welter et al. (2004) reported that stimulation at frequencies over 40 Hz decreased firing frequency and increased burst-like activity of STN neurons in patients with PD. Montgomery (2006) reported on microelectrode recordings in the posterior VO nucleus of the thalamus during high frequency GPi DBS in a patient with dystonia. Eighty-eight percent of neurons showed brief but highly consistent increased firing in the first 1ms following stimulation. This was followed by inhibition in about half of the neurons, which occurred at about 3.5 to 5 ms, and a post-inhibitory rebound of enhanced activity in 25% of neurons.

The importance of stimulus intensity in determining effects on neuronal firing was demonstrated by Maurice et al. (2003) who reported that the firing rate of the SNr neurons increased with high intensity, and decreased with low intensity STN DBS. This observation suggests that the fibers connecting STN to SNr neurons may carry inhibitory or excitatory inputs depending on the firing frequency. Sterio et al. (2002b) demonstrated that the STN neurons were activated by stimuli applied to the GPi, with two different main effects: reduction of firing rate in neurons of the dorsal region of the STN, and facilitation in those of the ventral region of the STN. The latter had a behavior similar to that of the SNr neurons. The authors point out that this finding is just one example of the complexity of the basal ganglia loops, which overshadows the relatively simple and linear, although still useful, schematic connections predicted after the classical circuitry (Alexander and Crutcher, 1990; Wichmann and DeLong, 1996).

2.1.4 Effects of disease and treatment on neuronal activity in the basal ganglia

The possible association between characteristics of the neuronal firing in the STN and GPi and tremor, dyskinesias and other movement dysfunctions of PD patients has been studied by many authors in 'off' and 'on' medication state. The high frequency STN rhythm at about 300 Hz described by Foffani et al. (2003) was dopamine-dependent. It was more robust and larger after apomorphine, suggesting that modulation of this high frequency band may be underlying beneficial therapeutic effects in PD. The authors suggested that an absent 300-Hz STN rhythm during movement could be a pathophysiological clue for PD. Priori et al. (2004) reported that the main effects of L-Dopa and apomorphine were an increase in the power of the low frequency bands (2-7 Hz), and a decrease in the power of low-beta activity (13-20 Hz). Their findings were compatible with at least two STN neuronal oscillatory rhythms, separately modulated by antiparkinsonian medication: one at low frequencies and one in the beta range. Alonso-Frech et al. (2006) found basically the same results and suggested that the increase in the power of the 4-10 Hz frequency band could account for dopamine-induced dyskinesias in PD patients. This has been also pointed out more recently by Lee et al. (2007) who observed that a decrease in neuronal firing rate in the GPi preceded the onset of dyskinesias induced by the administration of apomorphine.

Kuhn et al. (2006b) calculated in 9 PD patients the STN LFP power over the frequencies of the most prominent spectral peak within the 8-35 Hz frequency band and of any peak in the 60-90 Hz band. They observed a dopamine-related reduction in peak activity in the 8-35 Hz band, which was positively correlated with the contralateral hemibody improvement on motor aspects of the unified Parkinson's disease rating scale (UPDRS) and with hemibody subscores of akinesia-rigidity, but not tremor. They also found a trend for negative correlations between peak 60-90 Hz LFP power and UPDRS hemibody score, suggesting that positive correlations were relatively frequency specific. Peak amplitude or power of the frequency band may be not the only relevant aspect for the function of basal ganglia.

A few authors have examined whether STN DBS have the same effects as dopamine on neuronal firing and LFP oscillations. This has been assessed immediately after switching off the stimulator, when patients still benefit from STN DBS but there is no ongoing stimulation (Foffani et al., 2003; Priori et al., 2006). In those studies, the effects were limited to an increase in the power of very low frequency bands (1-1.5 Hz), while no effects were seen in the low beta band (13-20 Hz), high beta band (20-35 Hz), gamma band (60-90 Hz) or in the 300 Hz oscillations. However, Wingeier et al. (2006) were able to document in two patients a significant attenuation of the power of the beta band oscillatory activity recorded from the STN immediately after DBS, an effect that lasted for 15-25 s after DBS had been turned off. Therefore, more work is needed in this area to establish whether or not the effects induced by DBS on the neuronal oscillatory activity of the STN are the same or not as those induced by dopaminergic treatment.

The mechanisms by which DBS is effective in the symptomatic treatment of PD remain not fully elucidated. A prevailing theory is that, instead of just blocking the activity, the electrical stimuli interfere with the output from the STN, in such a way that the pathological activity is jammed. Carlson et al. (2010) found results consistent with this hypothesis when recording from the STN during therapeutically effective stimulation. These authors saw that the spontaneous firing was not arrested but the firing patterns were altered, with a predominant shift toward random firing.

2.1.5 Discussion

Neurophysiological recordings during surgery are routine practice for most departments carrying out stereotactic procedures for treatment of Parkinson's disease. Recording neuronal spikes helps in the assessment of the trajectory and, together with the magnetic resonance imaging (MRI) correlate of the electrode and the relevant anatomical structures, has provided cues for the assessment of the electrode position with most effective clinical results. Although landmarks have been defined and are helpful for orientation of the target, modification of the first tract is done in about 1/3 of patients in order to reach better outcomes for the specific individual. The relationship between movements of specific body parts and STN neuronal activity has led to recognize topographic specificity of neuronal groups within the STN, which may lead in the future to modification of the target to better suit specific purposes. One example is speech, a complex function that is not always improved and many times even worsens when the STN DBS has been implanted in the best location for improvement of motor function (Rodriguez-Oroz et al., 2005; Tornqvist et al., 2005). At present, when morbidity is low and patients can be relatively assured of an outstanding clinical benefit, the challenge for specialized teams is to search for alternatives that lead to still larger benefit by improving as many functions as possible and avoiding unwanted effects. The neurophysiological mapping of neuronal groups in the STN and other target nuclei could help to better locate the leads in the somatosensory area of the STN, avoiding associative and limbic areas.

Unfortunately, the findings on frequency of spike recordings, band power of LFPs, or even cortico-STN oscillations cannot have a direct correlation with the pathophysiological mechanisms of the disease, since the setup in which these features are recorded implies the presence of interfering factors such as anesthetics, surgery-related stress, and others that may influence brain activity in general. However, measurements of neuronal firing and

LFPs allow for understanding better the effects of medication and repetitive stimulation on the behaviour of local neuronal activity and oscillatory loops. Many authors agree in that frequency bands at about the beta range decrease with dopamine. However, it is not always clear whether repetitive STN DBS modifies the recordings in the same way, and further work is certainly needed in this regard.

2.2 Intracranial recording through the implanted electrode
2.2.1 Characteristics of the evoked potentials
Intracranial electrodes can be used to record relatively large volume conduction action potentials from distant sources. The electrodes inserted in the thalamus, mainly with the purposes of arresting tremor in patients with PD or severe ET, are likely the most appropriate for recording the evoked potentials (EP) after somatosensory stimuli (). In general, the EPs recorded from DBS electrodes are polyphasic and of a latency 2 to 3 ms shorter than the cortical EPs (Figure 2). In most occasions, the subcortical EPs have been recorded from the thalamic Vim, where the electrodes are close to the source of activity. Klosterman et al. (2003) recorded the median nerve EPs from various sites along the pathway of the electrode. When recording from sites along the tract to the STN or the Vim, the EPs were of low amplitude with no high frequency oscillations (HFO). These characteristics did not change when the electrode entered the STN, while entering the Vim it

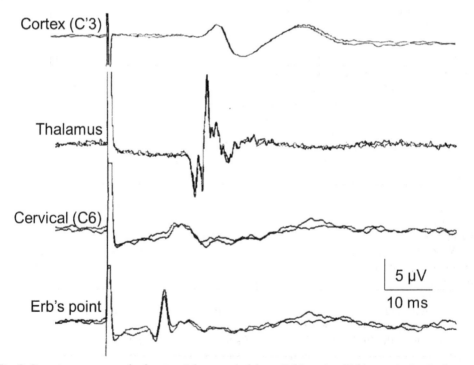

Fig. 2. Somatosensory evoked potentials recorded from Erb's point (Erb), cervical spinal cord (cervical), the nucleus ventral intermedius of the thalamus (thalamus) and the cortex to median nerve stimulation at the wrist.

was recognized by a sharp amplitude increase and the observation of HFOs. The latter were characterized by Hanajima et al. (2004a), who identified them with intrathalamic neuronal firing at intervals between 0.8 and 1.2 ms (a frequency of about 1000 Hz) and found the site of phase reversal at about the nucleus ventralis caudalis. The same authors (Hanajima et al., 2004b) recorded from the thalamic electrode a large somatosensory EP with a mean latency of 17.9+/-1.7 ms, which had a phase reversal at the level of the inter-commissural line. Assessment of phase reversal with bipolar recordings from two electrode leads may be potentially useful intraoperatory to establish the optimal position of the contacts relative to the sensory pathways, contributing to the choice of contacts for chronic stimulation. Laser stimulation has been reported recently to induce also intrathalamic evoked potentials (Kobayashi et al., 2009; Valeriani et al., 2009).

The small EPs recorded from the STN or along the tract are likely to be volume conduction from non-local generators, although Pesenti et al. (2003) proposed that the STN EPs can also be due to local field potentials elicited by muscle afferent inputs to the STN or to activity in thalamo-subthalamic projections. A few articles have been published on intracerebral recording from other nuclei than the thalamus. However, Kitagawa et al. (2007) recorded the somatosensory EPs from the thalamus and the subthalamic area, indicating that this could be a way to refine target localization. Balaz et al. (2008) recorded the P300 wave from the STN, suggesting that this nucleus is involved in cognitive executive functions.

2.2.2 Efferent and afferent gating in subcortical structures

Efferent or centrifugal gating is understood as the modulatory effect of movement on incoming sensory volleys (Grunewald et al., 1984; Cohen and Starr, 1987), while afferent or centripetal gating is understood as the competition between incoming afferent volleys to the brain (Schmidt et al., 1990; Nakajima et al., 2005). Both types of gating of EPs in humans have been documented to occur in part in subcortical structures by recording from the DBS electrodes. However, all authors agree in that a significantly larger effect is seen in scalp recordings than in subcortical recordings.

Regarding efferent gating, Valeriani et al. (2001) recorded the subcortical EPs during voluntary movement of the stimulated foot and saw a significant reduction of amplitude in all DBS recordings and in cortical somatosensory EP components following the P30 potential at the vertex but not at the contralateral temporal and ipsilateral parietal recordings. The authors speculated on the possibility that posterior tibial nerve stimulation generates two differently oriented dipoles in the contralateral hemisphere, one perpendicular to the mesial cortex and another radial to the convexity. Insola et al (2004) also reported that the movement-induced gating of somatosensory EPs occurs at a subcortical level by recording from the STN and GPi electrodes in 9 PD patients. The EPs recorded in those nuclei were triphasic (P1-N1-P2) and their latency ranged from 14 to 22 ms. When they were recorded during voluntary flexo-extension movements of the stimulated wrist, the subcortical EPs significantly decreased in the same way as the scalp N20, P22 and N30 potentials, while the response recorded in the Erb's point remained unchanged. Klosterman et al. (2002) investigated gating of intrathalamic somatosensory EPs in 10 PD patients during the surgical procedure. These authors applied median nerve stimuli to record EPs simultaneously with the intrathalamic and scalp electrodes in patients anesthetized with propofol. They compared conditions before and after application of the depolarising muscle blocker succinylcholine, i.e., with and without reafferent somatosensory inflow from background muscular tone and the repetitive muscle twitches caused by the median nerve stimulation needed to induce the EPs. The authors found no changes in the sensory nerve action potentials recorded at the upper arm, but the primary cortical component (N20) was significantly increased under succinylcholine (+17%). This cortical release from gating was not paralleled, however, by an increased thalamic response; rather, the primary thalamic response (P16) showed a significant (-9%) amplitude reduction. Thus, the findings reported by these authors suggest a thalamo-cortical dissociation in the phenomenon of gating, when tested by causing muscle relaxation, with significantly more effect in the primary somatosensory cortex than in the thalamus.

Regarding afferent gating, Hsieh et al. (1995) performed a very early study in 5 patients with PD and one with Meige's syndrome undergoing thalamotomy. These authors examined the afferent gating induced by simultaneous stimulation of two fingers. Apart from intrathalamic recordings, these authors obtained direct recordings also from the sensory and motor cortices, and the cuneate nucleus. Electrical stimulation was applied to the II, III or V fingers individually, and also to pairs of either the II and III fingers or the II and V fingers simultaneously. The authors calculated the interaction between afferent volleys as the ratio of amplitude attenuation of the EP caused by the simultaneous stimulation to two fingers compared with the amplitude of the arithmetically summed EPs to the individual stimulation of each finger. The largest interaction was observed in the responses recorded in the scalp (P25 and P22), but a significant effect was also seen in the thalamic recordings. We have examined another form of afferent gating, i.e., the simultaneous activation of fibers by two different stimulus modalities: mechanical taps to the muscle and electrical stimulation to the digital nerves. Interactions between inputs of different sensory modality occur along the sensory pathway, including the thalamus. We investigated the interactions between mechanical taps and electrical nerve stimuli in 8 patients who had an implanted electrode for deep brain stimulation for symptomatic treatment of ET or PD (Costa et al., 2008). A hand-held electronic reflex hammer was used to deliver a mechanical tap to the skin overlying the first dorsal interosseous muscle, and trigger an ipsilateral digital median nerve electrical stimulus time-locked to the mechanical tap with a variable delay of 0 to 50ms. There were significant time-dependent interactions between the two sensory volleys at subcortical level. Thalamic SEPs were decreased in amplitude at inter-stimulus intervals (ISIs) from 10 to 40ms with maximum effect at 20ms, with no changes in peripheral responses. Our results are in line with those reported in other forms of gating and indicate that gating among two different somatosensory afferent volleys occurs at various levels of the central nervous system, and although it is predominating in cortical circuits there is already a significant effect taking place at a subcortical level.

2.2.3 Discussion

Having electrodes implanted in the basal ganglia and particularly in thalamic nuclei called for investigating physiological mechanisms involving sensory events. Most of the research in this area has dealt with thalamic EPs. Although the Vim does not contain the second order neurons activated by somatosensory inputs, the EPs to median or tibial nerve stimulation show consistently reproducible HFOs thought to reflect neuronal activity in the nearby nucleus ventralis caudalis of the thalamus. A few authors have used the electrodes in the STN or GPi to record EPs. In most instances, the authors agree in the fact that the EPs recorded in these nuclei have the same characteristics as those recorded outside the thalamus and are probably volume-conducted from distant sources.

Many investigators have devoted their efforts to examine the phenomenon of gating at the thalamic level. All authors coincide in that the two main forms of gating reported in the EPs (afferent and efferent) can already be demonstrated at thalamic level. However, gating increases in more rostral structures, in such a way that the EPs recorded from scalp electrodes show more effect than those of the thalamus. The whole picture indicates that gating is a multilevel effect that begins at a point caudal to the thalamus and increases along the path up to the site of generation of the scalp EPs.

Interestingly, while nerve stimulation causes well defined EPs in the Vim, we were unable to record such EPs to mechanical muscle taps. Only a slow shift of the baseline time-locked to the mechanical stimulus was apparent in some recordings, indicating that the afferent volley has reached a central nervous system structure where it generated an action potential that is volume conducted towards the electrode. A series of studies may be necessary to determine, for instance, whether or not direct electrical stimulation of muscle afferents does or does not generate Vim EPs. It would be interesting also to use other more natural forms of stimulation to assess their effects on thalamic neurons either by direct recording of EPs or by assessing the effects that such stimuli may induce in thalamic EPs generated by electrical stimuli. In the same line, research has not been done yet in other afferent pathways, such as visual or auditory. Challenges for future investigations using intrathalamic electrodes involve not only deepening in the mechanisms of gating but also in the role of the thalamus in mediating and processing the input from different sources of information.

3. Stimulation

3.1 Experimental procedures
3.1.1 Effects due to activation of circuits and tracts

Because patients are kept awake during most of the surgical time during implantation of electrodes for DBS, the immediate beneficial effects of electrical stimulation can be evaluated in situ by clinical neurological observations and tests. Nevertheless, Liu et al. (2005) have drawn the attention to the usefulness of monitoring the effects of DBS with surface electromyography from the affected muscles to assist electrode implantation and lesioning. According to the authors, there are several potential uses of intraoperative EMG monitoring. EMG can be used as the reference signal for other events, such as the oscillatory LFPs simultaneously recorded via the implanted electrodes, to quantify the effects of acute electrical stimulation on the motor symptoms and to detect unwanted muscle responses induced by direct stimulation of the motor tract.

The effects of stimulation through the DBS electrode may be evaluated in a neurophysiological environment that is more convenient than the operating room if the electrodes are left available for a few days for further testing before implantation of the stimulator. It is understood that the electric field generated by the current delivered through the electrode spreads beyond the target nuclei and affects surrounding structures (McIntyre et al., 2004; Butson et al., 2007). According to the general principles of the effects of stimulation of the neuropil (Nowak and Bullier 1998; Ashby et al., 1999), electrical stimuli are more likely to activate axons than cell bodies, fibers near the cathode than those near the anode, and fiber tracts that run parallel rather than those that run perpendicular to the electrode. Indeed, the effects obtained with just a single stimulus at the weakest possible intensity are usually those due to activation of axons in long tracts located in the vicinity of the target nuclei. Ashby and Rothwell (2000) have summarized nicely the possibilities for neurophysiological studies using deep brain electrodes. Two structures have been used for recording: the brain and the muscle.

3.1.2 Effects on cortical activity

The EEG activity is modulated by stimuli applied through the electrodes inserted in the STN (Ashby et al., 2001). Single stimuli elicited a negative potential with an onset latency of approximately 3 ms, followed by later potentials at 5 and 8 ms, which were usually largest over the frontal region in 9 out of 11 sides. Medium latency (18-25 ms) and long latency (longer than 50 ms) responses were also reported. Short latency EPs had short chronaxie and refractory period, implying that they arose from the activation of low threshold neural elements, possibly myelinated axons. They were maintained without blocking at stimulation frequencies as high as 100 Hz. Cortical responses likely due to direct stimulation of axons running close to the electrode were reported by Baker et al. (2002) with latencies ranging from 8 to 400 ms. Medium-latency EPs, with an average onset of 14 +/- 3 ms and peak at 23 +/- 4 ms, were reported by MacKinnon et al. (2005) to low frequency STN stimulation (5-10 Hz). These authors showed that the distribution of the EPs recorded by scalp electrodes to stimuli applied through the STN electrode was similar to that of the EPs elicited by median nerve stimuli. One likely axonal bundle that may generate the EEG potentials after electrical stimulation through the electrode inserted in the STN is the pallido-thalamic tract, which contains highly myelinated axons and traverses the dorsal aspect of the STN. These authors, did not find a positive correlation between the cathodal contact that produced the largest EEG response and the one that produced the optimal clinical benefit, suggesting that the neural elements mediating the medium-latency EP are different from those responsible for clinical effects. However, Kuriakose et al. (2010) have recently suggested that one of the mechanisms by which the STN DBS causes a beneficial effect is through cortical activation. These authors examined the time course of cortical activation after controlled stimulation at the STN and suggested that cortical activation could be due to short-latency antidromic stimulation of cortico-subthalamic projections and the medium-latency facilitatory basal ganglia-thalamo-cortical interactions. No significant changes were observed in event related potentials in regard to amplitude in a standard oddball auditory paradigm (Kovacs et al., 2008), in spite of the improvement in the accuracy of the task. Interestingly, the P300 was recorded from the STN or its vicinity in 8 out of 14 leads examined by Balaz et al. (2008).

A few other observations of the effects of DBS have been reported in circuits involving the cortex. Fraix et al. (2008) reported a tendency to normalization of the contralateral silent period to TMS and short-interval intracortical facilitation during STN DBS. Herzog et al. (2008) reported improvement of integration of sensory inputs from the bladder with STN DBS 'on'. Using positron emission computed tomography (PET) they showed that urinary bladder filling led to an increased regional cerebral blood flow (rCBF) in the periaqueductal grey, the posterior thalamus, the insular cortex as well as in the right frontal cortex and the cerebellum bilaterally. These authors suggest that STN DBS facilitates the discrimination of different bodily states by supporting sensory perception and the underlying neural mechanisms.

Neuroimaging techniques have given some cues for understanding the relationship between basal ganglia nuclei and regions of the cortex using functional MRI (fMRI) (Jech et al., 2001; Perlmutter et al., 2002; Karimi et al., 2008) or rCBF with PET (Payoux et al., 2004, Grafton et al., 2006; Thobois et al., 2002; Strafella et al., 2003; Vafaee et al., 2004). In these studies, high frequency stimulation decreased the abnormal hyperactivity of the motor cortex at rest and increased activity in premotor areas during movement in PD patients. Measuring rCBF,

Payoux et al. (2009) showed opposite effects of GPi and GPe over the ipsilateral primary sensorimotor cortex. Using PET, Arai et al. (2008) observed effects of unilateral thalamic stimulation on the motor cortex of the side stimulated and on the GPi of the contralateral side, which could underline the observation of bilateral improvement after unilateral stimulation.

3.1.3 Muscle responses

Ashby et al. (1998; 1999) were the first to report the effects of controlled external stimuli using the artifact of the implanted stimulator, picked up by cutaneous electrodes, as the trigger of the recording device a few months after the stimulator had been implanted. Single stimuli modulated voluntary EMG activity of contralateral muscles, inducing a short-latency facilitation, followed by a longer latency inhibition. The authors hypothesized that facilitation was due to activation of descending axons in the corticospinal tract of the capsula interna, which lies at a mean distance of about 4.5 mm in the mediolateral plane and 2 mm in the antero-posterior plane from the tip of the electrode implanted in the STN (Schaltenbrand and Wahren, 1977; Voges et al., 2002; Molinuevo et al., 2003). Ashby et al. (1999) reported also an inhibitory effect of DBS on the ongoing voluntary activity, revealed by a decrease ('dip') in the level of EMG activity. This silent period (SP) was thought to arise from the activation of large-diameter inhibitory thalamo-cortical fibres running parallel to the electrode. Hanajima et al., (2004c) observed that 3 ms after STN stimulation, the Motor Evoked Potential (MEP) amplitudes produced by TMS-induced anterior-posterior directed currents were significantly larger than control responses, while the responses to lateral-medial currents were unchanged. Similar facilitation also occurred after GPi stimulation, but not with thalamic stimulation. Therefore, single pulse STN DBS had a short latency facilitatory effect on motor cortex, which may be due to antidromic excitation of the cortico-STN fibers or transmission through the basal ganglia-thalamocortical pathway.

Kuhn et al. (2004) compared motor effects of activation of corticospinal neurons using either subcortical (direct electrical stimulation through the DBS electrode) or cortical (indirect stimulation of cortical neurons by TMS) stimuli. The study was done in 8 dystonic patients that underwent GPi DBS, using again the artifact of the stimuli issued by the implanted electrodes as triggers for the recording. Single pulse DBS activated a fast conducting monosynaptic pathway to alpha motoneurones. The contralateral MEPs had a significantly shorter onset latency and shorter duration compared to the responses induced by TMS. They reported the observation of a contralateral SP of short duration and no ipsilateral facilitatory or inhibitory motor effects. These results suggest that DBS of the GPi activates the corticospinal neurons at the level of the internal capsule to account for the MEP, and the thalamic fasciculus or cerebellothalamic fibers to account for the SP (see also Strafella et al., 1997 and Ashby et al., 1999). The absence of ipsilateral inhibition is consistent with a transcallosal pathway for the ipsilateral SP. In contrast, our group (Compta et al., 2006), who used the electrode implanted in the STN, reported ipsilateral SP with two short duration phases. This challenged the possibility that the ipsilateral SP is mediated through the corpus callosum since the stimuli were applied caudal to the transcallosal fibers. However, the possibility still exists that some parts of the ipsilateral SP are indeed mediated through transcallosal collaterals activated antidromically.

We found a long duration contralateral SP that had the peculiarity of having a burst separating it into two parts (Figure 3). The characteristics of the contralateral SP were explained on the bases of collision between the antidromic impulses generated through the DBS electrode and the descending volleys related to voluntary activity. Collision would have freed some neurons from antidromic invasion of inhibitory collaterals and precisely the firing of these neurons with new premotor inputs would account for the burst of EMG activity breaking through the SP. Methodological differences could account for the different results reported by Kuhn et al. (2004) and our group (Compta et al., 2006). Kuhn et al. (2004) used electrodes inserted in the GPi, which is slightly more rostral, anterior and lateral than the STN, and could activate a different bunch of corticospinal axons than the electrode inserted in the STN. The same differences apply to the volley reaching the axons responsible for inhibitory effects via the thalamus. Whereas Compta et al. (2006) studied patients with Parkinson's disease, Kuhn et al. (2004) studied patients with generalized dystonia who are known to have a disorder of inhibition and an abnormally shorter SP (Ridding et al., 1995; Chen et al., 1997). Finally, Kuhn et al. (2004) applied the stimuli at a frequency of 5 Hz from the implanted generators, which allows for a relatively short time for analysis between two consecutive stimuli.

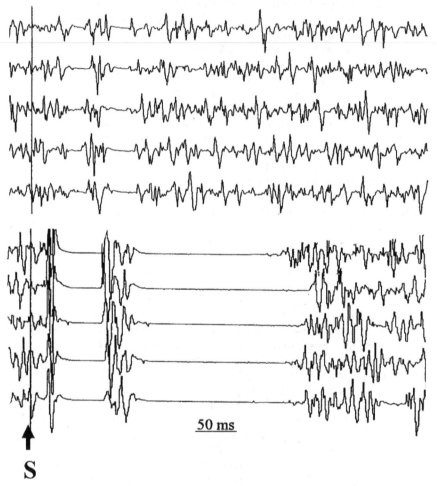

Fig. 3. Contralateral and ipsilateral silent periods induced by a single unilateral suprathreshold stimulus through the electrode inserted in the STN

Obviously, MEPs are not only obtained in hand muscles but in all muscles receiving innervation through fibers running in the capsula interna. This includes the cortico-bulbar tract. Fibers of the cortico-bulbar tract run in the genu of the capsula interna and are readily accessible to stimuli applied through the DBS electrode. Our knowledge of the distribution of cortical innervation to muscles innervated by cranial nerves is less accurate than for limb muscles because of various drawbacks of cortical stimulation such as the generation of large artefacts and the unavoidable elicitation of direct and reflex responses to activation of cranial nerves in the posterior fossa. We studied responses of cranial nerve innervated muscles to single STN DBS in 14 PD patients (Costa et al., 2007). The stimulus intensity used was 130% the resting threshold for an MEP in the thenar muscles. The inhibitory effects were also examined during sustained voluntary contraction of about 20% of maximum. As expected, unilateral stimuli induced strictly contralateral responses in thenar muscles at a mean latency of 20.1±2.0 ms. The MEPs obtained in the trapezius, deltoid and biceps muscles were also present in only the contralateral side, but the same stimulus induced always (i.e., a probability of 100%) bilateral MEPs in orbicularis oculi, orbicularis oris, masseter and sternocleidomastoid. The mean MEP latency ranged from 6.0 to 9.1 ms. The MEP latencies were significantly longer in facial nerve innervated muscles than in masseter and sternocleidomastoid muscles (Figure 4).

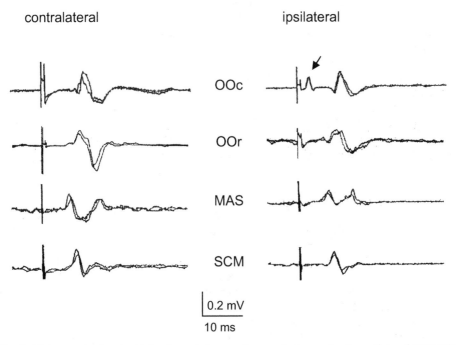

Fig. 4. Motor evoked potentials of cranial nerve innervated muscles to unilateral STN DBS electrode stimulation. Responses in the contralateral muscles are on the left side column while those of the ipsilateral muscles are on the right side column. OOc= Orbicularis oculi; OOr=Orbicularis oris; MAS= Maseter; SCM= sternocleidomastoid. Note the small short latency potential in the ipsilateral orbicularis oculi (inclined arrow)

Well defined SPs to single unilateral STN stimuli were present in both sides in the orbicularis oculi and masseter muscles in all patients, probably due to transient alpha motoneuron refractoriness after synchronized firing, blocking of the arrival of excitatory inputs to the motoneurons (Compta et al., 2006), and activation of thalamocortical inhibitory projections (Strafella et al., 1997). The amplitude of the MEP elicited during contraction was higher, and the duration of the SP was significantly longer, in the contralateral with respect to the ipsilateral sides. However, duration of the SP had no significant correlation with amplitude of the MEP.

3.1.4 Discussion

It seems obvious that chronic high frequency DBS causes its therapeutic effects by changing neuronal excitability in the area covered by the electrical field. Therefore, several authors have studied the effect in neurons in the vicinity. However, the mechanism of action of high frequency DBS is far from being clarified. Instead, the analysis of the effects of stimulation through one electrode lead and recording with a nearby electrode has brought new evidences for interconnections between nuclei of the basal ganglia. As expected, the observations suggest a more complex circuitry than a simple chain of nuclei with excitatory and inhibitory connections. In at least some connections, the frequency of inputs determines the sign of the effect while in others the exact site of the nucleus receiving the inputs is what makes a difference. This is likely reflecting that we are beginning to establish the temporal and spatial characteristics of the connectivity between basal ganglia nuclei and from the basal ganglia to output structures.

STN DBS induces consistent changes in cortical metabolism that can be summarized as a decrease of motor cortical activity at rest and an increase in cortical activity of the supplementary motor area and premotor cortex during active movements. However, the changes in metabolism do not necessarily show the function of the neurons undergoing such change, because they may involve both facilitatory and inhibitory neurons. Unfortunately, a good correlation between neuroimaging studies reflecting changes in metabolism and neurophysiology studies showing changes in cortical excitability has not yet been done.

There are effects of STN DBS on tracts with long projections that run close to the position of the electrode. We do not know if activation of those tracts contributes somehow to the clinical effects of DBS. Corticonuclear and corticospinal fiber tracts can be activated at relatively low intensity through the electrodes inserted in the STN or in the GPi. It is noteworthy that the effects on the motor tract of stimuli applied through the STN electrode seem not to be the same as those induced by stimuli applied through the GPi electrode (Kuhn et al., 2004; Compta et al., 2006). If these differences hold true in future works, they may be a hint to further understand the differential mechanisms of action of electrodes inserted in the two nuclei.

As with the MEPs elicited in hand muscles, the most likely physiological mechanism accounting for the generation of the MEPs in cranial nerve innervated muscles is activation of axons of the corticonuclear tracts within the internal capsule. However, in the case of the facial nucleus, Morecraft et al. (2001) have reported up to 5 projections from motor cortical areas to subsectors of the facial nucleus. Therefore, the MEPs obtained in cranial nerve innervated muscles by single pulse STN DBS could result from activation of just one of the many descending corticonuclear pathways, the function of which is largely unknown.

3.2 Effects of DBS on neurophysiological tests of clinical use

Several studies have demonstrated that high frequency DBS improves the symptoms of PD patients. These effects have been documented and quantified using clinical scales. For instance, a clinical significant effect of the treatment is usually considered when there is more than 30% improvement in the UPDRS score. However, researchers have been interested in knowing how DBS modifies certain clinical neurophysiological abnormalities that may not have a direct clinical correlate but support in part pathophysiological mechanisms underlying parkinsonian symptoms and signs (Hallett, 1998; Rossini et al., 1998; Deecke, 2001; Valls-Solé and Valldeoriola, 2002). This has a double advantage: One is the quantitation and documentation of improvement through objective scales; the other is the determination of the neurophysiological abnormalities that are more closely related to clinical changes. Usually, the clinical and neurophysiological effects of DBS are compared with those of dopaminergic medication in a quadruple comparison: 'on' vs. 'off' medication and 'on' vs. 'off' stimulation.

3.2.1 Cortical physiology

One of the first observations on the neurophysiological effects of DBS was the change in contingent negative variation reported by Gerschlager et al. (1999) with bilateral STN DBS in PD patients. The contingent negative variation is a slow negative potential shift reflecting cognitive processes associated with the preparation and/or anticipation of a response that has been found to be reduced over the frontal and frontocentral regions in PD (Deecke, 2001). The increase in amplitude of the contingent negative variation with STN DBS 'on' (Gerschlager et al., 1999) suggests improvement of the impaired cortical functioning in PD, particularly within the frontal and premotor areas.

In a series of works on ERD preceding movement and ERS at movement termination, Devos et al. (2003, 2004, 2006) showed that STN DBS had also effects on the abnormally reduced and delayed cortical oscillatory activity patterns of PD patients, which have been considered a correlate of bradykinesia (Magnani et al., 1998; Brown and Marsden, 1999). The effects shown by Devos et al. with STN DBS (2003, 2004) were similar to those of an acute administration of L-Dopa. Interestingly, when recording ERD and ERS from the electrode inserted in the STN, the contacts that produced the best clinical results were also those showing the earliest mu and beta ERD and the strongest beta and gamma ERS.

The effects of STN or GPi DBS on motor cortex excitability have been studied by many authors. Chen et al. (2001) reported the effects of GPi DBS on several brain circuits that may exhibit functional abnormalities when examined with neurophysiological methods in PD patients. These included motor threshold, MEP recruitment curve, SP duration, short interval intracortical inhibition (SICI), long interval intracortical inhibition, and intracortical facilitation. The stimulators were set at the optimal parameters, at half the optimal stimulus intensity or switched off, in random order, while patients remained in their usual medication condition. No significant differences were found in most tests among the three conditions, the only exception being a reduction in the SP duration. Similar absence of modification of SICI was reported by Kuhn et al. (2003) during GPi DBS in patients with dystonia. However, switching off GPi stimulation led to an increase in motor threshold, and reduced the size of contralateral responses in the stimulus-response curves in relaxed muscles. On top of that, the authors reported no STN DBS related changes in spinal excitability, assessed by the H-reflex in the forearm muscles.

A different result was reported by Cunic et al. (2002) who examined the effects of STN DBS on cortical excitability in 9 PD patients, using the same protocol that Chen et al. (2001) and Kuhn et al. (2003) used for the GPi. These authors found that resting SICI, studied with paired-pulse TMS at the interstimulus interval of 2 ms, was restored to normal levels in the 'on' condition. Opposite to the results reported with GPi DBS, STN DBS did not induce changes in SP duration, motor threshold or MEP recruitment curve. Thus, in parallel to the differences found when recording hand muscle responses (Kuhn et al., 2004; Compta et al., 2006), it seems that the effects of STN DBS are different from those of the GPi DBS on motor cortex excitability changes accessible to neurophysiological testing with TMS. The effects of STN DBS on resting SICI were confirmed by Pierantozzi et al. (2002), who found an increase in SICI at intervals of 2 ms with STN and 2 and 3 ms with GPi. The improvement was similar to the one provided by apomorphine infusion. The authors suggest that improvement of SICI may be related to a recovery in modulation of thalamo-cortical motor pathway.

3.2.2 Subcortical circuits

Tisch et al. (2006a) measured changes in the excitability of the blink reflex after GPi DBS in 10 patients with dystonia. The abnormally enhanced excitability recovery after a conditioning stimulus (Kimura, 1973) was found to decrease progressively at intervals of 1, 3, and 6 months after surgery, suggesting that GPi DBS results in functional reorganization of the nervous system and a long-term increase in brainstem inhibition. Another dysfunction seen in the recording of the blink reflexes in PD patients is reduced prepulse inhibition (Schicatano et al., 2000; Valls-Solé et al., 2004). The pathophysiology of this phenomenon is not clarified but the abnormalities observed in PD may be due to a dysfunction in the connections between the basal ganglia and the brainstem nuclei, particularly the PPN (Pahapill and Lozano, 2000). We investigated the prepulse effects of single electrical STN DBS on the blink reflex induced in orbicularis oculi muscle by supraorbital electrical nerve stimulation in 7 PD patients (Costa et al., 2006). Five of them had an abnormally reduced prepulse inhibition to auditory and somatosensory stimuli. In all 7 patients, stimuli applied through the STN electrodes induced significant inhibition of the R2 at inter-stimuli intervals between 10 and 30 ms, with a mean percentage inhibition of 92% at 20 ms. Therefore, dysfunction of auditory and somatosensory prepulses in PD patients cannot be due to the machinery activated by DBS. We proposed that either the abnormal reduction in prepulse inhibition lies in a point of the circuit before reaching the structures activated by DBS, or STN DBS causes the prepulse by a different circuit than auditory and somatosensory stimuli.

The effects of DBS on spinal cord excitability have been reported for propriospinal circuits in the forearm (Tisch et al., 2006b) and in the leg (Potter et al., 2004). Tisch et al. (2006) reported a progressive improvement of the reciprocal inhibitory effect of a radial nerve stimulus on the median nerve H reflex, at 1,3, and 6 months of GPi DBS in patients with dystonia, and suggested that DBS causes functional reorganization of the nervous system that includes the spinal machinery. Potter et al. (2004) reported an increase of autogenic inhibition of the soleus H reflex, a propriospinal inhibitory phenomenon that has been found to be abnormal in PD (Delwaide et al., 1991). The authors measured the soleus H-reflex alone or conditioned by previous gastrocnemius nerve stimulation at ISIs of 2 to 10 ms in 10 PD patients. STN DBS induced an increase in the inhibitory effect of the conditioning stimulus that was significantly correlated with the clinical improvement of gait and posture. In a more recent work, the same group (Tisch et al., 2007) reported the absence of long-term potentiation-like effect in patients with dystonia and GPi DBS. This has been considered a sign of abnormal plasticity in patients with dystonia (Quartarone et al., 2003). Therefore, this negative result could be reflecting the mechanism of action of pallidal DBS in dystonia.

Activity in descending tracts facilitates the soleus H reflex but such facilitation is abnormally decreased in patients with PD. This has been shown for auditory stimuli (Delwaide et al., 1993) and for TMS (Valls-Sole and Valldeoriola, 2002). Potter-Nerger et al. (2008) reported an improvement of the descending modulation of the H reflex by continuous high frequency STN DBS. Using single pulse STN DBS, we found in 11 PD patients that it modulates the amplitude of the soleus H reflex and therefore the net influence of the various mechanisms determining the excitability of the spinal alpha-motoneuron pool (Costa et al., 2011). Furthermore, the modulation of the H reflex was different according to the site of stimulation (ipsilateral vs. contralateral). In the case of contralateral single pulse STN DBS, the modulation of the soleus H reflex is distributed in an early and late facilitation phases, while in the case of ipsilateral single pulse STN DBS, there is a single early facilitation phase. Whether the modulation of the H reflex by STN DBS is the consequence of direct or indirect effects on the reticulospinal motor system is presently unknown.

The work of Tisch et al. and Potter et al. are just illustrative studies of one of the many positive effects reported during continuous high frequency STN DBS in the various abnormalities described in patients with PD, dystonia or ET (Sailer et al., 2007 for afferent inhibition; Potter et al., 2008 for audiospinal reactions; Yugeta et al., 2010, for the initiation and inhibition of saccades; Kronenbuerger et al., 2010 for eyeblink conditioning).

3.2.3 Discussion

In general terms, DBS causes changes in neurophysiological tests of clinical use that consist in a tendency to normalization, although in many occasions differences remain between patients with DBS 'on' and control subjects. This is consistent with clinical observations and points to a good correlate of some neurophysiological tests. This is particularly true for those tests related to planning and execution of voluntary movements such as the ERD or the cognitive negative variation. Changes in these tests demonstrate the influence of basal ganglia on cortical reactivity.

Less straightforward are the results of the assessment of motor cortical excitability at rest or during tonic voluntary contraction. Although there is no complete agreement among all authors, changes in SICI and in the SP duration seem not to result from activation of the same structure since most studies show that when there is reduction in SICI there is no effect on SP duration and viceversa. Interestingly, GPi and STN seem to give different results, reinforcing the possibility to identify distinctive neurophysiological outcome from the two nuclei.

The effects of DBS on subcortical circuits, including the brainstem and spinal levels, indicate a tendency to normalization of the results of neurophysiological tests. One of the subcortical circuits of interest in PD is the one responsible for prepulse inhibition (Fendt et al., 2001). The abnormally reduced prepulse inhibition in PD patients (Schicatano et al., 2000; Valls-Solé et al., 2004) reflects in part disturbed sensorimotor integration, but the normality of the effects when DBS is used as prepulse indicate that the defect does not lie ahead of the structures activated by the stimulus. We cannot assume that the circuit of prepulse inhibition is the same with DBS and with auditory or somatosensory stimuli. Actually, the STN is not part of the circuit of the prepulse. However, fibers connecting the GPi and the

PPN run close to the STN (Swerdlow et al., 2001) and might have been activated by the stimulus through the STN electrode. If this was the case, two explanations should be considered: One is that the dysfunction responsible for the loss of prepulse inhibition by acoustic and somatosensory inputs lies in circuits rostral to the PPN. One such possibility is the nucleus reticularis pontis caudalis, which receives inputs from the acoustic and somatosensory stimuli, and has reciprocal connections to the PPN. Another is that STN DBS induces its effects at a point beyond the PPN in the prepulse circuit. In favour of the first hypothesis is the fact that PD patients have an abnormal startle reaction due to dysfunction in nuclei of the reticular formation. In favour of the second hypothesis is the fact that STN DBS is known to cause inhibitory effects by way of activating afferents to the thalamic nuclei. Only further work in the area may help in answering the questions that remain unsolved by the findings reported so far.

4. Conclusion and future perspectives

The outstanding clinical neurophysiological investigation that is currently ongoing makes probably superfluous the task of guessing what can be expected in future years in this field. Nevertheless, the rapid growing understanding of both, the physiology and pathophysiology mechanisms of the different subcortical-cortical circuits, as well as the underlying clinical neurophysiological mechanisms of DBS, points to the possibility in the near future to: (1) Change the paradigm of DBS to another one were patients are treated with electrodes placed simultaneous in different nuclei (e.g. STN and PPN); (2) Allow for the simultaneous assessment of neuronal activity through recording of LFPs from DBS electrode leads and the consequent change in DBS stimulation parameters delivered by other DBS electrode leads, in a kind of real time individualised DBS therapy; (3) Begin to explore the possibility of improving non-motor symptoms through identification of new targets and stimulation parameters.

Many more studies than those reported here dealing with the effects of DBS have been published, bringing small or large pieces of information to increase our understanding of how the basal ganglia participate in the very many tasks that they are assigned. In this review, we attempted to focus on neurophysiological aspects of DBS not necessarily correlated with therapeutic effects. Understanding the physiological mechanisms accounting for some of the events seen with DBS is a growing field in which relevant contributions appear often in the literature and some of them might have done so while this chapter was in the review or publication processes. We hope, however, that this review reflects the state of our knowledge at the beginning of a new era in neurophysiology: that of direct recording and stimulation from deep brain electrodes. We hope also that it stimulates research in the field, the only way to eventually understand at least partially the function of the basal ganglia and subcortical motor circuits.

5. References

Alegre M, Alonso-Frech F, Rodriguez-Oroz MC, Guridi J, Zamarbide I, Valencia M, Manrique M, Obeso JA, Artieda J. Movement-related changes in oscillatory activity in the human subthalamic nucleus: ipsilateral vs. contralateral movements. Eur J Neurosci 2005;22:2315-2324.

Alegre M, Rodríguez-Oroz MC, Valencia M, Pérez-Alcázar M, Guridi J, Iriarte J, Obeso JA, Artieda J. Changes in subthalamic activity during movement observation in Parkinson's disease: is the mirror system mirrored in the basal ganglia? Clin Neurophysiol 2010;121:414-425.

Alessandro S, Ceravolo R, Brusa L, Pierantozzi M, Costa A, Galati S, Placidi F, Romigi A, Iani C, Marzetti F, Peppe A. Non-motor functions in parkinsonian patients implanted in the pedunculopontine nucleus: focus on sleep and cognitive domains. J Neurol Sci 2010;289:44-48.

Alexander GE, Crutcher MD. Functional architecture of basal ganglia circuits: neural substrates of parallel processing. Trends Neurosci 1990;13:266-271.

Alonso-Frech F, Zamarbide I, Alegre M, Rodriguez-Oroz MC, Guridi J, Manrique M, Valencia M, Artieda J, Obeso JA. Slow oscillatory activity and levodopa-induced dyskinesias in Parkinson's disease. Brain 2006;129:1748-1757.

Androulidakis AG, Kühn AA, Chen CC, Blomstedt P, Kempf F, Kupsch A, Schneider GH, Doyle L, Dowsey-Limousin P, Hariz MI, Brown P. Dopaminergic therapy promotes lateralized motor activity in the subthalamic area in Parkinson's disease. Brain 2007;130:457-468.

Arai N, Yokochi F, Ohnishi T, Momose T, Okiyama R, Taniguchi M, Takahashi H, Matsuda H, Ugawa Y. Mechanisms of unilateral STN-DBS in patients with Parkinson's disease: a PET study. J Neurol 2008;255:1236-1243.

Ashby P, Strafella A, Dostrovsky JO, Lozano A, Lang AE. Immediate motor effects of stimulation through electrodes implanted in the human globus pallidus. Stereotact Funct Neurosurg 1998;70:1-18.

Ashby P, Kim JY, Kumar R, Lang AE, Lozano AM. Neurophysiological effects of stimulation through electrodes in the human subthalamic nucleus. Brain 1999; 122: 1919-1931.

Ashby P, Rothwell JC. Neurophysiologic aspects of deep brain stimulation. Neurology 2000;55(Suppl 6):S17-20.

Ashby P, Paradiso G, Saint-Cyr JA, Chen R, Lang AE, Lozano AM. Potentials recorded at the scalp by stimulation near the human subthalamic nucleus. Clin Neurophysiol 2001;112:431-437.

Baker KB, Montgomery Jr EB, Rezai AR, Burgess R, Lüders HO. Subthalamic nucleus deep brain stimulus evoked potentials: Physiological and therapeutical implications. Mov Disord 2002;17:969-983.

Baláz M, Rektor I, Pulkrábek J. Participation of the subthalamic nucleus in executive functions: An intracerebral recording study. Mov Disord 2008;23:553-557.

Benabid AL, Chabardes S, Mitrofanis J, Pollak P. Deep brain stimulation of the subthalamic nucleus for the treatment of Parkinson's disease. Lancet Neurol 2009;8:67-81.

Benazzouz A, Breit S, Koudsie A, Pollak P, Krack P, Benabid AL. Intraoperative microrecordings of the subthalamic nucleus in Parkinson's disease. Mov Disord 2002;17 Suppl3:S145-149.

Bronte-Stewart H, Barberini C, Koop MM, Hill BC, Henderson JM, Wingeier B. The STN beta-band profile in Parkinson's disease is stationary and shows prolonged attenuation after deep brain stimulation.Exp Neurol 2009;215:20-28.

Brown P, Marsden CD. Bradykinesia and impairment of EEG desynchronization in Parkinson's disease. Mov Disord 1999;14:423-429.

Brown P, Williams D, Aziz T, Mazzone P, Oliviero A, Insola A, Tonali P, Di

Lazzaro V. Pallidal activity recorded in patients with implanted electrodes predictively correlates with eventual performance in a timing task. Neurosci Lett 2002;330:188-192.

Brown P. Oscillatory nature of human basal ganglia activity: relationship to the pathophysiology of Parkinson's disease. Mov Disord 2003;18:357-363.

Brown P, Williams D. Basal ganglia local field potential activity: character and functional significance in the human. Clin Neurophysiol 2005;116:2510-2519.

Burke D, Hicks RG. Surgical monitoring of motor pathways. J Clin Neurophysiol 1998;15:194-205.

Butson CR, Cooper SE, Henderson JM, McIntyre CC. Patient-specific analysis of the volume of tissue activated during deep brain stimulation. Neuroimage 2007;34:661-670.

Carlson JD, Cleary DR, Cetas JS, Heinricher MM, Burchiel KJ. Deep brain stimulation does not silence neurons in subthalamic nucleus in Parkinson's patients. J Neurophysiol 2010;103:962-967.

Cassidy M, Mazzone P, Oliviero A, Insola A, Tonali P, Di Lazzaro V, Brown P. Movement-related changes in synchronization in the human basal ganglia. Brain 2002;125:1235-1246.

Chen R, Wassermann EM, Canos M, Hallett M. Impaired inhibition in writer's cramp during voluntary muscle contraction. Neurology 1997; 49: 1054-1059.

Chen R, Garg RR, Lozano AM, Lang AE. Effects of internal globus pallidus stimulation on motor cortex excitability. Neurology 2001;56:716-723.

Chen H, Zhuang P, Miao SH, Yuan G, Zhang YQ, Li JY, Li YJ. Neuronal firing in the ventrolateral thalamus of patients with Parkinson's disease differs from that with essential tremor. Chin Med J 2010;123:695-701.

Chu Chen C, Kuhn AA, Trottenberg T, Kupsch A, Schneider GH, Brown P. Neuronal activity in globus pallidus interna can be synchronized to local field potential activity over 3-12 Hz in patients with dystonia. Exp Neurol 2006;202:480-486.

Cohen LG, Starr A. Localization, timing and specificity of gating of somatosensory evoked potentials during active movement in man. Brain 1987;110:451-467.

Compta Y, Valls-Sole J, Valldeoriola F, Kumru H, Rumia J. The silent period of the thenar muscles to contralateral and ipsilateral deep brain stimulation. Clin Neurophys 2006;117:2512-2520.

Costa J, Valls-Sole J, Valldeoriola F, Pech C, Rumia J. Single subthalamic nucleus deep brain stimuli inhibit the blink reflex in Parkinson's disease patients. Brain 2006;129:1758-1767.

Costa J, Valls-Sole J, Valldeoriola F, Rumia J, Tolosa E. Motor responses of muscles supplied by cranial nerves to subthalamic nucleus deep brain stimuli. Brain 2007;130:245-255.

Costa J, Valls-Solé J, Valldeoriola F, Rumià J. Subcortical interactions between somatosensory stimuli of different modalities and their temporal profile. J Neurophysiol 2008;100:1610-1621.

Costa J, Guzmán J, Valldeoriola F, Rumià J, Tolosa E, Casanova-Molla J, Valls-Solé J. Modulation of the soleus H reflex by electrical subcortical stimuli in humans. Exp Brain Res 2011 (in press).

Cunic D, Roshan L, Khan FI, Lozano AM, Lang AE, Chen R. Effects of subthalamic nucleus stimulation on motor cortex excitability in Parkinson's disease. Neurology 2002;58:1665-1672.

Danish SF, Moyer JT, Finkel LH, Baltuch GH, Jaggi JL, Priori A, Foffani G. High-frequency oscillations (>200 Hz) in the human non-parkinsonian subthalamic nucleus. Brain Res Bull 2007;74:84-90.

Danish SF, Baltuch GH, Jaggi JL, Wong S. Determination of subthalamic nucleus location by quantitative analysis of despiked background neural activity from microelectrode recordings obtained during deep brain stimulation surgery. J Clin Neurophysiol 2008;25:98-103.

Deecke L. Clinical neurophysiology of Parkinson's disease. Bereitschaftspotential and contingent negative variation. Adv Neurol 2001;86:257-271.

Deletis V, Sala F. Intraoperative neurophysiological monitoring of the spinal cord during spinal cord and spine surgery: a review focus on the corticospinal tracts. Clin Neurophysiol 2008;119:248-264.

Delwaide PJ, Pepin JL, Maertens de Noordhout A. Short-latency autogenic inhibition in patients with Parkinsonian rigidity. Ann Neurol 1991;30:83-89.

Delwaide PJ, Pepin JL, Maertens de Noordhout A. The audiospinal reaction in Parkinsonian patients reflect functional changes in reticular nuclei. Ann Neurol 1993; 33: 63–9.

Devos D, Labyt E, Cassim F, Bourriez JL, Reyns N, Touzet G, Blond S, Guieu JD, Derambure P, Destée A, Defebvre L. Subthalamic stimulation influences postmovement cortical somatosensory processing in Parkinson's disease. Eur J Neurosci 2003;18:1884-1888.

Devos D, Labyt E, Derambure P, Bourriez JL, Cassim F, Reyns N, Blond S, Guieu JD, Destée A, Defebvre L. Subthalamic nucleus stimulation modulates motor cortex oscillatory activity in Parkinson's disease. Brain 2004;127:408-419.

Devos D, Szurhaj W, Reyns N, Labyt E, Houdayer E, Bourriez JL, Cassim F, Krystkowiak P, Blond S, Destée A, Derambure P, Defebvre L. Predominance of the contralateral movement-related activity in the subthalamo-cortical loop. Clin Neurophysiol 2006;117:2315-2327.

Di Lazzaro V, Pilato F, Oliviero A, Dileone M, Saturno E, Mazzone P, Insola A, Profice P, Ranieri F, Capone F, Tonali PA, Rothwell JC. Origin of facilitation of motor-evoked potentials after paired magnetic stimulation: direct recording of epidural activity in conscious humans. J Neurophysiol 2006;96:1765-771.

Dostrovsky JO, Levy R, Wu JP, Hutchison WD, Tasker RR, Lozano AM. Microstimulation-induced inhibition of neuronal firing in human globus pallidus. J Neurophysiol 2000;84:570-574.

Fendt M, Li L, Yeomans JS. Brain stem circuits mediating prepulse inhibition of the startle reflex. Psychopharmacology 2001;156:216-224.

Filali M, Hutchison WD, Palter VN, Lozano AM, Dostrovsky JO. Stimulation-induced inhibition of neuronal firing in human subthalamic nucleus. Exp Brain Res 2004;156:274-281.

Foffani G, Priori A, Egidi M, Rampini P, Tamma F, Caputo E et al. 300-Hz subthalamic oscillations in Parkinson's disease. Brain 2003;126:2153-2163.

Foffani G, Bianchi AM, Baselli G, Priori A. Movement-related frequency modulation of beta oscillatory activity in the human subthalamic nucleus. J Physiol 2005;568:699-711.

Foltynie T, Hariz MI. Surgical management of Parkinson's disease. Expert Rev Neurother 2010;10:903-914.

Fraix V, Pollak P, Vercueil L, Benabid AL, Mauguière F. Effects of subthalamic nucleus stimulation on motor cortex excitability in Parkinson's disease. Clin Neurophysiol. 2008;119:2513-2518.

Galati S, Scarnati E, Mazzone P, Stanzione P, Stefani A. Deep brain stimulation promotes excitation and inhibition in subthalamic nucleus in Parkinson's disease. Neuroreport 2008;19:661-666.

Gaynor LM, Kühn AA, Dileone M, Litvak V, Eusebio A, Pogosyan A, Androulidakis AG, Tisch S, Limousin P, Insola A, Mazzone P, Di Lazzaro V, Brown P. Suppression of beta oscillations in the subthalamic nucleus following cortical stimulation in humans. Eur J Neurosci. 2008;28:1686-1695.

Gerschlager W, Alesch F, Cunnington R, Deecke L, Dirnberger G, Endl W, Lindinger G, Lang W. Bilateral subthalamic nucleus stimulation improves frontal cortex function in Parkinson's disease. An electrophysiological study of the contingent negative variation. Brain 1999;122:2365-2373.

Giannicola G, Marceglia S, Rossi L, Mrakic-Sposta S, Rampini P, Tamma F, Cogiamanian F, Barbieri S, Priori A. The effects of levodopa and ongoing deep brain stimulation on subthalamic beta oscillations in Parkinson's disease. Exp Neurol 2010;226:120-127.

Grafton ST, Turner RS, Desmurget M, Bakay R, Delong M, Vitek J, Crutcher M. Normalizing motor-related brain activity: subthalamic nucleus stimulation in Parkinson disease. Neurology 2006;66:1192-1199.

Grunewald G, Grunewald-Zuberbier E, Schuhmacher H, Mewald J, Noth J. Somatosensory evoked potentials to mechanical disturbances of positioning movements in man: gating of middle-range components. Electroencephalogr Clin Neurophysiol 1984;58:525-536.

Guehl D, Edwards R, Cuny E, Burbaud P, Rougier A, Modolo J, Beuter A. Statistical determination of the optimal subthalamic nucleus stimulation site in patients with Parkinson disease. J Neurosurg 2007;106:101-110.

Hallett M. The neurophysiology of dystonia. Arch Neurol 1998;55:601-603.

Hanajima R, Chen R, Ashby P, Lozano AM, Hutchison WD, Davis KD, Dostrovsky JO. Very fast oscillations evoked by median nerve stimulation in the human thalamus and subthalamic nucleus. J Neurophysiol 2004a;92:3171-3182.

Hanajima R, Dostrovsky JO, Lozano AM, Hutchison WD, Davis KD, Chen R, Ashby P. Somatosensory evoked potentials (SEPs) recorded from deep brain stimulation (DBS) electrodes in the thalamus and subthalamic nucleus (STN). Clin Neurophysiol 2004b;115:424-434.

Hanajima R, Ashby P, Lozano AM, Lang AE, Chen R. Single pulse stimulation of the human subthalamic nucleus facilitates the motor cortex at short intervals. J Neurophysiol 2004c;92:1937-1943.

Herzog J, Hamel W, Wenzelburger R, Pötter M, Pinsker MO, Bartussek J, Morsnowski A, Steigerwald F, Deuschl G, Volkmann J. Kinematic analysis of thalamic versus subthalamic neurostimulation in postural and intention tremor. Brain 2007;130:1608-1625.

Herzog J, Weiss PH, Assmus A, Wefer B, Seif C, Braun PM, Pinsker MO, Herzog H, Volkmann J, Deuschl G, Fink GR. Improved sensory gating of urinary bladder afferents in Parkinson's disease following subthalamic stimulation. Brain 2008;131:132-145.

Horikoshi T, Omata T, Uchida M, Asari Y, Nukui H. Usefulness and pitfalls of intraoperative spinal motor evoked potential recording by direct cortical electrical stimulation. Acta Neurochir 2000;142:257-262.

Hsieh CL, Shima F, Tobimatsu S, Sun SJ, Kato M. The interaction of the somatosensory evoked potentials to simultaneous finger stimuli in the human central nervous system. A study using direct recordings. Electroencephalogr Clin Neurophysiol 1995;96:135-142.

Hutchison WD, Levy R, Dostrovsky JO, Lozano AM, Lang AE. Effects of apomorphine on globus pallidus neurons in parkinsonian patients. Ann Neurol 1997;42:767-775.

Hutchison WD, Allan RJ, Opitz H, Levy R, Dostrovsky JO, Lang AE, Lozano AM. Neurophysiological identification of the subthalamic nucleus in surgery for Parkinson's disease. Ann Neurol 1998;44:622-628.

Hutchison WD, Lang AE, Dostrovsky JO, Lozano AM. Pallidal neuronal activity: implications for models of dystonia. Ann Neurol 2003;53:480-488.

Ince NF, Gupte A, Wichmann T, Ashe J, Henry T, Bebler M, Eberly L, Abosch A. Selection of optimal programming contacts based on local field potential recordings from subthalamic nucleus in patients with Parkinson's disease.Neurosurgery 2010;67:390-397.

Insola A, Le Pera D, Restuccia D, Mazzone P, Valeriani M. Reduction in amplitude of the subcortical low- and high-frequency somatosensory evoked potentials during voluntary movement: an intracerebral recording study. Clin Neurophysiol 2004;115:104-111.

Jech R, Urgosik D, Tintera J, Nebuzelsky A, Krasensky J, Liscak R, Roth J, Růzicka E. Functional magnetic resonance imaging during deep brain stimulation: a pilot study in four patients with Parkinson's disease. Mov Disord 2001;16:1126-1132.

Karimi M, Golchin N, Tabbal SD, Hershey T, Videen TO, Wu J, Usche JW, Revilla FJ, Hartlein JM, Wernle AR, Mink JW, Perlmutter JS. Subthalamic nucleus stimulation-induced regional blood flow responses correlate with improvement of motor signs in Parkinson disease. Brain 2008;131:2710-2719.

Kimura J. Disorder of interneurons in Parkinsonism. The orbicularis oculi reflex to paired stimuli. Brain 1973; 96: 87-96.

Kitagawa M, Murata J, Uesugi H, Hanajima R, Ugawa Y, Saito H. Characteristics and distribution of somatosensory evoked potentials in the subthalamic region. J Neurosurg 2007;107:548-554.

Klostermann F, Gobbele R, Buchner H, Curio G. Dissociation of human thalamic and cortical SEP gating as revealed by intrathalamic recordings under muscle relaxation. Brain Res 2002; 958: 146-151.

Klostermann F, Vesper J, Curio G. Identification of target areas for deep brain stimulation in human basal ganglia substructures based on median nerve sensory evoked potential criteria. J Neurol Neurosurg Psychiatry 2003;74:1031-1035.

Kobayashi K, Winberry J, Liu CC, Treede RD, Lenz FA.A painful cutaneous laser stimulus evokes responses from single neurons in the human thalamic principal somatic sensory nucleus ventral caudal (Vc). J Neurophysiol 2009;101:2210-2217.

Kovacs N, Balas I, Kellenyi L, Janszky J, Feldmann A, Llumiguano C, Doczi TP, Ajtay Z, Nagy F. The impact of bilateral subthalamic deep brain stimulation on long-latency event-related potentials. Parkinsonism Relat Disord 2008;14:476-480.

Kronenbuerger M, Tronnier VM, Gerwig M, Fromm C, Coenen VA, Reinacher P, Kiening KL, Noth J, Timmann D. Thalamic deep brain stimulation improves eyeblink conditioning deficits in essential tremor. Exp Neurol. 2008;211:387-396.

Kuhn AA, Meyer BU, Trottenberg T, Brandt SA, Schneider GH, Kupsch A. Modulation of motor cortex excitability by pallidal stimulation in patients with severe dystonia. Neurology 2003;60:768-774.

Kuhn AA, Brandt SA, Kupsch A, Trottenberg T, Brocke J, Irlbacher K et al. Meyer BU. Comparison of motor effects folllowing subcortical electrical stimulation through electrodes in the globus pallidus internus and cortical transcranial magnetic stimulation. Exp Brain Res 2004; 155: 48-55.

Kuhn AA, Trottenberg T, Kivi A, Kupsch A, Schneider GH, Brown P. The relationship between local field potential and neuronal discharge in the subthalamic nucleus of patients with Parkinson's disease. Exp Neurol 2005a;194:212-220.

Kuhn AA, Hariz MI, Silberstein P, Tisch S, Kupsch A, Schneider GH, Limousin-Dowsey P, Yarrow K, Brown P. Activation of the subthalamic region during emotional processing in Parkinson disease. Neurology 2005b;65:707-713.

Kuhn AA, Doyle L, Pogosyan A, Yarrow K, Kupsch A, Schneider GH, Schneider GH, Hariz MI, Trottenberg T, Brown P. Modulation of beta oscillations in the subthalamic area during motor imagery in Parkinson's disease. Brain 2006a;129:695-706.

Kuhn AA, Kupsch A, Schneider GH, Brown P. Reduction in subthalamic 8-35 Hz oscillatory activity correlates with clinical improvement in Parkinson's disease. Eur J Neurosci 2006b;23:1956-1960.

Kühn AA, Kempf F, Brücke C, Gaynor Doyle L, Martinez-Torres I, Pogosyan A, Trottenberg T, Kupsch A, Schneider GH, Hariz MI, Vandenberghe W, Nuttin B, Brown P. High-frequency stimulation of the subthalamic nucleus suppresses oscillatory beta activity in patients with Parkinson's disease in parallel with improvement in motor performance. J Neurosci 2008;28:6165-6173.

Kuriakose R, Saha U, Castillo G, Udupa K, Ni Z, Gunraj C, Mazzella F, Hamani C, Lang AE, Moro E, Lozano AM, Hodaie M, Chen R. The nature and time course of cortical activation following subthalamic stimulation in Parkinson's disease. Cereb Cortex 2010;20:1926-36.

Lafreniere-Roula M, Hutchison WD, Lozano AM, Hodaie M, Dostrovsky JO. Microstimulation-induced inhibition as a tool to aid targeting the ventral border of the subthalamic nucleus. J Neurosurg 2009;111:724-728.

Lafreniere-Roula M, Kim E, Hutchison WD, Lozano AM, Hodaie M, Dostrovsky JO. High-frequency microstimulation in human globus pallidus and substantia nigra. Exp Brain Res 2010;205:251-261.

Lalo E, Thobois S, Sharott A, Polo G, Mertens P, Pogosyan A, Brown P. Patterns of bidirectional communication between cortex and basal ganglia during movement in patients with Parkinson disease. J Neurosci. 2008;28:3008-3016.

Lanotte MM, Rizzone M, Bergamasco B, Faccani G, Melcarne A, Lopiano L. Deep brain stimulation of the subthalamic nucleus: anatomical, neurophysiological, and outcome correlations with the effects of stimulation. J Neurol Neurosurg Psychiatry 2002;72:53-58.

Lee JI, Verhagen Metman L, Ohara S, Dougherty PM, Kim JH, Lenz FA. Internal pallidal neuronal activity during mild drug-related dyskinesias in Parkinson's Disease: decreased firing rates and altered firing patterns. J Neurophysiol 2007;97:2627-2641.

Levy R, Dostrovsky JO, Lang AE, Sime E, Hutchison WD, Lozano AM. Effects of apomorphine on subthalamic nucleus and globus pallidus internus neurons in patients with Parkinson's disease. J Neurophysiol 2001;86:249-260.

Levy R, Hutchison WD, Lozano AM, Dostrovsky JO. Synchronized neuronal discharge in the basal ganglia of parkinsonian patients is limited to oscillatory activity. J Neurosci 2002;22:2855-2861.

Limousin P, Martinez-Torres I. Deep brain stimulation for Parkinson's disease. Neurotherapeutics 2008;5:309-319.

Liu X, Aziz TZ, Bain PG. Intraoperative monitoring of motor symptoms using surface electromyography during stereotactic surgery for movement disorders. J Clin Neurophysiol 2005;22:183-191.

Liu X, Yianni J, Wang S, Bain PG, Stein JF, Aziz TZ. Different mechanisms may generate sustained hypertonic and rhythmic bursting muscle activity in idiopathic dystonia. Exp Neurol 2006;198:204-213.

Lozano AM, Snyder BJ. Deep brain stimulation for parkinsonian gait disorders. J Neurol. 2008;255 Suppl 4:30-31.

MacKinnon CD, Webb RM, Silberstein P, Tisch S, Asselman P, Limousin P, Rothwell JC. Stimulation through electrodes implanted near the subthalamic nucleus activates projections to motor areas of cerebral cortex in patients with Parkinson's disease. Eur J Neurosci 2005; 21: 1394-1402.

Magnani G, Cursi M, Leocani L, Volonte MA, Locatelli T, Elia A, Comi G. Event-related desynchronization to contingent negative variation and self-paced movement paradigms in Parkinson's disease. Mov Disord 1998;13:653-660.

Maks CB, Butson CR, Walter BL, Vitek JL, McIntyre CC. Deep brain stimulation activation volumes and their association with neurophysiological mapping and therapeutic outcomes. J Neurol Neurosurg Psychiatry 2009;80:659-66.

Marceglia S, Foffani G, Bianchi AM, Baselli G, Tamma F, Egidi M, Priori A. Dopamine-dependent non-linear correlation between subthalamic rhythms in Parkinson's disease. J Physiol 2006;571:579-591.

Marceglia S, Servello D, Foffani G, Porta M, Sassi M, Mrakic-Sposta S, Rosa M, Barbieri S, Priori A. Thalamic single-unit and local field potential activity in Tourette syndrome. Mov Disord. 2010;25:300-308.

Maurice N, Thierry AM, Glowinski J, Deniau JM. Spontaneous and evoked activity of substantia nigra pars reticulata neurons during high-frequency stimulation of the subthalamic nucleus. J Neurosci 2003;23:9929-9936.

McIntyre CC, Mori S, Sherman DL, Thakor NV, Vitek JL. Electric field and stimulating influence generated by deep brain stimulation of the subthalamic nucleus. Clin Neurophysiol 2004;115:589-595.

Miyagi Y, Okamoto T, Morioka T, Tobimatsu S, Nakanishi Y, Aihara K, Hashiguchi K, Murakami N, Yoshida F, Samura K, Nagata S, Sasaki T. Spectral analysis of field potential recordings by deep brain stimulation electrode for localization of subthalamic nucleus in patients with Parkinson's disease. Stereotact Funct Neurosurg 2009;87:211-218.

Molinuevo JL, Valldeoriola F, Valls-Solé J. Usefulness of neurophysiologic techniques in stereotactic subthalamic nucleus stimulation for advanced Parkinson's disease. Clinical Neurophysiology 2003;114:1793-1799.

Montgomery EB Jr. Effects of GPi stimulation on human thalamic neuronal activity. Clin Neurophysiol 2006; 117: 2691-2702.

Morecraft RJ, Louie JL, Herrick JL, Stilwell-Morecraft KS. Cortical innervation of the facial nucleus in the non-human primate: a new interpretation of the effects of stroke and related subtotal brain trauma on the muscles of facial expression. Brain 2001;124: 176–208.

Mrakic-Sposta S, Marceglia S, Egidi M, Carrabba G, Rampini P, Locatelli M, Foffani G, Accolla E, Cogiamanian F, Tamma F, Barbieri S, Priori A. Extracellular spike microrecordings from the subthalamic area in Parkinson's disease. J Clin Neurosci 2008;15:559-567.

Nakajima T, Endoh T, Sakamoto M, Komiyama T. Nerve specific modulation of somatosensory inflow to cerebral cortex during submaximal sustained contraction in first dorsal interosseous muscle. Brain Res 2005;1053:146-53.

Novak P, Klemp JA, Ridings LW, Lyons KE, Pahwa R, Nazzaro JM. Effect of deep brain stimulation of the subthalamic nucleus upon the contralateral subthalamic nucleus in Parkinson disease. Neurosci Lett 2009;463:12-16.

Nowak LG, Bullier J. Axons, but not cell bodies, are activated by electrical stimulation in cortical gray matter I. Evidence from chronaxie measurements. Exp Brain Res 1998;118: 477–88.

Pahapill PA, Lozano AM. The pedunculopontine nucleus and Parkinson's disease. Brain 2000; 123: 1767-1783.

Paradiso G, Saint-Cyr JA, Lozano AM, Lang AE, Chen R. Involvement of the human subthalamic nucleus in movement preparation. Neurology 2003;61:1538-1545.

Payoux P, Remy P, Damier P, Miloudi M, Loubinoux I, Pidoux B, Gaura V, Rascol O, Samson Y, Agid Y. Subthalamic nucleus stimulation reduces abnormal motor cortical overactivity in Parkinson disease. Arch Neurol 2004;61:1307-1313.

Payoux P, Remy P, Miloudi M, Houeto JL, Stadler C, Bejjani BP, Yelnik J, Samson Y, Rascol O, Agid Y, Damier P. Contrasting changes in cortical activation induced by acute high-frequency stimulation within the globus pallidus in Parkinson's disease. J Cereb Blood Flow Metab 2009;29:235-243.

Penfield W, Jasper HH. Epilepsy and the functional anatomy of the human brain. Boston: Little Brown, 1954.

Perlmutter JS, Mink JW, Bastian AJ, Zackowski K, Hershey T, Miyawaki E, Koller W, Videen TO. Blood flow responses to deep brain stimulation of thalamus. Neurology 2002;58:1388-1394.

Pesenti A, Priori A, Locatelli M, Egidi M, Rampini P, Tamma F, Caputo E, Chiesa V, Barbieri S. Subthalamic somatosensory evoked potentials in Parkinson's disease. Mov Disord 2003;18:1341-1345.

Pierantozzi M, Palmieri MG, Mazzone P, Marciani MG, Rossini PM, Stefani A, Giacomini P, Peppe A, Stanzione P. Deep brain stimulation of both subthalamic nucleus and internal globus pallidus restores intracortical inhibition in Parkinson's disease paralleling apomorphine effects: a paired magnetic stimulation study. Clin Neurophysiol 2002;113:108-113.

Potter M, Illert M, Wenzelburger R, Deuschl G, Volkmann J. The effect of subthalamic nucleus stimulation on autogenic inhibition in Parkinson disease. Neurology 2004;63:1234-1239.

Pötter M, Herzog J, Siebner HR, Kopper F, Steigerwald F, Deuschl G, Volkmann J. Subthalamic nucleus stimulation modulates audiospinal reactions in Parkinson disease. Neurology. 2008;70:1445-1451.

Pötter-Nerger M, Ilic TV, Siebner HR, Deuschl G, Volkmann J. Subthalamic nucleus stimulation restores corticospinal facilitation in Parkinson's disease. Mov Disord 2008;23:2210-2215.

Pralong E, Pollo C, Coubes P, Bloch J, Roulet E, Tetreault MH, Debatisse D, Villemure JG. Electrophysiological characteristics of limbic and motor globus pallidus internus (GPI) neurons in two cases of Lesch-Nyhan syndrome. Neurophysiol Clin 2005;35:168-173.

Pralong E, Pollo C, Villemure JG, Debatisse D. Opposite effects of internal globus pallidus stimulation on pallidal neurones activity. Mov Disord 2007;22:1879-1884.

Priori A, Foffani G, Pesenti A, Tamma F, Bianchi AM, Pellegrini M, Locatelli M, Moxon KA, Villani RM. Rhythm-specific pharmacological modulation of subthalamic activity in Parkinson's disease. Exp Neurol 2004;189:369-379.

Priori A, Ardolino G, Marceglia S, Mrakic-Sposta S, Locatelli M, Tamma F, Rossi L, Foffani G. Low-frequency subthalamic oscillations increase after deep brain stimulation in Parkinson's disease. Brain Res Bull 2006;71:149-154.

Purzner J, Paradiso GO, Cunic D, Saint-Cyr JA, Hoque T, Lozano AM, Lang AE, Moro E, Hodaie M, Mazzella F, Chen R. Involvement of the basal ganglia and cerebellar motor pathways in the preparation of self-initiated and externally triggered movements in humans. J Neurosci 2007;27:6029-6036.

Quartarone A, Bagnato S, Rizzo V, Siebner HR, Dattola V, Scalfari A, Morgante F, Battaglia F, Romano M, Girlanda P. Abnormal associative plasticity of the human motor cortex in writer's cramp. Brain 2003; 126, 2586–2596.

Rainov NG, Fels C, Heidecke V, Burkert W. Epidural electrical stimulation of the motor cortex in patients with facial neuralgia. Clin Neurol Neurosurg 1997;99:205-209.

Ridding MC, Sheean G, Rothwell JC, Inzelberg R, Kujirai T. Changes in the balance between motor cortical excitation and inhibition in focal, task specific dystonia. J Neurol Neurosurg Psychiatry 1995; 59: 493-498

Rodriguez-Oroz MC, Rodriguez M, Guridi J, Mewes K, Chockkman V, Vitek J, DeLong MR, Obeso JA. The subthalamic nucleus in Parkinson's disease: somatotopic organization and physiological characteristics. Brain 2001;124:1777-1790.

Rodriguez-Oroz MC, Obeso JA, Lang AE, Houeto JL, Pollak P, Rehncrona S, Kulisevsky J, Albanese A, Volkmann J, Hariz MI, Quinn NP, Speelman JD, Guridi J, Zamarbide I, Gironell A, Molet J, Pascual-Sedano B, Pidoux B, Bonnet AM, Agid Y, Xie J, Benabid AL, Lozano AM, Saint-Cyr J, Romito L, Contarino MF, Scerrati M, Fraix V, Van Blercom N. Bilateral deep brain stimulation in Parkinson's disease: a multicentre study with 4 years follow-up. Brain 2005;128:2240-2249.

Rossini PM, Filippi MM, Vernieri F. Neurophysiology of sensorimotor integration in Parkinson's disease. Clin Neurosci 1998;5:121-130.

Sailer A, Cunic DI, Paradiso GO, Gunraj CA, Wagle-Shukla A, Moro E, Lozano AM, Lang AE, Chen R. Subthalamic nucleus stimulation modulates afferent inhibition in Parkinson disease. Neurology 2007;68:356-363.

Saint-Cyr JA, Hoque T, Pereira LC, Dostrovsky JO, Hutchison WD, Mikulis DJ, Abosch A, Sime E, Lang AE, Lozano AM. Localization of clinically effective stimulating electrodes in the human subthalamic nucleus on magnetic resonance imaging. J Neurosurg 2002;97:1152-1166.

Sanghera MK, Grossman RG, Kalhorn CG, Hamilton WJ, Ondo WG, Jankovic J. Basal ganglia neuronal discharge in primary and secondary dystonia in patients undergoing pallidotomy. Neurosurgery 2003;52:1358-1370.

Sani S, Ostrem JL, Shimamoto S, Levesque N, Starr PA. Single unit "pauser" characteristics of the globus pallidus pars externa distinguish primary dystonia from secondary dystonia and Parkinson's disease. Exp Neurol 2009;216:295-299.

Sauleau P, Eusebio A, Thevathasan W, Yarrow K, Pogosyan A, Zrinzo L, Ashkan K, Aziz T, Vandenberghe W, Nuttin B, Brown P. Involvement of the subthalamic nucleus in engagement with behaviourally relevant stimuli. Eur J Neurosci 2009;29:931-942.

Schaltenbrand G, Wahren W. Atlas for stereotaxy of the human brain. 2nd ed. Stuttgart, Germany. Thieme Medical Publishers, 1977.

Schicatano EJ, Peshori KR, Gopalaswamy R, Sahay E, Evinger C. Reflex excitability regulates prepulse inhibition. J Neurosci 2000;20:4240-4247.

Schmidt RF, Torebjork HE, Schady WJ. Gating of tactile input from the hand. II. Effects of remote movements and anaesthesia. Exp Brain Res 1990;79:103-108.

Schrock LE, Ostrem JL, Turner RS, Shimamoto SA, Starr PA. The subthalamic nucleus in primary dystonia: single-unit discharge characteristics. J Neurophysiol 2009;102:3740-3752.

Shimamoto SA, Larson PS, Ostrem JL, Glass GA, Turner RS, Starr PA. Physiological identification of the human pedunculopontine nucleus. J Neurol Neurosurg Psychiatry 2010;81:80-86.

Silberstein P, Kuhn AA, Kupsch A, Trottenberg T, Krauss JK, Wohrle JC, Mazzone P, Insola A, Di Lazzaro V, Oliviero A, Aziz T, Brown P. Patterning of globus pallidus local field potentials differs between Parkinson's disease and dystonia. Brain 2003;126:2597-2608.

Snellings A, Sagher O, Anderson DJ, Aldridge JW. Identification of the subthalamic nucleus in deep brain stimulation surgery with a novel wavelet-derived measure of neural background activity. J Neurosurg 2009;111:767-774.

Starr PA, Christine CW, Theodosopoulos PV, Lindsey N, Byrd D, Mosley A et al. Implantation of deep brain stimulators into the subthalamic nucleus: technical approach and magnetic resonance imaging-verified lead locations. J Neurosurg 2002;97:370-387.

Sterio D, Zonenshayn M, Mogilner AY, Rezai AR, Kiprovski K, Kelly PJ, Beric A. Neurophysiological refinement of subthalamic nucleus targeting. Neurosurgery 2002a;50:58-67.

Sterio D, Rezai A, Mogilner A, Zonenshayn M, Gracies JM, Kathirithamby K, Berić A. Neurophysiological modulation of the subthalamic nucleus by pallidal stimulation in Parkinson's disease. J Neurol Neurosurg Psychiatry 2002b;72:325-328.

Strafella A, Ashby P, Munz M, Dostrovsky JO, Lozano AM, Lang AE. Inhibition of voluntary activity by thalamic stimulation in humans: Relevance for the control of tremor. Mov Disord 1997;12:727-737.

Strafella AP, Dagher A, Sadikot AF. Cerebral blood flow changes induced by subthalamic stimulation in Parkinson's disease. Neurology 2003;60:1039-1042.

Swerdlow NR, Geyer MA, Braff DL. Neural circuit regulation of prepulse inhibition of startle in the rat: current knowledge and future challenges. Psychopharmacology 2001;156:194-215.

Tang JK, Moro E, Mahant N, Hutchison WD, Lang AE, Lozano AM, Dostrovsky JO. Neuronal firing rates and patterns in the globus pallidus internus of patients with cervical dystonia differ from those with Parkinson's disease. J Neurophysiol 2007;98:720-729.

Thobois S, Dominey P, Fraix V, Mertens P, Guenot M, Zimmer L, Pollak P, Benabid AL, Broussolle E. Effects of subthalamic nucleus stimulation on actual and imagined movement in Parkinson's disease: a PET study. J Neurol 2002;249:1689-1698.

Tisch S, Limousin P, Rothwell JC, Asselman P, Quinn N, Jahanshahi M, Bhatia KP, Hariz M. Changes in blink reflex excitability after globus pallidus internus stimulation for dystonia. Mov Disord 2006a;21:1650-1655.

Tisch S, Limousin P, Rothwell JC, Asselman P, Zrinzo L, Jahanshahi M, Bhatia KP, Hariz MI. Changes in forearm reciprocal inhibition following pallidal stimulation for dystonia. Neurology 2006b;66:1091-1093.

Tisch S, Rothwell JC, Bhatia KP, Quinn N, Zrinzo L, Jahanshahi M, Ashkan K, Hariz M, Limousin P. Pallidal stimulation modifies after-effects of paired associative stimulation on motor cortex excitability in primary generalised dystonia. Exp Neurol 2007;206:80-85.

Tornqvist AL, Schalen L, Rehncrona S. Effects of different electrical parameter settings on the intelligibility of speech in patients with Parkinson's disease treated with subthalamic deep brain stimulation. Mov Disord 2005;20:416-423.

Vafaee MS, OStergaard K, Sunde N, Gjedde A, Dupont E, Cumming P. Focal changes of oxygen consumption in cerebral cortex of patients with Parkinson's disease during subthalamic stimulation. Neuroimage 2004;22:966-974.

Valeriani M, Insola A, Restuccia D, Le Pera D, Mazzone P, Altibrandi MG, Tonali P. Source generators of the early somatosensory evoked potentials to tibial nerve stimulation: an intracerebral and scalp recording study. Clin Neurophysiol 2001;112:1999-2006.

Valeriani M, Truini A, Le Pera D, Insola A, Galeotti F, Petrachi C, Mazzone P, Cruccu G. Laser evoked potential recording from intracerebral deep electrodes. Clin Neurophysiol 2009;120:790-795.

Valls-Sole J, Valldeoriola F. Neurophysiological correlate of clinical signs in Parkinson's disease. Clin Neurophysiol 2002;113:792-805.

Valls-Sole J, Munoz JE, Valldeoriola. Abnormalities of prepulse inhibition do not depend on blink reflex excitability: a study in Parkinson's disease and Huntington's disease. Clinical Neurophysiology 2004;115:1527-1536.

Valls-Solé J, Compta Y, Costa J, Valldeoriola F, Rumià J. Human central nervous system circuits examined through the electrodes implanted for deep brain stimulation. Clin Neurophysiol 2008;119:1219-31.

Vitek JL, Chockkan V, Zhang JY, Kaneoke Y, Evatt M, DeLong MR et al, Mewes K, Hashimoto T, Bakay RAE. Neuronal activity in the basal ganglia in patients with generalized dystonia and hemiballismus. Ann Neurol 1999; 46:22-35.

Voges J, Volkmann J, Allert N, Lehrke R, Koulousakis A, Freund HJ, Sturm V. Bilateral high frequency stimulation in the subthalamic nucleus for the treatment of Parkinson's disease: correlation of therapeutic effect with anatomical electrode position. J Neurosurg 2002; 96:269-279.

Weinberger M, Mahant N, Hutchison WD, Lozano AM, Moro E, Hodaie M, Lang AE, Dostrovsky JO. Beta oscillatory activity in the subthalamic nucleus and its relation to dopaminergic response in Parkinson's disease. J Neurophysiol 2006;96:3248-3256.

Weinberger M, Hamani C, Hutchison WD, Moro E, Lozano AM, Dostrovsky JO. Pedunculopontine nucleus microelectrode recordings in movement disorder patients. Exp Brain Res 2008;188:165-174.

Weinberger M, Hutchison WD, Lozano AM, Hodaie M, Dostrovsky JO. Increased gamma oscillatory activity in the subthalamic nucleus during tremor in Parkinson's disease patients. J Neurophysiol 2009;101:789-802.

Welter ML, Houeto JL, Bonnet AM, Bejjani PB, Mesnage V, Dormont D, Navarro S, Cornu P, Agid Y, Pidoux B. Effects of high-frequency stimulation on subthalamic neuronal activity in parkinsonian patients. Arch Neurol 2004;61:89-96.

Wichmann T, DeLong MR. Functional and pathophysiological models of the basal ganglia. Curr Opin Neurobiol 1996; 6:751-758.

Williams D, Tijssen M, Van Bruggen G, Bosch A, Insola A, Di Lazzaro V, Mazzone P, Oliviero A, Quartarone A, Speelman H, Brown P. Dopamine-dependent changes in the functional connectivity between basal ganglia and cerebral cortex in humans. Brain 2002;125:1558-1569.

Wingeier B, Tcheng T, Koop MM, Hill BC, Heit G, Bronte-Stewart HM. Intra-operative STN DBS attenuates the prominent beta rhythm in the STN in Parkinson's disease. Exp Neurol 2006;197:244-251.

Woolsey CN, Erickson TC, Gilson WE. Localization in somatic sensory and motor areas of human cerebral cortex as determined by direct recording of evoked potentials and electrical stimulation. J Neurosurg 1979;51:476-506.

Yugeta A, Terao Y, Fukuda H, Hikosaka O, Yokochi F, Okiyama R, Taniguchi M, Takahashi H, Hamada I, Hanajima R, Ugawa Y. Effects of STN stimulation on the initiation and inhibition of saccade in Parkinson disease. Neurology 2010;74:743-748.

Zaidel A, Spivak A, Grieb B, Bergman H, Israel Z. Subthalamic span of beta oscillations predicts deep brain stimulation efficacy for patients with Parkinson's disease. Brain 2010;133:2007-2021.

Zhuang P, Hallett M, Zhang X, Li J, Zhang Y, Li Y. Neuronal activity in the globus pallidus internus in patients with tics. J Neurol Neurosurg Psychiatry 2009;80:1075-1081.

Electrical Stimulation of Primary Motor Cortex for Parkinson's Syndrome

Naoki Tani[1] and Youichi Saitoh[1,2]
[1]Department of Neurosurgery,
Osaka University Graduate School of Medicine,
[2]Department of Neuromodulation and Neurosurgery,
Osaka University,
Japan

1. Introduction

Deep brain stimulation (DBS) of several nuclei at the basal ganglia, mainly globus pallidus interna (GPi), and subthalamic nucleus (STN) is highly effective in controlling motor symptoms in patients with advanced Parkinson's disease (PD) (Krack et al., 1998; Limousin et al., 1998) However, several complications have been published by different groups with a large experience in DBS (Lyons et al., 2004; Umemura et al., 2003), and patients with poor response to levodopa or those with cognitive impairment, advanced age, considerable brain atrophy, cerebral ischemic foci in the white matter or Unified Parkinson's Disease Rating Scale (UPDRS) part III < 30 to 40 in the *off* condition are considered unsuitable patients for DBS, because of the increased surgical risk (Lopiano et al., 2002; Pahwa et al., 2005). On the other hand, STN DBS may improve axial symptoms at the beginning, but results are less rewarding at long-term follow-up (Bejjani et al., 2000; Kleiner-Fisman et al., 2003).

At the early of the 1990s, Tsubokawa introduced electrical motor cortex stimulation (EMCS) for the relief of central pain (Tsubokawa et al., 1991a, b). Its use has been extended to peripheral neuropathic pain conditions, and very recently to patients with movement disorders. EMCS might represent an alternative in patients who would not fulfill all DBS inclusion criteria. There has been some evidence that EMCS may relieve motor symptoms of patients with PD (Canavero et al., 2002; Pagni et al., 2005). However, there have also been a number of contradictory reports regarding the efficacy of EMCS in patients with PD. A number of reasons could account for the apparent discrepancies among different studies which may include different selection criteria, different surgical (i.e. extradural vs. subdural electrode) or methodological (i.e. stimulation frequencies) approaches, and importantly, different way of motor performance assessments. This report attempts to summarize current evidence on these topics.

2. Transcranial magnetic stimulation on primary motor cortex

Several studies have shown the transient benefit of the stimulation of primary motor cortex (M1) using repetitive transcranial magnetic stimulation (rTMS) for the symptoms of patients with PD, such as akinesia, tremor, rigidity and depression. The benefits depend on stimulus frequency and the site of the stimulation; high frequency rTMS of M1 (5-25 Hz) improved the motor performance (Khedr et al., 2006; Lefaucheur et al., 2004), rTMS of the supplementary motor area (SMA) worsened performance of motor tasks at high frequencies (5-10 Hz) or improved UPDRS (Hamada et al, 2008) but reduced levodopa-induced dyskinesias at low frequency (1 Hz) (Boylan et al., 2001; Koch et al., 2005), and 5 Hz rTMS of the dorsolateral prefrontal cortex (DLPFC) demonstrated the benefit on depression of patients with PD (Pal et al., 2010). Recently, rTMS on M1 is expected to predict the efficacy of EMCS for patients with PD, for instance, we experienced a patient with akinesia in whom high frequency rTMS on M1 showed similar beneficial effect on motor symptom to the subsequent EMCS. In the patients with intractable pain, Andre-Obadia demonstrated that 20 Hz rTMS on M1 predicted the efficacy of subsequent EMCS for pain reduction (Andre-Obadia et al., 2006) and Hosomi et al reported that there is good correlation between the pain reduction with 5 Hz rTMS and that with EMCS (Hosomi et al, 2008). Thus, the rTMS technique might be used to better define the targets and the parameters of stimulation subsequently applied in chronic EMCS.

3. Surgical procedure

Basically, the surgical procedure of EMCS for Parkinson's Syndrome is same as that for intractable pain. Because of the small number of the reported case of EMCS for PD, there is still controversy, such as unilateral stimulation or bilateral stimulation, epidural electrode or subdural electrode. Detailed procedure of EMCS will be mentioned in this session. Previously the detailed methods were reported (Saitoh and Hosomi, 2009).

3.1 Pre-surgical preparation

Prior to the surgical procedure, the hand motor area is identified as a target of EMCS using fMRI or anatomical MRI. Because the lower limb motor area locates in the inter-hemispheric fissure, implanting an electrode on the lower limb motor area is difficult. Functional MRI (fMRI) (Figure 1) is useful to precisely localize the site of the M1, otherwise some anatomical landmarks can help to identify the central sulcus. The central sulcus is characterized by the lack of sulcal branches, and lies just anterior to the pars marginalis of the cingulate sulcus on the interhemispheric surface (Naidich et al., 2001; Naidich et al., 1995). The precentral knob sign corresponding to the hand motor area is easily identified on surface view of MRI (Figure 2).

3.2 Neuronavigation

After the identification of targeted area, neuronavigation is used to precisely identify M1 intraoperatively. Several kinds of navigation systems for neurosurgical assistance can be used to estimate the position of the central sulcus from skin surface (Tirakotai et al., 2007). Neuronavigation combined with fMRI data help to decide the best position for craniotomy and for placement of the stimulating paddle (Rasche et al., 2006). A drawback of neuronavigation is the requirement that the patient's head be fixed in a 3-point pin holder or vacuum headrest (Tirakotai et al., 2007), which several patients may not tolerate under local anesthesia. For this reason, other surgeons prefer not to fix the patient's head and operate without neuronavigation, and use the Taylor-Haughton instead of neuronavigation lines (Figure 3) (Greenberg, 2010).

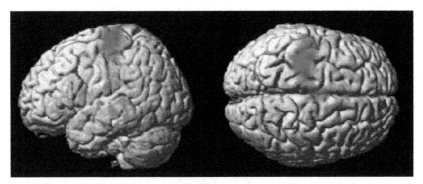

Fig. 1. Motor cortex localization using fMRI. During the acquisition of fMRI data (echo planar imaging), the patient perfomed twelve 30-second epocks of right hand grasp with identical rest epochs. Data analysis was performed in MATLAB 2008a (Math Works, Inc., Natick, MA) using Statistical Parametric Mapping software (SPM@; Wellcome Department of Imaging Neuroscience, London, England).

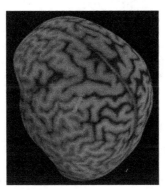

Fig. 2. Brain surface view of MRI. Red arrow indicates the left primary motor cortex hand area.

3.3 Anethesia

Implantation of electrode is done under local anesthesia or general anesthesia. General anesthesia is induced with a loading dose of Remifentanil 3-4 ng/ml in continuous infusion followed after 5-8 min by Propofol 5.5 µg/ml as induction dose (Total intravenous anesthesia, TIVA). Endotracheal intubation is facilitated by vecuronium bromide 0.1 mg/kg; no further doses of muscle relaxants are administered throughout surgery. The lungs are mechanically ventilated with a 50% O_2 in air mixture, in order to maintain end tidal concentrations of CO_2 (ETCO2) at 30–35 mmHg. Anesthesia is maintained with Remifentanil (5–6 ng/ml, up to 7-8 ng/ml if necessary) and Propofol (2.5-3.0 µg/ml). At the end of the surgical procedure, all patients are awakened within 15–30 min from cessation of TIVA.

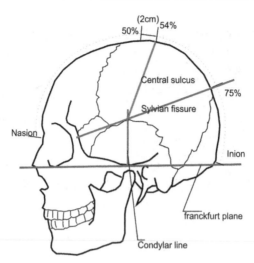

Fig. 3. Taylor-Haughton line indicates the position of the central sulcus from the scalp. The Frankfurt plane is the line from the inferior margin of the orbit through the upper margin of the external auditory meatus. The distance from the nasion to the inion is measured across the top of the calvaria and is divided into quarters. The condylar line runs perpendicular to the baseline through the mandibular condyle (intersecting the line representing the sylvian fissure). The Sylvian fissure is approximated by a line connecting the lateral canthus to the point 3/4 of the way posterior along the arc running over convexity from nasion to inion. Central sulcus is drawn from 54% point on naso-inoin line to the point where the Sylvian line cuts the condylar line.

3.4 Electrophysiological localization of hand motor area

For localizing central sulcus, most neurosurgeons employ somatosensory evoked potential (SSPE) using contralateral median nerve stimulation. The phase reversal of the N20 (sensory cortex) /P20 (motor cortex) waves is used to confirm the location of the central sulcus (Wood et al., 1988), using a multi-contact grid and the central scalp EEG leads or directly using the definitive 4-contact strip overlying the dura matter (Figure 4). Recently, an enlarged and displaced motor map for the hand area was described in patients with PD. Map shifts were found in the majority of the patients (Thickbroom et al., 2006). Therefore, electrode placement only with SSEP is often inadequate or impossibles. According to Velasco et al. (Velasco et al., 2002), recording corticocortical evoked responses (CCER) is simple and reliable and superior to SSEPs. M1 stimulation elicits negative CCER over the frontal scalp, whereas the stimulation of primary sensory cortex (S1) elicits positive responses over parietal and occipital scalp regions.

Most neurosurgeons attempt intraoperative test stimulation by using the quadripolar or the grid electrodes. Test bipolar stimulation (210-1000 μs –generally 400-500-μs, 1-5 Hz up to 500Hz, at increasing voltage or intensity –up to 50 mA, anodally, but also cathodally) is applied by means of the contacts situated over M1. In general, the amplitude needed to produce motor responses is higher using epidural rather than subdural stimulation. Motor contraction can be elicited at relatively lower amplitudes when general anesthesia is not employed. 1Hz stimulation is preferred to higher frequencies, since the former does not habituate and has less potential to trigger seizures. Muscle responses are recorded from muscle bellies of the contralateral upper limb, with EMG electrodes or visually.

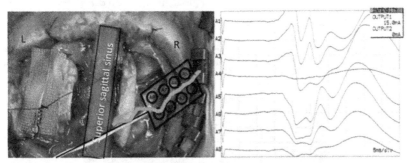

Fig. 4. SSEP recording on the right central sulcus using an eight contact subdural electrode. An eight-polar plate electrode (Specify Lead, 3998; Medtronic, Minneapolis, MN) was placed on the right central sulcus. Left median nerve was stimulated at wrist with stimuli consist of single shocks (0.5 ms, 4.7 Hz, 20 mA) to produce a small, but consistent contraction of the thumb. SSEPs were recorded from each cortical electrode referenced to the ipsilateral ear lobe. Individual SSEP signals were differentially amplified and filtered: 200 were averaged through a digital signal analyzer with sample interval of 100 msec. Blue line indicates the central sulcus confirmed by SSPE.

3.5 Electrode implantation

For EMCS, the great majority of investigators prefer epidural electrode to subdural electrode. This attitude is attributed largely to the greater risk of developing complications with subdural EMCS, such as cerebrospinal fluid leakage, difficulty in fixing the electrode, hemorrhage, and iatrogenic seizures. However, according to the physical model suggested by Holsheimer et al. (Holsheimer et al., 2007) and Manola et al. (Manola et al., 2007), subdural EMCS appears to be more energy-efficient, as compared with epidural EMCS. In some patients with brain atrophy, the cortical surface and the dura mater are wide apart, in which case patients may fail to respond to extradural stimulation: a subdural approach may be considered in selected cases.

There is no direct comparison study between unilateral EMCS and bilateral EMCS. Some investigator reported the bilateral effects in clinical outcome by unilateral EMCS (Cilia et al., 2008; Pagni et al., 2005). These bilateral effects of unilateral cortical stimulation are probably due to bilateral afferent and efferent connections between cortical and subcortical structures (Leichnetz, 1986).

The four-contact electrode array or 2 side-by-side 4-contact electrode strips is placed on the hand motor area. Some surgeons place the electrode perpendicular to the central sulcus above the precentral (cathode) and postcentral (anode) gyri for the supposed improved selectivity (Nguyen et al., 1999), others in a parallel fashion, i.e. with all contacts on the M1 or S1 (Canavero and Bonicalzi, 2002; Rasche et al., 2006). Moreover, no polarity-related difference in pain relief is seen for most patients with epidural electrodes (Katayama et al., 1998).

3.5.1 Epidural electrode

Canavero (Canavero et al., 2002, 2003) makes an oblique linear skin incision (6-10cm) parallel to and 1 cm ahead of or behind the projection of the central sulcus and then drills two burr holes at a distance of 2-4 cm (plus a bony groove parallel to the paddle to accommodate the connector between the looping lead and the extension). A stimulating paddle is inserted from the edge of one burr hole into the epidural space overlying the precentral gyrus contralateral to more disabled side for movement disorders. The bony bridge between the two holes will then hold the plate in place and simultaneously reduce the durocortical gap (Figure 5). This technique entails no risk of epidural hematoma, and accidental displacement of the electrode has never been observed (S Canavero, personal communication)

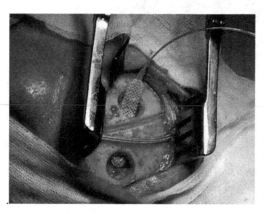

Fig. 5. Two burr-hole surgery is shown. The locations of burr holes are marked on the scalp depending on the anatomical landmarks (courtesy of Prof. Canavero).

3.5.2 Subdural electrode

In patients with advanced cortical atrophy, epidural stimulation may fail due to the duro-cortical separation. The cortical surface and interhemispheric surfaces subdurally may be elected as targets for stimulation. However, large bridging veins sometimes interfere with implantation on the interhemispheric surface. We performs bilateral craniotomy over superior sagittal sinus. After the opening of dura mater, the location of central sulcus is confirmed using phase reverse of the N20 component upon stimulation of the median nerve. A subdural quadripolar electrodes (Resume II, model 3587A; Medtronic, Minneapolis, MN) are then placed bilaterally on the M1 adjacent to the superior sagittal sinus. At the end of surgery, the lead extension is fixed to the dura or the border of the burr hole with a silk suture to prevent dislocation. However, migration of the electrodes seems to be more of a problem with a subdural than an extradural approach. A meticulous, watertight dural closure is mandatory to minimize the risk of cerebrospinal fluid leakage.

3.6 Test stimulation

After closure of the craniotomy, the electrode cable(s) is/are connected to trial stimulator. After 3 to 14 days period of test stimulation, the best stimulation parameters and electrodes are decided. There is considerable variation in the stimulation parameters; amplitudes range from 2 V to 6 V, rates from 10 Hz to 130 Hz, and pulse widths from 60 μsec to 450 μsec (Canavero et al., 2003; Canavero et al., 2002; Cilia et al., 2007; Cilia et al., 2008; Fasano et al., 2008; Gutierrez et al., 2009; Pagni et al., 2005; Strafella et al., 2007; Tani et al., 2007). The best location and orientation of the electrode array are generally determined in such a way that bipolar stimulation with an appropriate pair of electrodes. Once the pulse width and frequency have been optimized, most investigators will increase stimulus intensities during the trial using a percentage of the motor threshold as a guide. Many investigators begin by increasing the intensity by 20% of the motor threshold and then increase by 20% increments thereafter to 80% of motor threshold.

3.7 Implantation of IPG

If the test stimulation improves the motor symptom, patients would be returned to the operating room and the electrode(s) is/are connected to implanted pulse generator(s) (Itrel III IPG; Medtronic Inc., Minneapolis, MN, USA), usually placed subcutaneously over the pectoralis muscle under general anesthesia (Figure 6).

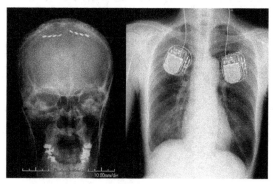

Fig. 6. Subdural electrodes implanted bilaterally on the primary motor cortex and pulse generators. The two Resume II electrodes are connected to pulse generators (Itrel III; Medtronic) that are implanted in the bilateral anterior chests.

4. Clinical outcome

Clinical outcomes from several studies were summerised in Table 1. Variable clinical outcomes after EMCS have been reported in the patients with PD. The limited case series available on literature and the differences in patient selection criteria and stimulus parameters may partly account for the variable clinical benefit reported so far. Basically, the degree of the clinical improvement obtained with EMCS is lower than that reported with DBS (Cilia et al., 2008; Gutierrez et al., 2009). Most of EMCS studies did not find significant mean changes between stimulation-on and stimulation-off in UPDRS part II and III (Cilia et al., 2008; Gutierrez et al., 2009; Strafella et al., 2007). On the other hand, motor evaluation in individual patients revealed clinical improvement during stimulation in comparison to STIM-OFF condition (Cilia et al., 2008; Fasano et al., 2008; Gutierrez et al., 2009; Strafella et al., 2007; Tani et al., 2007). These published data must be interpreted very cautiously, because they are from open labelled studies that involved only small numbers of patients from a few centres. The clinical benefits from EMCS were observed mainly in axial symptoms, such as gait, stooped posture and postural instability. Because axial symptom has small proportion in UPDRS-III (20/108), the benefit of EMCS for axial symptom does not change a lot in UPDRS-III score. Additionally, clinical improvement by EMCS occurs

Authors	Cases	Stimulation condition	clinical outcome
Cilla	6	epidural, unilateral, monopolar, 40-60 Hz, 3.0 ± 0.67 V, 180 -210 μsec	No significant mean changes in UPDRS-II (40% improvement), UPDRS-III (20% improvement), as well as medication dose (15% reduction) between baseline, 6-month STIM-ON and 6-month STIM-OFF. Objective motor benefit was observed mainly in axial symptoms, such as gait, stooped posture and postural instability.
Pagni	6	epidural, unilateral, bipolar, 25-40 Hz, 2.5-6 V, 100-180 μsec	UPDRS: tremor;bilateraly more than 80% reduction in 3 of 4 cases, rigidity; more than 50% reduction in 5 of 6 cases in contralateral side and in 4 of 6 cases in ipsilateral side, activityies of daily living; more than 50 % reduction in 3 of 6 cases, axial symptom.; more than 50% reduction in 3 of 6 cases, dyskinesia; more than 50% reduction in 4 of 5 cases, 11-70 % reduction of L-dapa daily dose
Strafella	4	subdural, unilateral, 50 or 130 Hz, 3-5 V, 60-90 μsec	No reduction of daily L-dopa dose, no significant difference in the UPDRS motor score between OFF stimulation (43.0 ± 7.9) and ON stimulation (39.5 ±12.5).
Gutierrez	6	epidural, unilateral, bipolar, 10-30 Hz, 3-4.5 V, 330-450 μsec	Mild improvement in 2 of 6 cases (14.7% and 7.3% improvement in UPDRS-III)(on stimulation on medication vs off stimulation on medication), 17.1 ± 11.1% reduction of L-dopa daily dose.
Canavero	3	epidural, unilateral, bipolar, 20-31 Hz, 2-3.5 V, 90-330 μsec	Case 1; independent walk, absence of rigidity, trochlea, and tremor to all four limbs, 80% reduction of L-dopa daily dose. Case 2; 50% improvement of UPDRS-III, absense of freezing gait, tremor, improvement of bradykinesia, 70% reduction of L-dopa daily dose. Case 3; absence of tremor, rigidity, improvement of gait and speech.
Fasano	1	epidural, bilateral, bipolar, 130 Hz, subthreshold intensity, 120 μsec	20% improvement of UPDRS-III, mainly in Axial score (UPDRS items 27-30).
Tani	1	subdural, bilateral, bipolar, 100 Hz, 1.8 V, 210 μsec	50% improvement of UPDRS-III and dramatic improvement in walking

Table 1. Summery of clinical outcomes

after a variable time interval - most often several days up to 4 weeks - after stimulation parameters modifications (Cilia et al., 2008). Several investigators reported that rigidity and tremor were abolished within several minutes of stimulation, but the full effect on bradykinesia and axial symptom, especially gait disturbance, were appreciated only after a longer period of stimulation, with a slow worsening over more than 2 days period after stimulation-off (Canavero et al., 2002; Cilia et al., 2008; Pagni et al., 2003; Tani et al., 2007). In some studies, the motor symptom assessments were done in shorter period after the modification of stimulation parameter, so the benefit in motor symptom could be underestimated.

5. Mechanisms of action

The exact mechanisms of action of EMCS are poorly understood. It is noteworthy that, whereas the effects of EMCS on rigidity and tremor are almost immediate (observed within the first minute of stimulation), the clinical benefit on akinesia and axial symptom necessitate a longer stimulation time to become detectable. The latency of the clinical effects of high-frequency STN-DBS is also known to vary from one type of parkinsonian motor symptoms to another with short latency benefit (less than 1 min) observed for rigidity and tremor and longer time delay (a few minutes, up to a few days) observed for other symptoms such as bradykinesia and akinesia (Krack et al., 2002). As discussed by others, the delays of clinical benefits observed with EMCS may be due to synaptic plasticity, long-term potentiation, long-term depression, expression of secondary messengers or polarization of brain tissue (Drouot et al., 2004; Krack et al., 2002; Priori and Lefaucheur, 2007), and the immediate effects may be due to the dual effect - imposing a specific pattern of activity and suppress abnormal, disease-associated rhythmicity of oscillation in corticobasal ganglia-cortical circuit (Brown, 2006; Fasano et al., 2008; Garcia et al., 2003; Priori and Lefaucheur, 2007).

Studies of rTMS of M1 reveal that PD is associated with excess excitability or reduced inhibition at the M1 (Cantello et al., 2002), and rigidity and tremor might be caused by hyperactivity of the M1 (Haslinger et al., 2001; Rodriguez-Oroz et al., 2009). In the patients with PD, during production of a voluntary output, its activation is inadequately modulated, owing, for instance, to reduction of intracortical inhibitory mechanisms mediated by γ-aminobutyric acid A (GABA) and GABA receptors (Cantello et al., 2002). Canavero et al. suggests that EMCS increases the cortical GABA in patients affected by central pain syndromes (Canavero and Bonicalzi, 1995, 1998). EMCS might reduce cortical hyperactivity, increasing GABA concentration and activating inhibitory neurons (Hanajima et al., 2002). Indeed, ECD SPECT data demonstrated a resting state reduction of neuronal activity in motor cortical areas during EMCS (Cilia et al., 2008).

Finally, functional neuroimaging studies showed a significant increase of cerebral perfusion in the SMA and the DLPFC in STIM-ON condition (Drouot et al., 2004; Fasano et al., 2008; Tani et al., 2007). The SMA and the DLPFC are known to be under-active in patients with PD, probably underlying bradykinesia (Haslinger et al., 2001; Jahanshahi et al., 1995; Rascol et al., 1992), and these cortical metabolic abnormalities can be reversed by antiparkinsonian therapies such as dopaminergic treatment (Jenkins et al., 1992), pallidotomy (Grafton et al., 1995), STN-DBS (Limousin et al., 1997) or GPi-DBS (Fukuda et al., 2001). The similarity of these results suggests that these strategies may induce a similar therapeutic benefit in the patients with PD and might have some common mechanism.

Authors	Cases	Stimulation	Modality	Neuroimaging
Cilla	6	unilateral, 40-60 Hz	Tc-SPECT STIM-ON vs STIM-OFF under rest	Decrease in bilateral M1, bilateral premotor cortex, left DLPFC, right caudate nucleus and left middle occipital gyrus Increase in right cerebellar lobe, left inferior occipital gyrus, left cerevellar lobe and vermis.
Strafella	4	unilateral, 50 or 130 Hz	[^{15}O] H$_2$O PET movement vs rest	the changes in rCBF were not significantly different when comparing across different stimulation setting (OFF vs 50 Hz vs 130 Hz).
Canavero	3	unilateral, 20 - 31 Hz	IBZM-SPECT	Before EMCS, asymmetrical binding (right less than left) in the basal ganglia During EMCS, renormalization of basal ganglia anomalies
			ECD-SPECT	Before EMCS, bilateral parieto-temporal hypoperfusion. During EMCS, renormalization of cortical metabolism on the side of stimulation but not contralaterally.
Fasano	1	bilateral, 130 Hz	ECD-SPECT STIM-OFF vs STIM-ON (medication off)	increase in the right frontal, right parietal cortex and left frontal cortex.
Tani	1	bilateral, 100 Hz	[^{15}O] H$_2$O PET STIM-OFF vs STIM-ON (medication on)	increase in the left SMA and right DLPFC.

Table 2. Summery of the functional neuroimaging

6. Complication

The only complication reported concerning EMCS for PD was misplaced electrode (Pagni et al., 2005). Because of the small number of the cases of EMCS for PD, we summarize the reported complication of EMCS for intractable pain patients in this section.

While a majority of studies have reported no adverse events with EMCS (Gharabaghi et al., 2005; Saitoh et al., 2000; Tsubokawa et al., 1991b), serious complications have been reported. Montes et al. (Montes et al., 2002) analyzed event-related potentials (ERPs) and behavioral performance during an auditory target-detection task in 11 consecutive patients obtained during EMCS and 10 minutes after switching off stimulation. While sensory responses remained unaffected by EMCS, there was a significant delay of brain potentials reflecting target detection in the older patients, rapidly reversible after EMCS discontinuation. No effect was observed in patients younger than 50 years. Cognitive effects of EMCS appeared as mild and non-specific, directly related to the stimulation period (i.e. with no post-effect), in a manner reminding of cognitive effects reported during rTMS on M1. Thus, EMCS may interfere with relatively simple cognitive processes such as those underlying target detection, notably in the elderly and in the presence of preexistent cerebral lesions.

Occurrence of epileptic seizures has been reported during test stimulation in a minority of patients. The low rate of epileptic seizures during chronic stimulation (0.2%) means that stimulation of M1 within an appropriate range of parameters is reasonably safe. The most serious reported complications are epidural or subdural hematomas. These are definitely exceptional with an extradural approach, and some surgeons never observed one, making the risk of peri-operative hemorrhage much lower compared to DBS.

Some wound infections have been reported by most neurosurgeons. If the infection occurs, all devices including the paddle, extension leads, and pulse generators must be removed temporally. The implanted pulse generator (IPG) can accidentally turn off due to electromagnetic interference from household devices in close (<10 cm) proximity, such as electric appliances of any kind, but also anti-theft devices and metal detectors or magnets in loudspeakers.

At impedances >2000 Ω, a connection problem, such as a broken cable or a lead fracture, must be suspected. The operator should thus measure impedance in a unipolar configuration in order to assign a value to the single contact.

7. Conclusion

EMCS can provide some different benefit for the patients with PD from STN-DBS. Although the degree of clinical improvement of EMCS is lower than that of DBS, the fact that EMCS can improve axial symptom of PD, which is difficult even with STN-DBS, is an irreplaceable gift for some part of patients with PD, and its less surgical invasiveness than DBS can make the surgery safer for the patients with advanced age or sever brain atrophy.

8. References

Andre-Obadia, N., Peyron, R., Mertens, P., Mauguiere, F., Laurent, B., Garcia-Larrea, L. (2006). Transcranial magnetic stimulation for pain control. Double-blind study of different frequencies against placebo, and correlation with motor cortex stimulation efficacy. *Clin Neurophysiol*, 117, 1536-1544, ISSN 1388-2457

Bejjani, B.P., Gervais, D., Arnulf, I., Papadopoulos, S., Demeret, S., Bonnet, A.M., Cornu, P., Damier, P., Agid, Y. (2000). Axial parkinsonian symptoms can be improved: the role of levodopa and bilateral subthalamic stimulation. *J Neurol Neurosurg Psychiatry*, 68, 595-600, ISSN 0022-3050

Boylan, L.S., Pullman, S.L., Lisanby, S.H., Spicknall, K.E., Sackeim, H.A. (2001). Repetitive transcranial magnetic stimulation to SMA worsens complex movements in Parkinson's disease. *Clin Neurophysiol*, 112, 259-264, ISSN 1388-2457

Brown, P. (2006). Bad oscillations in Parkinson's disease. *J Neural Transm Suppl*, 27-30, ISSN 0303-6995

Canavero, S., Bonicalzi, V. (1995). Cortical stimulation for central pain. *J Neurosurg*, 83, 1117, ISSN 0022-3085

Canavero, S., Bonicalzi, V. (1998). The neurochemistry of central pain: evidence from clinical studies, hypothesis and therapeutic implications. *Pain*, 74, 109-114, ISSN 0304-3959

Canavero, S., Bonicalzi, V. (2002). Therapeutic extradural cortical stimulation for central and neuropathic pain: a review. *Clin J Pain*, 18, 48-55, ISSN 0749-8047

Canavero, S., Bonicalzi, V., Paolotti, R., Castellano, G., Greco-Crasto, S., Rizzo, L., Davini, O., Maina, R. (2003). Therapeutic extradural cortical stimulation for movement disorders: a review. *Neurol Res*, 25, 118-122, ISSN 0161-6412

Canavero, S., Paolotti, R., Bonicalzi, V., Castellano, G., Greco-Crasto, S., Rizzo, L., Davini, O., Zenga, F., Ragazzi, P. (2002). Extradural motor cortex stimulation for advanced Parkinson disease. Report of two cases. *J Neurosurg*, 97, ISSN 1208-1211

Cantello, R., Tarletti, R., Civardi, C. (2002). Transcranial magnetic stimulation and Parkinson's disease. *Brain Res Brain Res Rev*, 38, 309-327, ISSN 0165-0173

Cilia, R., Landi, A., Vergani, F., Sganzerla, E., Pezzoli, G., Antonini, A. (2007). Extradural motor cortex stimulation in Parkinson's disease. *Mov Disord*, 22, 111-114, ISSN 0885-3185

Cilia, R., Marotta, G., Landi, A., Isaias, I.U., Vergani, F., Benti, R., Sganzerla, E., Gerundini, P., Pezzoli, G., Antonini, A. (2008). Cerebral activity modulation by extradural motor cortex stimulation in Parkinson's disease: a perfusion SPECT study. *Eur J Neurol*, 15, 22-28, ISSN 1468-1331

Drouot, X., Oshino, S., Jarraya, B., Besret, L., Kishima, H., Remy, P., Dauguet, J., Lefaucheur, J.P., Dolle, F., Conde, F., Bottlaender, M., Peschanski, M., Keravel, Y., Hantraye, P., Palfi, S. (2004). Functional recovery in a primate model of Parkinson's disease following motor cortex stimulation. *Neuron*, 44, 769-778, ISSN 0896-6273

Fasano, A., Piano, C., De Simone, C., Cioni, B., Di Giuda, D., Zinno, M., Daniele, A., Meglio, M., Giordano, A., Bentivoglio, A.R. (2008). High frequency extradural motor cortex stimulation transiently improves axial symptoms in a patient with Parkinson's disease. *Mov Disord*, 23, 1916-1919, ISSN 1531-8257

Fukuda, M., Mentis, M., Ghilardi, M.F., Dhawan, V., Antonini, A., Hammerstad, J., Lozano, A.M., Lang, A., Lyons, K., Koller, W., Ghez, C., Eidelberg, D. (2001). Functional correlates of pallidal stimulation for Parkinson's disease. *Ann Neurol*, 49, 155-164, ISSN 0364-5134

Garcia, L., Audin, J., D'Alessandro, G., Bioulac, B., Hammond, C. (2003). Dual effect of high-frequency stimulation on subthalamic neuron activity. *J Neurosci*, 23, 8743-8751, ISSN 1529-2401

Gharabaghi, A., Hellwig, D., Rosahl, S.K., Shahidi, R., Schrader, C., Freund, H.J., Samii, M. (2005). Volumetric image guidance for motor cortex stimulation: integration of three-dimensional cortical anatomy and functional imaging. *Neurosurgery*, 57, 114-120; discussion 114-120, ISSN 1524-4040

Grafton, S.T., Waters, C., Sutton, J., Lew, M.F., Couldwell, W. (1995). Pallidotomy increases activity of motor association cortex in Parkinson's disease: a positron emission tomographic study. *Ann Neurol*, 37, 776-783, ISSN 0364-5134

Greenberg, M., (2010). *Handbook of neurosurgery*, (5 ed), Thieme, ISBN 1604063262, New York

Gutierrez, J.C., Seijo, F.J., Alvarez Vega, M.A., Fernandez Gonzalez, F., Lozano Aragoneses, B., Blazquez, M. (2009). Therapeutic extradural cortical stimulation for Parkinson's Disease: report of six cases and review of the literature. *Clin Neurol Neurosurg*, 111, 703-707, ISSN 1872-6968

Hamada, M., Ugawa, Y., Tsuji, S., (2008) High-frequency rTMS over supplementary motor area for treatment of Parkinson's disease. Mov Disord 23, 1524-1531

Hanajima, R., Ashby, P., Lang, A.E., Lozano, A.M. (2002). Effects of acute stimulation through contacts placed on the motor cortex for chronic stimulation. *Clin Neurophysiol*, 113, 635-641, ISSN 1388-2457

Haslinger, B., Erhard, P., Kampfe, N., Boecker, H., Rummeny, E., Schwaiger, M., Conrad, B., Ceballos-Baumann, A.O. (2001). Event-related functional magnetic resonance imaging in Parkinson's disease before and after levodopa. *Brain*, 124, 558-570, ISSN 0006-8950

Holsheimer, J., Nguyen, J.P., Lefaucheur, J.P., Manola, L. (2007). Cathodal, anodal or bifocal stimulation of the motor cortex in the management of chronic pain? *Acta Neurochir Suppl*, 97, 57-66, ISSN 0065-1419

Hosomi, K., Saitoh, Y., Kishima, H., Oshino, S., Hirata, M., Tani, N., Shimokawa, T., Yoshimine, T. (2008). Electrical stimulation of primary motor cortex within the central sulcus for intractable neuropathic pain. *Clin Neurophysiol*, 119, 993-1001, ISSN 1388-2457

Jahanshahi, M., Jenkins, I.H., Brown, R.G., Marsden, C.D., Passingham, R.E., Brooks, D.J. (1995). Self-initiated versus externally triggered movements. I. An investigation using measurement of regional cerebral blood flow with PET and movement-related potentials in normal and Parkinson's disease subjects. *Brain*, 118 (Pt 4), 913-933, ISSN 0006-8950

Jenkins, I.H., Fernandez, W., Playford, E.D., Lees, A.J., Frackowiak, R.S., Passingham, R.E., Brooks, D.J. (1992). Impaired activation of the supplementary motor area in Parkinson's disease is reversed when akinesia is treated with apomorphine. *Ann Neurol*, 32, 749-757, ISSN 0364-5134

Katayama, Y., Fukaya, C., Yamamoto, T. (1998). Poststroke pain control by chronic motor cortex stimulation: neurological characteristics predicting a favorable response. *J Neurosurg*, 89, 585-591, ISSN 0022-3085

Khedr, E.M., Rothwell, J.C., Shawky, O.A., Ahmed, M.A., Hamdy, A. (2006). Effect of daily repetitive transcranial magnetic stimulation on motor performance in Parkinson's disease. *Mov Disord*, 21, 2201-2205, ISSN 0885-3185

Kleiner-Fisman, G., Fisman, D.N., Sime, E., Saint-Cyr, J.A., Lozano, A.M., Lang, A.E. (2003). Long-term follow up of bilateral deep brain stimulation of the subthalamic nucleus in patients with advanced Parkinson disease. *J Neurosurg*, 99, 489-495, ISSN 0022-3085

Koch, G., Brusa, L., Caltagirone, C., Peppe, A., Oliveri, M., Stanzione, P., Centonze, D. (2005). rTMS of supplementary motor area modulates therapy-induced dyskinesias in Parkinson disease. *Neurology*, 65, 623-625, ISSN 1526-632X

Krack, P., Fraix, V., Mendes, A., Benabid, A.L., Pollak, P. (2002). Postoperative management of subthalamic nucleus stimulation for Parkinson's disease. *Mov Disord*, 17 Suppl 3, S188-197, ISSN 0885-3185

Krack, P., Pollak, P., Limousin, P., Hoffmann, D., Xie, J., Benazzouz, A., Benabid, A.L. (1998). Subthalamic nucleus or internal pallidal stimulation in young onset Parkinson's disease. *Brain*, 121 (Pt 3), 451-457, ISSN 0006-8950

Lefaucheur, J.P., Drouot, X., Von Raison, F., Menard-Lefaucheur, I., Cesaro, P., Nguyen, J.P. (2004). Improvement of motor performance and modulation of cortical excitability by repetitive transcranial magnetic stimulation of the motor cortex in Parkinson's disease. *Clin Neurophysiol*, 115, 2530-2541, ISSN 1388-2457

Leichnetz, G.R. (1986). Afferent and efferent connections of the dorsolateral precentral gyrus (area 4, hand/arm region) in the macaque monkey, with comparisons to area 8. *J Comp Neurol*, 254, 460-492, ISSN 0021-9967

Limousin, P., Greene, J., Pollak, P., Rothwell, J., Benabid, A.L., Frackowiak, R. (1997). Changes in cerebral activity pattern due to subthalamic nucleus or internal pallidum stimulation in Parkinson's disease. *Ann Neurol*, 42, 283-291, ISSN 0364-5134

Limousin, P., Krack, P., Pollak, P., Benazzouz, A., Ardouin, C., Hoffmann, D., Benabid, A.L. (1998). Electrical stimulation of the subthalamic nucleus in advanced Parkinson's disease. *N Engl J Med*, 339, 1105-1111, ISSN 0028-4793

Lopiano, L., Rizzone, M., Bergamasco, B., Tavella, A., Torre, E., Perozzo, P., Lanotte, M. (2002). Deep brain stimulation of the subthalamic nucleus in PD: an analysis of the exclusion causes. *J Neurol Sci*, 195, 167-170, ISSN 0022-510X

Lyons, K.E., Wilkinson, S.B., Overman, J., Pahwa, R. (2004). Surgical and hardware complications of subthalamic stimulation: a series of 160 procedures. *Neurology*, 63, 612-616, ISSN 1526-632X

Manola, L., Holsheimer, J., Veltink, P., Buitenweg, J.R. (2007). Anodal vs cathodal stimulation of motor cortex: a modeling study. *Clin Neurophysiol*, 118, 464-474, ISSN 1388-2457

Montes, C., Mertens, P., Convers, P., Peyron, R., Sindou, M., Laurent, B., Mauguiere, F., Garcia-Larrea, L. (2002). Cognitive effects of precentral cortical stimulation for pain control: an ERP study. *Neurophysiol Clin*, 32, 313-325, ISSN 0987-7053

Naidich, T.P., Blum, J.T., Firestone, M.I. (2001). The parasagittal line: an anatomic landmark for axial imaging. *AJNR Am J Neuroradiol*, 22, 885-895, ISSN 0195-6108

Naidich, T.P., Valavanis, A.G., Kubik, S. (1995). Anatomic relationships along the low-middle convexity: Part I--Normal specimens and magnetic resonance imaging. *Neurosurgery*, 36, 517-532, ISSN 0148-396X

Nguyen, J.P., Lefaucheur, J.P., Decq, P., Uchiyama, T., Carpentier, A., Fontaine, D., Brugieres, P., Pollin, B., Feve, A., Rostaing, S., Cesaro, P., Keravel, Y. (1999). Chronic motor cortex stimulation in the treatment of central and neuropathic pain. Correlations between clinical, electrophysiological and anatomical data. *Pain*, 82, 245-251, ISSN 0304-3959

Pagni, C.A., Zeme, S., Zenga, F. (2003). Further experience with extradural motor cortex stimulation for treatment of advanced Parkinson's disease. Report of 3 new cases. *J Neurosurg Sci*, 47, 189-193, ISSN 0390-5616

Pagni, C.A., Zeme, S., Zenga, F., Maina, R. (2005). Extradural motor cortex stimulation in advanced Parkinson's disease: the Turin experience: technical case report. *Neurosurgery*, 57, E402; discussion E402, ISSN 1524-4040

Pahwa, R., Wilkinson, S.B., Overman, J., Lyons, K.E. (2005). Preoperative clinical predictors of response to bilateral subthalamic stimulation in patients with Parkinson's disease. *Stereotact Funct Neurosurg*, 83, 80-83, ISSN 1011-6125

Pal, E., Nagy, F., Aschermann, Z., Balazs, E., Kovacs, N. (2010). The impact of left prefrontal repetitive transcranial magnetic stimulation on depression in Parkinson's disease: a randomized, double-blind, placebo-controlled study. *Mov Disord*, 25, 2311-2317, ISSN 1531-8257

Priori, A., Lefaucheur, J.P. (2007). Chronic epidural motor cortical stimulation for movement disorders. *Lancet Neurol*, 6, 279-286, ISSN 1474-4422

Rasche, D., Ruppolt, M., Stippich, C., Unterberg, A., Tronnier, V.M. (2006). Motor cortex stimulation for long-term relief of chronic neuropathic pain: a 10 year experience. *Pain*, 121, 43-52, ISSN 0304-3959

Rascol, O., Sabatini, U., Chollet, F., Celsis, P., Montastruc, J.L., Marc-Vergnes, J.P., Rascol, A. (1992). Supplementary and primary sensory motor area activity in Parkinson's disease. Regional cerebral blood flow changes during finger movements and effects of apomorphine. *Arch Neurol*, 49, 144-148, ISSN 0003-9942

Rodriguez-Oroz, M.C., Jahanshahi, M., Krack, P., Litvan, I., Macias, R., Bezard, E., Obeso, J.A. (2009). Initial clinical manifestations of Parkinson's disease: features and pathophysiological mechanisms. *Lancet Neurol*, 8, 1128-1139, ISSN 1474-4465

Saitoh, Y., Shibata, M., Hirano, S., Hirata, M., Mashimo, T., Yoshimine, T. (2000). Motor cortex stimulation for central and peripheral deafferentation pain. Report of eight cases. *J Neurosurg*, 92, 150-155, ISSN 0022-3085

Saitoh Y, Hosomi K: Chapter 2. From localization to surgical implantation. In Textbook of therapeutic cortical stimulation Ed: Sergio Canavero, Nova Science Publishers, Inc. Hauppauge NY, 2009

Strafella, A.P., Lozano, A.M., Lang, A.E., Ko, J.H., Poon, Y.Y., Moro, E. (2007). Subdural motor cortex stimulation in Parkinson's disease does not modify movement-related rCBF pattern. *Mov Disord*, 22, 2113-2116, ISSN 0885-3185

Tani, N., Saitoh, Y., Kishima, H., Oshino, S., Hatazawa, J., Hashikawa, K., Yoshimine, T. (2007). Motor cortex stimulation for levodopa-resistant akinesia: case report. *Mov Disord*, 22, 1645-1649, ISSN 0885-3185

Thickbroom, G.W., Byrnes, M.L., Walters, S., Stell, R., Mastaglia, F.L. (2006). Motor cortex reorganisation in Parkinson's disease. *J Clin Neurosci*, 13, 639-642, ISSN 0967-5868

Tirakotai, W., Hellwig, D., Bertalanffy, H., Riegel, T. (2007). Localization of precentral gyrus in image-guided surgery for motor cortex stimulation. *Acta Neurochir Suppl*, 97, 75-79, ISSN 0065-1419

Tsubokawa, T., Katayama, Y., Yamamoto, T., Hirayama, T., Koyama, S. (1991a). Chronic motor cortex stimulation for the treatment of central pain. *Acta Neurochir Suppl (Wien)*, 52, 137-139, ISSN 0065-1419

Tsubokawa, T., Katayama, Y., Yamamoto, T., Hirayama, T., Koyama, S. (1991b). Treatment of thalamic pain by chronic motor cortex stimulation. *Pacing Clin Electrophysiol*, 14, 131-134, ISSN 0147-8389

Umemura, A., Jaggi, J.L., Hurtig, H.I., Siderowf, A.D., Colcher, A., Stern, M.B., Baltuch, G.H. (2003). Deep brain stimulation for movement disorders: morbidity and mortality in 109 patients. *J Neurosurg*, 98, 779-784, ISSN 0022-3085

Velasco, M., Velasco, F., Brito, F., Velasco, A.L., Nguyen, J.P., Marquez, I., Boleaga, B., Keravel, Y. (2002). Motor cortex stimulation in the treatment of deafferentation pain. I. Localization of the motor cortex. *Stereotact Funct Neurosurg*, 79, 146-167, ISSN 1011-6125

Wood, C.C., Spencer, D.D., Allison, T., McCarthy, G., Williamson, P.D., Goff, W.R. (1988). Localization of human sensorimotor cortex during surgery by cortical surface recording of somatosensory evoked potentials. *J Neurosurg*, 68, 99-111, ISSN 0022-3085

11

Estimation of Electrode Position with Fused Images of Preoperative MRI and Postoperative CT Using the Mutual Information Technique After STN DBS in Patients with Advanced Parkinson's Disease

Sun Ha Paek

Movement Disorder Center, Department of Neurosurgery, Seoul National University Hospital, Seoul National University College of Medicine, South Korea

1. Introduction

Since the introduction of deep brain stimulation (DBS) by Benabid and colleagues in 1987, this technique has become the preferred treatment for patients with various movement disorders including Parkinson's disease (Benabid et al., 1987). Patients with advanced Parkinson's disease (PD) who have intolerable drug-induced side effects or motor complications following the long-term use of dopaminergic drugs have shown significant improvement in symptoms such as motor fluctuation and dyskinesia following subthalamic nucleus (STN) deep brain stimulation (DBS), facilitating reductions in dosages of levodopa (Limousin et al., 1998). Significant improvements in motor function have been documented in both short-term and long-term periods (Krack et al., 2003; Benabid et al., 2005; Lyons & Pahwa, 2005; Rodriguez-Oroz et al., 2005; Deuschl et al., 2006; Kleiner-Fisman et al., 2006; Tsai et al., 2009). However, variable improvement of symptoms has been observed after STN DBS even in well-selected patients with advanced PD (Paek et al., 2008). Such individual variation was not predictable before surgery and its cause is not obvious. Differences in the extent of disease progression or constitutional differences in response to STN DBS might lead to such variation; alternatively, it might be caused by differences in the accuracy of electrode positioning in relation to the STN.

The precise positioning of the electrodes in the STN is considered an important factor in achieving good clinical outcome following STN DBS. To achieve precise targeting of electrodes, many approaches have been taken; these include direct targeting based on fused images of CT-MRI, MRI-MRI, and MRI-brain atlas, as well as intra-operative microelectrode recording and intra-operative stimulation (Bejjani et al., 2000; Benazzou et al., 2002; Hamid et al., 2005; Godinho et al., 2006; Cho et al., 2010). However, many unexpected factors, such as possible brain shift due to CSF leakage, electrode artifacts in the MRI, and error in the manipulation of instruments, make it difficult to precisely position electrodes in the center of the STN (Martinez-Santiesteban et al., 2007; Miyagi et al., 2007; Halpern et al., 2008; Khan et al., 2008). Thus, following surgery, not all patients have electrodes positioned exactly in the STN. This might lead to different clinical outcomes following STN DBS in advanced PD patients. However, the existing literature contains few reports on the possible correlation between clinical outcome and electrode position confirmed at a stable period after bilateral STN stimulation.

The foregoing considerations suggest that it is necessary to determine the exact location of DBS electrodes after surgery in order to accurately predict clinical outcomes and to program appropriate stimulation parameters for STN DBS. The Movement Disorder Center of Seoul National University Hospital (SNUH MDC) was launched in March, 2005; at that time, DBS began to be covered by the National Health Insurance system in Korea. During the past six years, we have systematically approached the analysis of clinical outcome in terms of electrode position after bilateral STN stimulation (Heo et al., 2008; Kim et al., 2008a; Kim et al., 2008b; Lee et al., 2008; Kim et al., 2009; Kim et al., 2010; Lee et al., 2010a; Lee et al., 2010b; Paek et al., 2010).

In this chapter, I would like to briefly touch on these issues based on a review of the literature as well as on our own experience. I would also like to introduce the DBS Electrode Localization Analysis System (DELAS), an internet on-line service to estimate electrode positions with fused images of pre-operative MRI and post-operative CT using mutual information technique following STN DBS surgery in patients with advanced Parkinson's disease.

2. Image fusion using the mutual information technique and plotting of electrode positions with reference to the human brain atlas of Schaltenbrand and Wahren

2.1 Image-to-image registration using the mutual information technique

The mutual information technique is a commonly used image registration technique (Wells et al., 1996; Christensen et al., 1997; Maes et al., 1997). Fig. 1 (Lucion, Cybermed Inc., Korea) shows an instance of accurate registration between CT and MR images. The first image was obtained by preoperative MRI and the second by postoperative CT. The process of image-to-image registration using the mutual information technique can be briefly described as follows. Consider the 2D histogram of 3D images A and B for a given transform T between the two images: if the images have their discrete values m and n in [0...M], the 2D histogram is a function h(m,n) from [0...M]x[0...N] to ln that associates every pair of image values (m,n) with the number of occurrences in which image A equals n at the same spatial point x in 3D (for the given transform T, the number of such occurrences depends on parameters p:m=a(x) and n=B(T(x)). If we consider 3D images A and B to be from the same modality, then when the images are registered, the histogram h(m,n) is an array that has accumulation points on the line m=n. These accumulation points are therefore very concentrated.

A possible way to characterize the complexity of a 2D histogram is to consider entropy. Entropy, e(p), is minimal when the histogram is concentrated on very few accumulation points. It is given by the following equation:

$$e(p) = -\int P(m,n)\ln(P(m,n))dm\,dn \qquad (1)$$

When images are registered, the entropy will be minimized. Equation 1.1 is now replaced by the expression of mutual information, which has to be maximized, as follows:

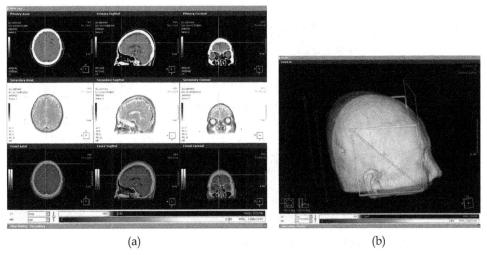

(a)   (b)

Fig. 1. Registration of multimodality images using entropy-based methods. (a) The different
CT slices are shown with the edges of the registered and reformatted MR data overlaid. (b)
A rendering of the 3D models constructed from different MR acquisitions that were
registered together: anatomic information (the skin, the brain, the vessels, the ventricles)
was generated from the post-contrast gradient echo (SPGR) MR images.

$$h(m,n) = -\int_S P(m)\ln(P(m))dm - \int_S P(n)\ln(P(n))dn + \int P(m,n)\ln(P(m,n))dm\,dn \qquad (2)$$

The method of Wells et al. (1996) implements this principle very efficiently. In practice,
images do not need to be of the same modality; they merely need to "look similar."
Obviously, there are some limitations to the method and many aspects remain to be
explored; however, the technique has yielded very efficient results in a variety of instances
(Pluim et al., 2003).

2.1.1 Calculation of mutual information (MI)

Calculation of MI is performed by employing formula (3) below. First, we need to obtain the
mutual histogram, $g(a,b)$, of two volumetric images; then, by using the following equation,
the normalized mutual information is obtained. As the optimization procedure proceeds,
the value of MI gradually decreases. The optimization procedure terminates when the
change in the MI value is below a threshold,

$$MI = \sum_{a,b} p_{u,v}(a,b)\log_2 \frac{p_{uv}(a,b)}{p_u(a)p_v(b)} , \text{ where}$$

$$p_u(x) = \sum_b p_{uv}(x,b) , \; p_v(y) = \sum_a p_{uv}(a,y) , \text{ and } p_{uv}(x,y) = \frac{g(x,y)}{\sum_{a,b} g(a,b)} . \qquad (3)$$

In this equation, $g(a,b)$ represents the mutual histogram, x represents the intensity index of
the primary image, and y represents the intensity index of the secondary image.

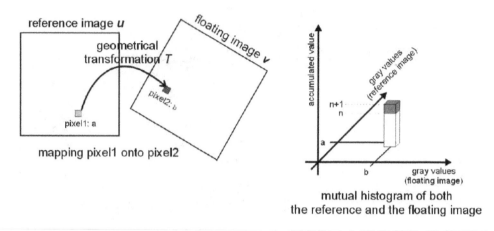

Fig. 2. Mutual histogram of two different images.

When the final screw vector is obtained, we can register the two volumetric images by applying the transformation to the secondary volume.

2.2 Image fusion of preoperative brain MRI and postoperative brain CT/MRI images and plotting of electrode positions with reference to the human brain atlas

Image fusions are performed using the mutual information technique with the preoperative brain MRI and the brain CT/MRI images taken after STN DBS. Window level and width are adjusted to best visualize the STN in the T2-weighted MRI and to best visualize the electrodes in the CT/MRI. The preoperative T2-weighted axial images are fused with the postoperative 3-D spiral CT scan images or T2-weighted axial images at the data set of 1-mm thickness reformatted images, aligned to the anterior commissure-posterior commissure

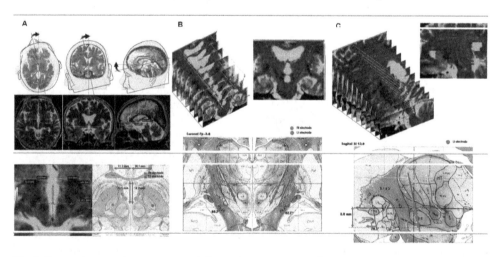

Fig. 3. Image fusion of preoperative MRI and postoperative brain CT.

(AC-PC) line. For the correction of head-rotation error, the midline of the reformatted coronal images is positioned to intersect the midsagittal plane. The length of the AC-PC line and the width of the third ventricle are taken into consideration for the proportional localization of electrode position with reference to the human brain atlas of Schaltenbrandt and Wahren (1998). In the reformatted axial images, the lateral distance from the midline and the antero-posterior distance from the mid-commissural line to each electrode are measured (Fig 3-A). In the reformatted coronal images in which the electrode trajectory is best visualized, the lateral angles of the electrode trajectory from the midline are measured for each electrode in every patient (Fig 3-B). In the reformatted sagittal images in which the electrode trajectory is best shown, the antero-posterior angle of the electrode trajectory from the line perpendicular to the AC-PC line and the depth of the electrodes are also measured for each electrode in every patient (Fig 3-C).

3. Comparison study of estimated electrode locations obtained using various image fusion techniques

3.1 Comparison study of CT and MRI for the localization of electrodes following subthalamic nucleus deep brain stimulation

Despite the wide use of MRI in stereotactic neurosurgical procedures, the potential for distortion of normal anatomical structures in MRI in comparison with brain CT scans has been noted. Several studies focused on the reliability of MRI in target localization and concluded that though some differences were identified, they were not significant and that MRI alone may be used for target localization (Kondziolka et al., 1992; Holtzheimer et al., 1999). Relatively less attention has been paid to the accuracy of MRI in localization of electrode position, and the results have been controversial. However, by calculating magnetic field perturbations using a Fourier-based method for various wire microelectrodes, one study showed that significant artifact is produced depending on the magnetic susceptibility of the material used and on the size, shape, and orientation of the electrodes with respect to the primary magnetic field (Martinez-Santiesteban et al., 2007). This study concluded that the platinum–iridium microwire commonly used for DBS shows a complete signal loss that covers a volume 400 times larger than the actual volume occupied by the microelectrode. Thus, artifacts caused by electrode interference with local magnetic fields can make it difficult to precisely localize the center of the electrodes in MRI.

We found that there is a considerable difference in the estimated electrode position obtained using postoperative CT and that obtained using MRI. Figure 4 shows fused images of a brain CT and a brain MRI from one patient, both taken 6 months after bilateral subthalamic stimulation. The fused images obtained from the MRI and the CT are aligned along the AC-PC line at the level of the AC and the PC in the axial, sagittal, and coronal planes. The red signal represents the position of the electrode extracted from brain CT images obtained six months after surgery, and the gray signal represents the position of the electrode extracted from brain MRI images obtained six months after surgery. The centers of the red and gray areas, representing the center of the electrode as extracted from brain CT and brain MRI images, respectively, do not coincide but instead show significant discrepancy in their positions in the axial, coronal, and sagittal planes of the fused images (Fig 4-A). With the adjustment of window level and width of the fused images, only the electrodes in red color are superimposed in 3-D reconstructive rendering brain MR images of the superior anterior view (Fig 4-B), the left anterior superior oblique view (Fig 4-C), and the anterior posterior view (Fig 4-D). The discrepancy in the electrode position extracted from the brain CT and the center of the electrode artifact from the brain MRI taken 6 months after surgery is remarkable in all three (axial, sagittal, and coronal) planes.

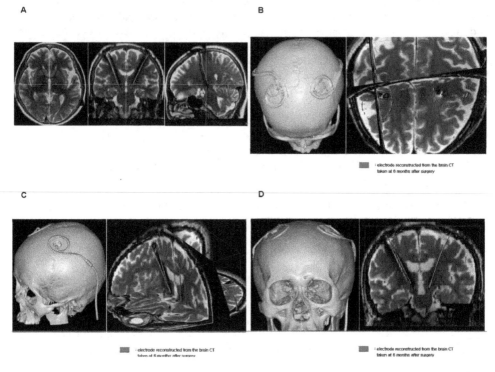

Fig. 4. Fused images of brain CT and brain MRI, both taken 6 months after bilateral subthalamic nucleus stimulation.

To validate the accuracy of MRI in electrode localization in comparison with CT scanning, we compared the X-, Y-, and Z- coordinates of the centers of the electrodes estimated by MRI and CT in 61 patients who received both MRI and CT at least six months after bilateral STN DBS (Lee et al., 2010b). The x- and y-coordinates of the centers of the electrodes shown by CT and MRI were compared in the fused images, and the average difference at five different levels was calculated. The difference in the location of the tips of the electrodes, designated as the z coordinate, was also calculated.

The average distance between the centers of the electrodes in the five levels estimated in the fused images of brain CT and MRI taken at least 6 months after STN DBS was 1.33 mm (0.1–5.8 mm). The average discrepancy of the x coordinates for all five levels between MRI and CT was 0.56±0.54 mm (0–5.7 mm); the discrepancy of the y coordinates was 1.06±0.59 mm (0–3.5 mm) and that of the z coordinates was 0.98±0.52 mm (0–3.1 mm) (all p values <0.001). Notably, the average discrepancy of x coordinates at 3.5 mm below the AC–PC level, i.e., at the level of the STN, was 0.59±0.42 mm (0–2.4) between MRI and CT; the discrepancy of the y coordinates at this level was 0.81±0.47 mm (0–2.9) (p values<0.001). It is suggested that the electrode location evaluated by postoperative MRI may show significant discrepancy with that estimated by brain CT scan.

3.2 Comparison of electrode location measured on the immediate postoperative day and six months after bilateral STN DBS

Despite the wide use of brain CT scans during and immediately after DBS surgery, unexpected circumstances during surgery, such as electrode bending and possible brain shift due to CSF leakage, have not been seriously considered in the estimation of electrode position using brain CT in the immediate postoperative period after DBS surgeries. One study, which used brain CT to evaluate and correct geometrical error due to brain shift during stereotactic brain surgery (van den Munckhof et al., 2010), showed that the stereotactically implanted DBS electrodes were displaced in an upward direction with time and that this displacement was significantly correlated with the amount of air in the subdural space. This study calculated the displacement of the electrode on the fusion image of preoperative and postoperative images. However, the fiducial points for the fusion of different images were not associated with brain structures but with the skull. The migration of metallic material in the parenchyma of the central nervous system has also been reported (Ott et al., 1976; Sorensen & Krauss, 1991). We observed considerable brain shift when comparing immediate postoperative CT scans and CT scans taken 6 months after surgery. We also found considerable discrepancy in the apparent electrode position on immediate postoperative CT scans and brain CT scans taken 6 months after surgery (Fig. 5).

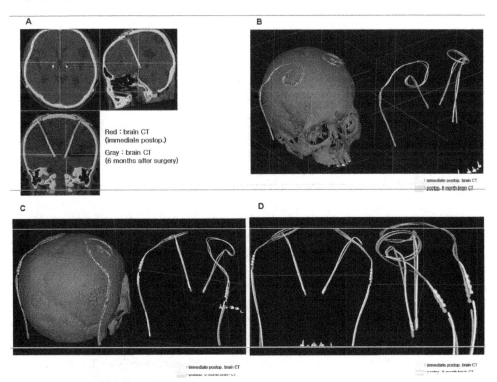

Fig. 5. Fused images of an immediate postoperative brain CT and a brain CT taken 6 months after bilateral subthalamic nucleus stimulation.

In Fig. 5, fused images obtained from two CT scans are aligned along the AC-PC line at the level of the AC and the PC in the axial, sagittal, and coronal planes. The red area represents the position of the electrode extracted from brain CT images obtained immediately after surgery, and the gray area represents the position of the electrode extracted from brain CT images taken six months after surgery. The red and the gray areas do not coincide, exhibiting significant discrepancy in their positions in the axial and coronal planes (Fig 5-A). With the adjustment of window level and width of the fused images, only the shadow of both electrodes is extracted in 3-D reconstructive rendering images of the right superior oblique view (Fig 5-B), the right posterior oblique view (Fig 5-C), and the AP and lateral views (Fig 5-D). In these views, the yellow area represents the position of the electrode extracted from brain CT images obtained immediately after surgery, and the sky-blue area represents the position of the electrode extracted from brain CT images taken six months after surgery. The discrepancy in the electrode position between the two CT scans is remarkable and significant.

We compared the positions of subthalamic nucleus (STN) deep brain stimulation (DBS) electrodes estimated during the immediate postoperative period with those estimated 6 months after surgery. Brain CT scans were taken immediately and 6 months after bilateral STN DBS in 53 patients with Parkinson's disease (Fig 5.). (Kim et al., 2010). The two images were fused using the mutual information technique. The discrepancies in electrode position in three coordinates were measured in the fused images, and the relationship with the pneumocephalus was evaluated.

The average discrepancies of the x- and y-coordinates of the electrode position at the level of the STN (3.5 mm below the anterior commissure–posterior commissure line) were 0.6± 0.5 mm (range, 0-2.1 mm) and 1.0±0.8 mm (range, 0~5.2 mm), respectively. The average discrepancy of the z-coordinate of the electrode tip in the fused images was 1.0±0.8 mm (range, 0.1~4.0 mm). The volume of pneumocephalus (range, 0-76 ml) was correlated with the y-coordinate discrepancies ($p<0.005$).

We found that there was significant discrepancy in the implanted electrode position measured during the immediate postoperative period and that measured 6 months after DBS surgery. The discrepancy was greatest when the amount of pneumocephalus measured in the immediate postoperative CT scan was large. We think that the stabilization of the electrode position may require at least one month following surgery.

4. Analysis of clinical outcome dependence on electrode position following subthalamic nucleus stimulation

4.1 Data management system in a movement disorder center

When evaluating patients with movement disorders such as Parkinson's disease (PD), most neurologists observe patients only during a limited period at the outpatient clinic. Such limited periods of observation may be less than optimal for precise evaluation of patients with varying and unexpected patterns of movement and for supporting the development of optimal treatment plans for such patients. In order to have a good DBS program, a system that can handle the vast amount of data generated by a DBS program is required (Lee et al., 2008). Data include information on patients' pre- and postoperative clinical condition (including videos), medications and stimulation-related parameters. For proper management of patients, easy access to these data is essential . For this reason, we designed a specialized monitoring unit and data management system with systematic storage and easy access for use in deep brain stimulation programs for patients with movement disorders (Paek et al., 2010). All patients were monitored and evaluated in a specialized 24-hour monitoring system, postoperatively as well as preoperatively, in order to provide information for making accurate diagnoses and thorough evaluation of surgical candidates, as well as to provide them with the best care based on a consistent management protocol and an organized follow-up system. We digitized all of the data and developed a data management system that allowed systematic storage and easy access to the data on demand by users in the offices and outpatient clinics. We describe our data management system and how it provides benefit to patients (Fig. 6), so that others may use it as a template for designing their own data management systems. The details have been described previously (Paek et al., 2010).

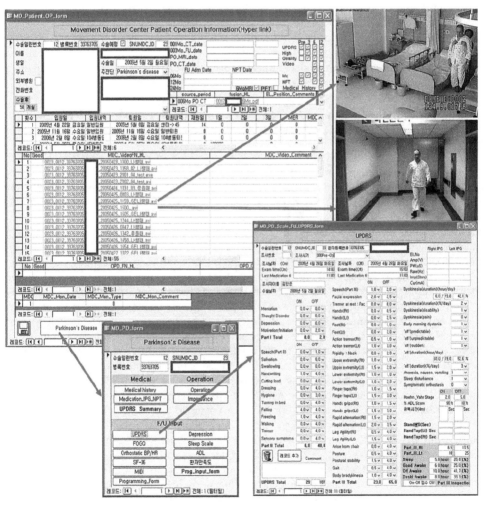

Fig. 6. Data management system in the Movement Disorder Center of SNUH.

The easy accessibility and the outstanding convenience for users of the stacked information in our data management system are useful in many ways.

First, they can improve the quality of patient management. Our specialized 24-hour monitoring system can provide more precise preoperative evaluation of patients with various movement disorders, including advanced PD, and can show various and unexpected side effects including the severe wearing-off phenomenon, dyskinesia and motor fluctuation during their 24-hour daily lives. The systematic management system can be useful not only for the selection of surgical candidates but also for dose adjustment of stimulation parameters before and after surgery.

Second, our data management system can be a useful tool for the education for patients and their caregivers. Many patients with PD have difficulty differentiating between off tremor, dystonia and dyskinesia. Video recordings were helpful in educating the patients about the conditions seen in the videos and in teaching them how to describe their symptoms correctly for future communication.

Third, we can use the data to continually review our performance and to perform standardized outcome analysis. With our data management system, we can access all the collected data representing integrated clinical information on all our patients and carry out a statistical evaluation of our performance.

4.2 Short-term outcome dependence on electrode position as determined by fused images of preoperative and postoperative brain MRI following bilateral subthalamic nucleus stimulation

STN DBS improves motor symptoms and daily activities in patients with advanced PD (Krack et al., 2003; Benabid et al., 2005; Lyons & Pahwa, 2005; Rodriguez-Oroz et al., 2005; Deuschl et al., 2006; Kleiner-Fisman et al., 2006; Tsai et al., 2009). However, variable improvement of symptoms has been observed after STN DBS, even in well-selected patients with advanced PD (Krack et al., 2003; Ford et al., 2004). Such individual variation was not predictable before surgery and no obvious explanation for it is evident; it might have resulted from differences in the extent of disease progression, constitutional differences in individual patients' responses to STN DBS, or the relative accuracy of electrode positioning. Many studies have discussed the technical details of electrode localization in postoperative magnetic resonance imaging (MRI) and have described the anatomical locations of clinically effective electrode contacts (Saint-Cyr et al., 2002; Schrader et al., 2002; Starr et al., 2002; Yelnik et al., 2003; Hamid et al., 2005; Plaha et al., 2006; Pollo et al., 2007). However, most reports do not include a comparison of electrode location and surgical outcome. Plaha et al. (2006) stated that electrodes located in the zona incerta resulted in greater improvement in contralateral motor scores than those located in the STN or dorsomedial/medial to the STN after STN DBS. These authors used guide tubes and plastic stylets implanted in the target point and performed intraoperative MRI to verify the electrode position. Postoperative confirmation of the electrode location was not carried out. McClelland et al. (2005) calculated the electrode tip coordinates in x, y, and z planes relative to the midcommissural point from fused MRI scans of postoperative and preoperative planning images in 26 consecutive patients and compared electrode tip location with clinical outcome. Yokoyama et al. (2006) compared the clinical improvement of Parkinsonian symptoms after monopolar stimulation using four electrode contacts, the locations of which were determined using intraoperative x-rays obtained after placing the DBS electrode in the STN. In both of these studies, the positions of the electrodes were determined by intraoperative x-ray or by using fused images from immediate pre- and postoperative MRI. Possible brain shift during the operation and/or the immediate postoperative period could be a concern regarding the accuracy of the electrode localization. Both studies assessed electrode position relative to the AC–PC line or to the midcommissural point, but neither demonstrated a 3-dimensional relationship between the electrode and the STN.

We evaluated the clinical outcomes of 53 advanced PD patients at three and six months after bilateral STN DBS with respect to electrode position estimated from fused pre- and postoperative magnetic resonance images (Paek et al., 2008). Patients were evaluated using the Unified Parkinson's Disease Rating Scale, Hoehn and Yahr staging, Schwab and England Activities of Daily Living, L-dopa equivalent dose, and the Short Form-36 Health Survey before surgery and at 3 and 6 months after surgery. Brain magnetic resonance imaging (1.5-T) was performed in all 53 patients at 6 months after STN DBS.

In this group of patients, the Unified Parkinson's Disease Rating Scale, Hoehn and Yahr staging, Schwab and England Activities of Daily Living, and Short Form-36 Health Survey scores all improved at 3 and 6 months after STN DBS, while the L-dopa equivalent dose decreased by 60%. The electrode position was classified according to its relationship to the STN and the red nucleus. The off-medication speech subscale score improved only in patients whose electrodes were correctly bilaterally positioned in the STN; however, the improvement of Parkinsonian symptoms other than speech and stimulation side effects did not vary with the variation of electrode locations found. It seems that there is a significant target volume in the region of the STN that provides equivalent clinical efficacy.

Despite these correlations, we found that there is a significant difference in electrode position determined from the fused images of postoperative MRI and CT scans taken six months after surgery and those measured immediately following bilateral STN DBS surgery. Thus, we again compared the clinical outcomes of 57 advanced PD patients at six and twelve months following bilateral STN DBS according to electrode positions estimated using fused preoperative magnetic resonance images and postoperative computed tomography obtained six months after surgery. Electrode positions were determined in the fused images of preoperative magnetic resonance images and postoperative computed tomography taken at six months after surgery. The patients were divided into three groups: group I, both electrodes in the subthalamic nucleus; group II, only one electrode in the subthalamic nucleus; group III, neither electrode in the subthalamic nucleus. Unified Parkinson's Disease Rating Scale, Hoehn and Yahr Stage, Schwab and England Activities of Daily Living were prospectively evaluated before and at 6 and 12 months after surgery.

In Groups I and II, the Unified Parkinson's Disease Rating Scale, the Hoehn and Yahr Stage, and the Schwab and England Activities of Daily Living scores significantly improved with a reduced l-dopa equivalent daily dose at 6 and 12 months after subthalamic nucleus stimulation. The patients of group I, especially those in whom the electrodes were located in the middle third of both subthalamic nuclei 3.5 mm below the anterior-posterior commissural line, had better outcome in speech with a smaller L-dopa equivalent daily dose than that of the two other groups.

The LEDD of 13 of the 57 patients was zero at their last follow up. The preoperative characteristics of this group were not different from those of the other patients. Their total UPDRS scores, H&Y Stage, SEADL, and dyskinesia disability scores improved dramatically at 12 months after STN DBS. Their off-time UPDRS part III subscores, including speech, were significantly improved at 12 months after surgery. On investigating electrode positioning in these patients, it was found that all had both electrodes positioned in or close to the middle one third of the STN on axial view, at a level of 3.5 mm below the AC-PC line. It is suggested that the best symptom relief, including improved speech with reduced LEDD, was observed in the patients whose electrodes were accurately positioned in both STN. Thus, a good long-term outcome of subthalamic nucleus stimulation is predicted when the electrodes are positioned in the middle third of the subthalamic nucleus (Fig. 7). However, the improvement of Parkinsonian symptoms, LEDD, neuropsychological changes other than speech, and stimulation side effects did not vary with the variation of electrode location found in this series of patients. This study thus supports the idea proposed by McClelland et al. (2005) that there is a significant target volume in the region of the STN that provides equivalent clinical efficacy.

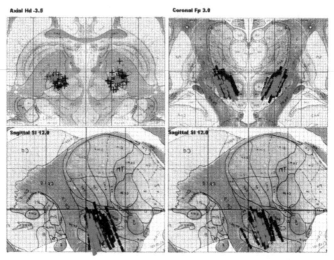

Fig. 7. Locations of the electrodes based on fused images obtained from 13 patients who showed significant clinical improvement in UPDRS part III including speech with nil LEDD (shown in red) and on fused images obtained from the remaining 44 patients (shown in black) at the last follow-up period more than one year after surgery. Most of the electrodes in the 13 patients who showed improvement are positioned in the middle one third of the subthalamic nucleus (in the axial view) at a level of 3.5 mm below the AC-PC line (upper left); they are also positioned in the subthalamic nucleus in the coronal view at a level of 3.0 mm posterior to the midcommissural point (upper right) and in the sagittal view at a level of 12 mm lateral to the midline (lower panels).

4.3 Three-year long-term outcome following bilateral STN DBS with respect to electrode position

Although many studies have addressed the relationship between patients' clinical outcomes and prognostic factors, few studies have analyzed the long-term clinical outcome of STN DBS as a function of inserted electrode positioning (Tsai et al., 2009). Many studies have shown stable improvement in patients' UDPRS scores after bilateral STN DBS (Krack et al., 2003; Liang et al., 2006; Ostergaard & Sunde., 2006; Piboolnurak et al., 2007; Wider et al., 2008; Tsai et al., 2009), although the scores were observed to diminish over time due to disease progression (Olanow et al., 1995; Louis et al., 1999; Jankovic et al., 2001; Krack et al.,

2003; Rodriguez-Oroz et al., 2005; Tsai et al., 2009). In a review of the literature, Benabid et al. (2009) found that improvements in UDPRS III scores after STN DBS were reasonably stable over time, decreasing from 66% improvement at one year to 54% improvement five years after surgery (Benabid et al., 2009). It is suggested that the progression of symptoms over time after STN DBS closely resembles the natural history of PD on medically-treated PD but motor complications, which was thought to represent disease progression. Piboolnurak et al. (2007) investigated the long-term levodopa response after bilateral STN DBS and the predictive value of preoperative L-dopa response in 33 patients with PD (Piboolnurak et al., 2007). They found a trend of decreasing DBS response and observed that preoperative L-dopa responsiveness was not predictive of long-term DBS benefit. Wider et al. (2008) have described the long-term outcomes of 50 consecutive PD patients up to five years after bilateral STN DBS. They noted that a highly significant improvement in UPDRS part III sub-scores with stimulation was maintained at five years; however, this tended to diminish over time due to disease progression. They suggest that the observation of worsening symptoms in these cases argues against the neuroprotective effect hypothesis of STN DBS and actually reflects disease progression (Olanow et al., 1995; Louis et al., 1999; Jankovic et al., 2001; Krack et al., 2003). Unfortunately, there is little information available in the literature on how patients' long-term outcomes relate to electrode position measured in a stable period following bilateral STN stimulation.

We investigated the three-year outcomes of 42 PD patients following bilateral STN DBS and related the outcomes to electrode position as determined by means of fused preoperative MRI and postoperative CT images. Forty-two advanced PD patients were followed for three years after bilateral STN DBS using a prospective protocol. Patients were evaluated before surgery and one, two, and three years after surgery using the Unified Parkinson's Disease Rating Scale, Hoehn and Yahr staging, Schwab and England Activities of Daily Living, and the Short Form-36 Health Survey. The patients were divided into two groups according to electrode position; group I included patients who had both electrodes in the STN (n=31), whereas group II included patients who did not have both electrodes in the STN (n=11).

The UPDRS, Hoehn & Yahr staging, Schwab and England Activities of Daily Living, and the Short Form-36 Health Survey scores showed significant improvements with decreased L-dopa equivalent daily doses (LEDDs) in both groups, as well as in the patient cohort as a whole, up to three years following bilateral STN DBS (Fig 8). However, for patients in group II, the off-medication UPDRS total and motor (part III) scores significantly deteriorated with increased LEDDs three years after STN DBS in comparison to patients in group I (Fig. 8).

It is suggested that electrode positioning influences the long-term outcome of advanced PD patients following STN DBS. Accurate electrode positioning and documentation thereof should be considered in long-term assessment following STN DBS.

5. Programming/reprogramming guided by the use of fused images from preoperative MRI and postoperative CT following STN DBS

5.1 DBS Electrodes Location Analysis System (DELAS)

We developed an on-line service called "DBS Electrode Localization Analysis System (DELAS)", (http://delas.ondemand3d.com) that can be used to estimate the location of an individual patient's electrodes following STN DBS. Based on our previous experience, estimation of electrode positions at a stable period (around one month) following STN DBS can provide a useful basis for predicting the surgical outcome of each patient and for programming appropriate IPG parameters for each advanced PD patient treated with STN DBS.

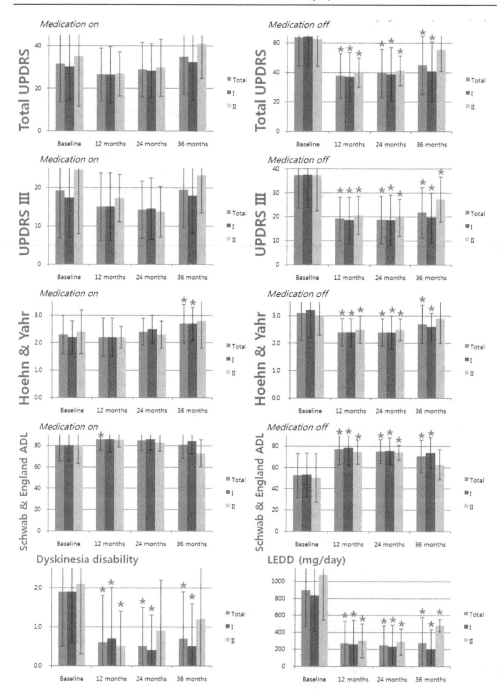

Fig. 8. On-time and off-time scores in 42 patients at 1, 2, and 3 years after subthalamic nucleus stimulation.

5.2 Programming/reprogramming guided by the use of fused images

An examination of the effectiveness and side effects of each of the four contacts of the electrodes used in DBS was performed using an N'vision® programmer (Medtronic, Minneapolis, WI) in all patients to select the best contact of the electrodes and electrical settings for chronic stimulation by the neurologist. After beginning stimulation at the minimal available level (around 1.0 volts), the medication and stimulation parameters were optimized to the demand for the best status of motor functions in harmony with the DBS programming via a 24-hour monitoring unit. Using this method and the electrode position identified by CT-MRI fused images, the stimulation parameters can be carefully adjusted with the selection of the best or the closest contacts of the stimulation electrodes.

5.2.1 Fusion-image-based programming

Subthalamic nucleus (STN) deep brain stimulation (DBS) is a standard therapy for patients with advanced Parkinson's disease (PD) and intolerance for long-term use of medication (Krack et al., 2003; Benabid et al., 2005; Lyons & Pahwa, 2005; Rodriguez-Oroz et al., 2005; Deuschl et al., 2006; Kleiner-Fisman et al., 2006; Tsai et al., 2009). DBS programming is a time-consuming task, however, that requires the patient to undergo a long period of adjustment after surgery (Moro et al., 2002; Deuschl et al., 2006a; Volkmann et al., 2006). Traditionally, DBS programming follows a standardized step-by-step approach (14, 19). The basic algorithm for DBS programming comprises (i) initial programming during the postoperative period; (ii) initiation of long-term stimulation; (iii) stimulation adjustment during the stabilization period (first 3–6 months after surgery) (Deuschl et al., 2006a; Volkmann et al., 2006). This approach tests each electrode individually to determine the most effective stimulation parameters. Generally, the starting point is set at a pulse width of 60 us and a frequency of 130 Hz. Subsequently, the amplitude thresholds for the induction of clinical responses and side effects are determined using monopolar stimulation for each electrode contact with stepwise increases in amplitude of 0.2–0.5 V. If clinical improvement is observed without side effects, the amplitude is increased further to determine the threshold of onset of adverse effects. If no beneficial or adverse effects are observed within the available amplitude range, the next contact is selected and tested. The electrode contact with the lowest threshold that induces a benefit and the largest therapeutic width (i.e., highest threshold for side effects) is selected for long-term stimulation.

We deemed that the determination of the best electrode contacts closest to the STN can be performed more easily and quickly via the use of fused preoperative magnetic resonance imaging (MRI) and postoperative computed tomography (CT) images. We proposed fusion-image-based programming to effectively adjust DBS parameters for patients with advanced Parkinson's disease (PD) after subthalamic nucleus (STN) deep brain stimulation (DBS) (Paek et al., 2011). Thirty-eight patients with advanced PD were consecutively treated with STN DBS between January 2007 and July 2008. The electrode positions and information regarding their contacts with the STN were determined via fusion of images obtained by preoperative magnetic resonance imaging (MRI) and postoperative computed tomography (CT) carried out 1 month after STN DBS (Fig. 9). Postoperative programming was performed using the information on electrode position acquired from the fused images.

All patients were evaluated using a prospective protocol of the Unified Parkinson's Disease Rating Scale, Hoehn and Yahr Staging, Schwab and England Activities of Daily Living, levodopa equivalent daily dose (LEDD), the Short Form-36 Health Survey, and neuropsychological tests prior to and at 3 and/or 6 months after surgery.

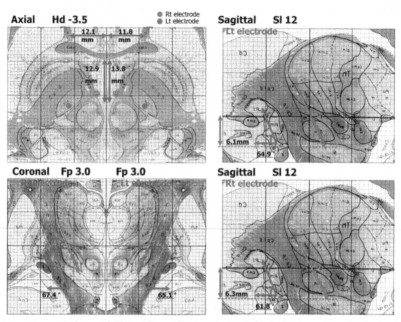

Fig. 9. Electrode positions plotted with reference to the human brain atlas of Schaltenbrandt and Wahren. The electrode positions are based on information obtained from fused images of preoperative MRI and postoperative CT taken one month after surgery.

After STN stimulation, there was rapid and significant improvement of motor symptoms, especially tremor and rigidity, with low morbidity. Stimulation led to an improvement in the off-medication UPRSR III scores of approximately 55% of the patients at 3 and 6 months after STN DBS. Dyskinesia was also significantly improved (74% at 3 months and 95% at 6 months) (Table 1).

In addition, LEDD values decreased to 50% of the level observed before surgery within 1 month after STN DBS surgery (Fig. 10).

When information from the fused images of preoperative MRI and postoperative CT was used to ascertain electrode position, the time spent selecting the stimulation contacts and appropriate stimulation parameters was markedly shortened, and patients were able to avoid prolonged experience of the unnecessary adverse effects caused by the selection of inappropriate contacts far from the STN target. With this approach, the selection of stimulation contacts with appropriate stimulation parameters can be achieved soon after surgery, in harmony with reduced dosages of antiparkinsonian drugs. When the fused images were used, the time and effort expended by physicians in the selection of the stimulation contacts and appropriate stimulation parameters were also markedly reduced, and the long-term trial-and-error rounds caused by the step-by-step selection of the contacts, which frequently occurred even with experienced specialists (Moro et al., 2002; Deuschl et al., 2006a; Volkmann et al., 2006), could be avoided. Thus, it is suggested that programming based on fused images of preoperative MRI and postoperative CT scans after STN DBS can often be carried out quickly, easily, and efficiently.

	Medication	DBS	Baseline	3 months	6 months	P-value 3 months vs. baseline	P-value 6 months vs. baseline
Total UPDRS	On	Off	30.8 ± 14.4				
	Off		65.7 ± 18.1				
	On	On		24.5 ± 12.8	25.3 ± 10.4	p=0.015	p=0.038
	Off			33.7 ± 16.4	33.4 ± 14.2	p<0.001*	p<0.001*
UPDRS III	On	Off	20.3 ± 11.7		33.4 ± 14.8		p<0.001*
	Off		40.9 ± 13.4		38.0 ± 13.6		P=0.203
	On	On		14.4 ± 8.3	14.5 ± 6.1	p=0.004*	p=0.005*
	Off			18.6 ± 8.4	18.1 ± 8.0	p<0.001*	p<0.001*
H & Y	On	Off	2.4 ± 0.5				
	Off		3.1 ± 0.9				
	On	On		2.4 ± 0.5	2.5 ± 0.5	p=0.729	p=0.337
	Off			2.6 ± 0.4	2.6 ± 0.5	p=0.001*	p<0.001*
SEADL	On	Off	83.3 ± 10.1				
	Off		64.2 ± 13.6				
	On	On		86.1 ± 9.9	86.6 ± 9.7	p=0.185	p=0.085
	Off			80.6 ± 13.7	80.5 ± 14.3	p<0.001*	p<0.001*
Dyskinesia disability			2.1 ± 1.5	0.5 ± 1.1	0.3 ± 0.8	p<0.001*	p<0.001*
LEDD (mg/day)			793.4 ± 527.0	285.3 ± 387.2	246.5 ± 322.1	p<0.001*	p<0.001*

Table 1. Clinical outcome in 38 patients after subthalamic nucleus stimulation. * Asterisks indicate p<0.01 and statistical significance with use of the Bonferroni correction method to avoid a Type I error when conducting multiple analyses over time.

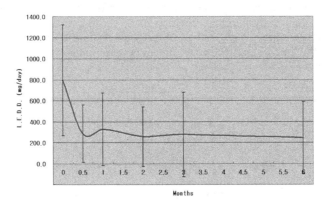

Fig. 10. Levodopa equivalent daily dose (LEDD) changes in 38 patients after subthalamic nucleus stimulation.

5.2.2 Fusion-image-based reprogramming

Published guidelines for DBS programming in PD recommend that the contact for chronic stimulation be selected after testing the efficacy of each electrode separately to evaluate its effective threshold and therapeutic width (Volkmann et al., 2002; Volkmann et al., 2006). Although the established guidelines provide a systematic approach, several practical difficulties are encountered in DBS programming. First, the responses from stimulating each contact serially at several-minute intervals can be confounded by the effects of the previously stimulated electrode. Second, it is time-consuming to stimulate each electrode separately and to evaluate the threshold of each parameter. Third, adequate patient cooperation, which can be easily affected by the patients' subjective feelings and motivation, is essential to determining the thresholds. The placebo effect is yet another difficulty. Therefore, the outcome of DBS programming is highly dependent on the physician's capability and the capacity of the DBS care facility (Moro et al., 2002; Moro et al., 2006).

We have developed a fusion method that combines images of pre-operative magnetic resonance imaging (MRI) and postoperative computed tomography (CT) (Kim et al., 2008a; Kim et al., 2008b; Lee et al., 2008; Kim et al., 2009; Kim et al., 2010; Paek et al., 2010). This fusion method enabled us to determine the 3-dimensional (3D) location of the leads and each contact in relation to the STN.

Assuming that use of this visual information would improve the outcomes of DBS programming, we reprogrammed the stimulator based on the fused images of MRI and CT in patients who had been stably managed on the STN-DBS for at least 6 months. To evaluate the usefulness of the visual information about the location of the contacts in deep brain stimulation (DBS) programming, we compared the outcomes of subthalamic nucleus (STN) stimulation before and after reprogramming guided by the fused images of MRI and CT (Lee et al., 2010a).

Of 65 patients with Parkinson's disease who underwent bilateral STN-DBS surgery between March 2005 and September 2006 and had been managed for at least 6 months with conventional programming based only on physiological responses from the patients, 54 patients were reprogrammed based on the 3D anatomical location of the contacts revealed by the fused images of preoperative MRI and post-operative CT scans taken 6 months after surgery. A total of 51 patients completed the evaluation after reprogramming.

Reprogramming significantly improved the patients' UPDRS part III scores during both on- and off-medication conditions. The daily levodopa-equivalent dose was significantly reduced. Improvement in the UPDRS part III scores after reprogramming was greater in the patients with electrodes in the STN than in patients with electrodes located outside the STN (Table 2).

Characteristics	Pre-reprogramming	Post-reprogramming	p-Value
Primary outcomes			
UPDRS – III (0–108)			
Off-medication	22.5 ± 10.5	19.1 ± 11.5	0.0137[†]
On-medication	17.0 ± 9.2	14.0 ± 7.9	0.0006[†]
Secondary outcomes			
UPDRS – I (0–16)			
Off-medication	4.5 ± 3.4	4.2 ± 2.5	0.5535
On-medication	2.8 ± 2.6	3.1 ± 2.3	0.2415
UPDRS – II (0–52)			
Off-medication	17.8 ± 7.9	16.3 ± 7.3	0.1455
On-medication	10.0 ± 6.4	12.3 ± 6.9	0.0130[†]
UPDRS – III subscores for axial symptoms (0–20)			
Off-medication	4.9 ± 2.2	5.0 ± 2.7	0.8645
On-medication	3.9 ± 2.0	4.0 ± 2.4	0.8812
Dyskinesia disability (0–4)	0.9 ± 1.3	0.6 ± 1.0	0.0598
Dyskinesia duration (0–4)	0.4 ± 0.6	0.3 ± 0.6	0.3991
Off-duration (0–4)	1.4 ± 1.1	1.1 ± 1.0	0.0549
Hoehn and Yahr stage (0–5)			
Off-medication	2.6 ± 0.5	2.6 ± 0.7	0.6465
On-medication	2.4 ± 0.6	2.5 ± 0.7	0.2620
LEDD (mg/day)	355.6 ± 321.3	276.7 ± 283.0	0.0155[†]

Table 2. Outcomes before and after reprogramming in 51 patients.

It is suggested that CT-MR fusion images helped physicians reprogram stimulation parameters with ease and confidence in a time-saving manner and resulted in further clinical improvement. This method could complement the conventional method of adjusting stimulation parameters after bilateral STN-DBS.

6. Conclusion

In STN DBS, precise positioning of electrodes within the STN is important for good clinical outcome after surgery. Many approaches, including image fusion of CT-MRI, MRI-MRI, use of an MRI brain atlas, intraoperative microelectrode recording, and stimulation, have been used in efforts to achieve precise targeting of electrodes. However, many unexpected factors such as possible brain shift due to CSF leakage, electrode artifacts in the MRI, and error in the manipulation of instruments, make it difficult to have electrodes precisely positioned in the center of the STN. Thus, not all patients have electrodes positioned exactly in the STN after surgery. This might result in different clinical outcomes following STN DBS in advanced PD patients. Knowledge of the exact location of DBS electrodes may be important in the prediction of clinical outcomes as well as in the programming of stimulation parameters following STN DBS.

We developed the DBS Electrode Localization Analysis System (DELAS) to estimate the location of electrodes following STN DBS. We demonstrated that electrode location can influence long-term clinical outcome in advanced PD patients following STN DBS. Hence, electrode positioning in relation with the STN and documentation thereof should be emphasized when adjusting long-term management plans and assessing the long-term effects of DBS on disease progression in advanced PD patients following STN DBS. We believe that the DELAS system makes it possible to try a new approach of programming or reprogramming after STN DBS that consists of fusing images of preoperative MRI and postoperative CT using the mutual information technique. This technique allows the identification of the 3-D location of the leads and of each contact in relation to the STN. Using information on the 3-D location of the electrodes and their contacts based on fused images of preoperative MRI and postoperative CT scans acquired 1 month after surgery, programming can be quickly, easily, and efficiently performed after STN DBS.

7. Acknowledgements

This work was supported by a grant from the Korea Healthcare Technology R&D Project, Ministry for Health, Welfare and Family Affairs, Republic of Korea (A092052-0911-000100).

8. References

Bejjani BP, Dormont D, Pidoux B, Yelnik J, Damier P, Arnulf I, Bonnet AM, Marsault C, Agid Y, Philippon J, Cornu P.(2000) Bilateral subthalamic stimulation for Parkinson's disease by using three-dimensional stereotactic magnetic resonance imaging and electrophysiological guidance. *J Neurosurg* 92(4):615-625. ISSN: 0022-3085

Benabid AL, Pollak P, Louveau A, Henry S, de Rougemont J. (1987) Combined (thalamotomy and stimulation) stereotactic surgery of the VIM thalamic nucleus for bilateral Parkinson disease. *Appl Neurophysiol* 50(1-6):344-346 ISSN: 0302-2773

Benabid AL, Chaardes S, Mitrofanis J, Pollak P. (2009) Deep brain stimulation of the subthalamic nucleus for the treatment of Parkinson's disease. *Lancet Neurol* 8 :67-81. ISSN: 1474-4422

Benabid AL, Chabardès S, Seigneuret E. (2005) Deep-brain stimulation in Parkinson's disease: Long-term efficacy and safety—What happened this year? *Curr Opin Neurol* 18:623–630. ISSN: 1350-7540

Benazzouz A, Breit S, Koudsie A, Pollak P, Krack P, Benabid AL. (2002) Intraoperative microrecordings of the subthalamic nucleus in parkinson's disease. *Mov Disord* 17:S145-149. ISSN: 0885-3185

Cho ZH, Min HK, Oh SH, Han JY, Park CW, Chi JG, Kim YB, Paek SH, Lozano AM, Lee KH. (2010) Direct visualization of deep brain stimulation targets in Parkinson disease with the use of 7-tesla magnetic resonance imaging. *J Neurosurg* 113(3):639-647. ISSN: 0022-3085

Christensen GE, Joshi SC, Miller MI. (1997) Volumetric transformation of brain anatomy. *IEEE Trans Med Imaging* 16:864–877. ISSN: 0278-0062

Deuschl G, Herzog J, Kleiner-Fisman G, Kubu C, Lozano AM, Lyons KE, Rodriguez-Oroz MC, Tamma F, Troster AI, Vitek JL, Volkmann J, Voon V. (2006a) Deep brain stimulation: postoperative issues. *Mov Disord* 21(Suppl 14):S219-S237. ISSN: 0885-3185

Deuschl G, Schade-Brittinger C, Krack P, Volkmann J, Schäfer H, Bötzel K, Daniels C, Deutschländer A, Dillmann U, Eisner W, Gruber D, Hamel W, Herzog J, Hilker R, Klebe S, Kloss M, Koy J, Krause M, Kupsch A, Lorenz D, Lorenzl S, Mehdorn HM, Moringlane JR, Oertel W, Pinsker MO, Reichmann H, Reuss A, Schneider GH, Schnitzler A, Steude U, Sturm V, Timmermann L, Tronnier V, Trottenberg T, Wojtecki L, Wolf E, Poewe W, Voges J; German Parkinson Study Group, Neurostimulation Section. (2006b) A randomized trial of deep-brain stimulation for Parkinson's disease. *N Engl J Med* 355:896–908. ISSN: 0028-4793

Ford B, Winfield L, Pullman SL, Frucht SJ, Du Y, Greene P, Cherinqal JH, Yu O, Cote LJ, Fahn S, McKhann GM 2nd, Goodman RR. (2004) Subthalamic nucleus stimulation in advanced Parkinson's disease: Blinded assessments at oneyear follow-up. *J Neurol Neurosurg Psychiatry* 75:1255–1259. ISSN: 0022-3050

Godinho F, Thobois S, Magnin M, Guenot M, Polo G, Benatru I, Xie J, Salvetti A, Garcia-Larrea L, Broussolle E, Mertens P. (2006) Subthalamic nucleus stimulation in Parkinson's disease: anatomical and electrophysiological localization of active contacts. *J Neurol* 253:1347-1355. ISSN: 0885-3185

Halpern CH, Danish SF, Baltuch GH, Jaggi JL. (2008) Brain shift during deep brain stimulation surgery for Parkinson's disease. *Stereotact Funct Neurosurg* 86:37-43. ISSN: 1011-6125

Hamid NA, Mitchell RD, Mocroft P, Westby GW, Milner J, Pall H. (2005) Targeting the subthalamic nucleus for deep brain stimulation: technical approach and fusion of pre-and postoperative MR images to define accuracy of lead placement. *J Neurol Neurosurg Psychiatry* 76:409-414. ISSN: 0022-3050

Heo JH, Lee KM, Paek SH, Kim MJ, Lee JY, Kim JY, Cho SY, Lim YH, Kim MR, Jeong SY, Jeon BS. (2008) The effects of bilateral Subthalamic Nucleus Deep Brain Stimulation (STN DBS) on cognition in Parkinson disease. J Neurol Sci. 273(1-2):19-24. ISSN: 0022-510X

Holtzheimer PE 3rd, Roberts DW, Darcey TM (1999) Magnetic resonance imaging versus computed tomography for target localization in functional stereotactic neurosurgery. *Neurosurgery* 45:290–297. ISSN: 0148-396X

Jankovic J & Kapadia AS. (2001) Functional decline in Parkinson disease. *Arch Neurol* 2001;58:1611–1615. ISSN: 0003-9942

Khan MF, Mewes K, Gross RE, Skrinjar O. (2008) Assessment of brain shift related to deep brain stimulation surgery. *Stereotact Funct Neurosurg* 86:44-53. ISSN: 1011-6125

Kim HJ, Lee JY, Kim JY, Kim DG, Paek SH, Jeon BS.(2008a) Effect of bilateral subthalamic deep brain stimulation on diphasic dyskinesia. *Clin Neurol Neurosurg* 110(4):328-332. ISSN: 0303-8467

Kim HJ, Paek SH, Kim JY, Lee JY, Lim YH, Kim MR, Kim DG, Jeon BS. (2008b) Chronic subthalamic deep brain stimulation improves pain in Parkinson disease. *J Neurol.* 255(12):1889-1894. ISSN: 0885-3185

Kim HJ, Paek SH, Kim JY, Lee JY, Lim YH, Kim DG, Jeon BS. (2009) Two-year follow-up on the effect of unilateral subthalamic deep brain stimulation in highly asymmetric Parkinson's disease. *Mov Disord* 15;24(3):329-335. ISSN: 0885-3185

Kim HJ, Jeon BS, Paek SH, Lee JY, Kim HJ, Kim CK, Kim DG. (2010) Bilateral subthalamic deep brain stimulation in Parkinson disease patients with severe tremor. *Neurosurgery* 67(3):626-632 ISSN: 0148-396X

Kim YH, Kim HJ, Kim C, Kim DG, Jeon BS, Paek SH. (2010) Comparison of electrode location between immediate postoperative day and 6 months after bilateral subthalamic nucleus deep brain stimulation. *Acta Neurochir (Wien)* 152(12):2037-2045. ISSN: 0001-6268

Kleiner-Fisman G, Herzog J, Fisman DN, Tamma F, Lyons KE, Pahwa R, Lang AE, Deuschl G. (2006) Subthalamic nucleus deep brain stimulation: summary and meta-analysis of outcomes. *Mov Disord* 21(Suppl.14): S290–S304. ISSN: 0885-3185

Kondziolka D, Dempsey PK, Lunsford LD, Kestle JR, Dolan EJ, Kanal E, Tasker RR (1992) A comparison between magnetic resonance imaging and computed tomography for stereotactic coordinate determination. *Neurosurgery* 30:402–406. ISSN: 0148-396X

Krack P, Batir A, Van Blercom N, Chabardes S, Fraix V, Ardouin C, Koudsie A, Limousin PD, Benazzouz A, Le Bas JF, Benabid AL, Pollak P. (2003) Five-year follow-up of bilateral stimulation of the subthalamic nucleus in advanced Parkinson's disease. *N Engl J Med* 349:1925–1934. ISSN: 0028-4793

Lee JY, Han JH, Kim HJ, Jeon BS, Kim DG, Paek SH. (2008) STN DBS of Advanced Parkinson's Disease Experienced in a Specialized Monitoring Unit with a Prospective Protocol J Korean Neurosurg Soc. 44(1):26-35. ISSN: 2005-3711

Lee JY, Jeon BS, Paek SH, Lim YH, Kim MR, Kim C. (2010a) Reprogramming guided by the fused images of MRI and CT in subthalamic nucleus stimulation in Parkinson disease. *Clin Neurol Neurosurg* 112(1):47-53. ISSN: 0303-8467

Lee JY, Kim JW, Lee JY, Lim YH, Kim C, Kim DG, Jeon BS, Paek SH. (2010b) Is MRI a reliable tool to locate the electrode after deep brain stimulation surgery? Comparison study of CT and MRI for the localization of electrodes after DBS. *Acta Neurochir (Wien)* 152(12):2029-2036. ISSN: 0001-6268

Liang GS, Chou KL, Baltuch GH, Jaggi JL, Loveland-Jones C, Leng L, Maccarone H, Hurtig HI, Colcher A, Stern MB, Kleiner-Fisman G, Simuni T, Siderowf AD. (2006) Long-term outcomes of bilateral subthalamic nucleus stimulation in patients with advanced Parkinson's disease. Stereotact Funct Neurosurg 84 :221-227. ISSN: 1011-6125

Limousin P, Krack P, Pollak P, Benazzouz A, Ardouin C, Hoffmann D, Benabid AL. (1998) Electrical stimulation of the subthalamic nucleus in advanced Parkinson's disease. N Engl J Med 339:1105–1111. ISSN: 0028-4793

Louis ED, Tang MX, Cote L, Alfaro B, Mejia H, Marder K. (1999) Progression of parkinsonian signs in Parkinson disease. Arch Neurol 56:334–337. ISSN: 0003-9942

Lyons KE, Pahwa R. (2005) Long-term benefits in quality of life provided by bilateral subthalamic stimulation in patients with Parkinson disease. J Neurosurg 103:252–255. ISSN: 0022-3085

Maes F, Collignon A, Vandermeulen D, Marchal G, Suetens P. (1997) Multimodality image registration by maximization of mutual information. IEEE Trans Med Imaging 16:187–198. ISSN: 0278-0062

Martinez-Santiesteban FM, Swanson SD, Noll DC, Anderson DJ. (2007) Magnetic field perturbation of neural recording and stimulating microelectrodes. Phys Med Biol 52:2073-2088. ISSN: 0031-9155

McClelland S 3rd, Ford B, Senatus PB, Winfield LM, Du YE, Pullman SL, Yu Q, Frucht SJ, McKhann GM 2nd, Goodman RR. (2005) Subthalamic stimulation for Parkinson disease: Determination of electrode location necessary for clinical efficacy. Neurosurg Focus 19:E12. ISSN: 1092-0684

Miyagi Y, Shima F, Sasaki T. (2007) Brain shift: an error factor during implantation of deep brain stimulation electrodes. J Neurosurg 107:989-997. ISSN: 0022-3085

Moro E, Esselink RJ, Xie J, Hommel M, Benabid AL, Pollak P. (2002) The impact on Parkinson's disease of electrical parameter settings in STN stimulation. Neurology 59:706-713. ISSN: 0028-3878

Moro E, Poon YW, Lozano AM, Saint-Cyr JA, Lang AE. (2006) Subthalamic nucleus stimulation; improvements in outcome with reprogramming. Arch Neurol 63:1266–1272. ISSN: 0003-9942

Olanow CW, Hauser RA, Gauger L, Malapira T, Koller W, Hubble J, Bushenbark K, Lilienfeld D, Esterlitz J. (1995) The effect of deprenyl and levodopa on the progression of Parkinson's disease. Ann Neurol 38:771–777. ISSN: 0364-5134

Ott K, Tarlov E, Crowell R, Papadakis N (1976) Retained intracranial metallic foreign bodies. Report of two cases. J Neurosurg 44:80-83. ISSN: 0022-3085

Ostergaard K, Sunde NA. (2006) Evolution of Parkinson's disease during 4 years of bilateral deep brain stimulation of the subthalamic nucleus. Mov Disord 21 :624-631. ISSN: 0885-3185

Paek SH, Han JH, Lee JY, Kim C, Jeon BS, Kim DG. (2008) Electrode position determined by fused images of preoperative and postoperative magnetic resonance imaging and surgical outcome after subthalamic nucleus deep brain stimulation. Neurosurgery 2008; 63:925-937. ISSN: 0148-396X

Paek SH, Kim JW, Lim YH, Kim MR, Kim DG, Jeon BS. (2010) Data Management System in a Movement Disorder Center: Technical Report. Stereotact Funct Neurosurg 88(4):216-223. ISSN: 1011-6125

Paek SH, Kim HJ, Yoon JY, Heo JH, Kim CY, Kim MR, Lim YH, Kim KR, Han JH, Kim DG, Jeon BS. (2011) Fusion image-based programming after subthalamic nucleus deep brain stimulation. World Neurosurgery [Epub ahead of print]. ISSN:1878-8750

Piboolnurak P, Lang AE, Lozano AM, Miyasaki JM, Saint-Cyr JA, Poon YY, Hutchison WD,
    Dostrovsky JO, Moro E (2007) Levodopa response in long-term bilateral
    subthalamic stimulation for Parkisnon's disease. Mov Disord 22 : 990-997. ISSN:
    0885-3185

Plaha P, Ben-Shlomo Y, Patel NK, Gill SS. (2006) Stimulation of the caudal zona incerta is
    superior to stimulation of the subthalamic nucleus in improving contralateral
    parkinsonism. Brain 129:1732–1747. ISSN: 0006-8950

Pluim JP, Maintz JB, Viergever MA. (2003) Mutual-information-based registration of
    medical images: a survey. IEEE Trans Med Imaging 22:986–1004. ISSN: 0278-0062

Pollo C, Vingerhoets F, Pralong E, Ghika J, Maeder P, Meuli R, Thiran JP, Villemure JG.
    (2007) Localization of electrodes in the subthalamic nucleus on magnetic resonance
    imaging. J Neurosurg 106:36–44. ISSN: 0022-3085

Rodriguez-Oroz MC, Obeso JA, Lang AE, Houeto JL, Pollak P, Rehncrona S, Kulisevsky J,
    Albanese A, Volkmann J, Hariz MI, Quinn NP, Speelman JD, Guridi J, Zamarbide I,
    Gironell A, Molet J, Pascual-Sedano B, Pidoux B, Bonnet AM, Agid Y, Xie J,
    Benabid AL, Lozano AM, Saint-Cyr J, Romito L, Contarino MF, Scerrati M, Fraix V,
    Van Blercom N. (2005) Bilateral deep brain stimulation in Parkinson's disease: a
    multicenter study with 4 years follow-up. Brain 128:2240–2249. ISSN: 0006-8950

Saint-Cyr JA, Hoque T, Pereira LC, Dostrovsky JO, Hutchison WD, Mikulis DJ, Abosch A,
    Sime E, Lang AE, Lozano AM. (2002) Localization of clinically effective stimulating
    electrodes in the human subthalamic nucleus on magnetic resonance imaging. J
    Neurosurg 97:1152–1166. ISSN: 0022-3085

Schaltenbrand G & Wharen W. (1998) Atlas of Stereotaxy of the Human Brain, 2nd ed. New
    York: Thieme. ISBN (Americas): 9780865770553, ISBN (EUR, Asia, Africa, AUS):
    9783133937023

Schrader B, Hamel W, Weinert D, Mehdorn HM. (2002) Documentation of electrode
    localization. Mov Disord 17 [Suppl 3]:S167–S174. ISSN: 0885-3185

Sorensen N & Krauss J (1991) Movement of hemostatic clips from the ventricles through the
    aqueduct to the lumbar spinal canal. Case report J Neurosurg 74:143–146. ISSN:
    0022-3085

Starr PA, Christine CW, Theodosopoulos PV, Lindsey N, Byrd D, Mosley A, Marks WJ Jr.
    (2002) Implantation of deep brain stimulators into the subthalamic nucleus:
    Technical approach and magnetic resonance imaging-verified lead locations. J
    Neurosurg 97:370–387. ISSN: 0022-3085

Tsai ST, Lin SH, Chou YC, Pan YH, Hung HY, Li CW, Lin SZ, Chen SY. (2009) Prognostic
    factors of subthalamic stimulation in Parkinson's disease: a comparative study
    between short- and long-term effects. Stereotact Funct Neurosurg 87:241-248. ISSN:
    1011-6125

van den Munckhof P, Contarino MF, Bour LJ, Speelman JD, de Bie RM, Schuurman PR
    (2010) Postoperative curving and upward displacement of deep brain stimulation
    electrodes caused by brain shift. Neurosurgery 67:49–53. ISSN: 0148-396X

Volkmann J, Herzog J, Kopper F, Deuschl G. (2002) Introduction to the programming of
    deep brain stimulators. Mov Disord 17:S181–S187. ISSN: 0885-3185

Volkmann J, Moro E, Pahwa R. (2006) Basic algorithms for the programming of deep brain
    stimulation in Parkinson's disease. Mov Disord 21:S284-S289. ISSN: 0885-3185

Wells WM 3rd, Viola P, Atsumi H, Nakajima S, Kikinis R. (1996) Multimodal volume
    registration by maximization of mutual information. *Med Image Anal* 1:35–51. ISSN:
    1361-8415
Wider C, Pollo C, Bloch J, Vingerhoets FJ. (2008) Long-term outcome of 50 consecutive
    Parkinson's diease patients treated with subthalamic deep brain stimulation.
    Parkinsonism and Relat Disord 14 :114-119. ISSN: 1353-8020
Yelnik J, Damier P, Demeret S, Gervais D, Bardinet E, Bejjani BP, Francois C, Houeto JL,
    Arnule I, Dormont D, Galanaud D, Pidoux B, Cornu P, Aqid Y. (2003) Localization
    of stimulating electrodes in patients with Parkinson disease by using a three-
    dimensional atlas-magnetic resonance imaging coregistration method. *J Neurosurg*
    99:89–99. ISSN: 0022-3085
Yokoyama T, Ando N, Sugiyama K, Akamine S, Namba H. (2006) Relationship of
    stimulation site location within the subthalamic nucleus region to clinical effects on
    parkinsonian symptoms. Stereotact Funct Neurosurg 84:170–175. ISSN: 1011-6125

12

Joint Replacement Surgery in Parkinson's Disease

Adrian J. Cassar Gheiti, Joseph F. Baker and Kevin J. Mulhall
Orthopaedic Research and Innovation Foundation
Republic of Ireland

1. Introduction

Parkinson Disease affects 4 million people worldwide and it is the second most common neurological disorder after Alzheimer disease (Huse et al. 2005). It occurs in 1% of the population over the age of 60 years (Adams et al. 1997). The annual incidence of Parkinson's disease is 20.5 per 100,000 (Rajput et al. 1984) and can result in numerous symptoms including tremor, muscular rigidity and abnormalities of gait, posture and facial expression. Despite optimal pharmacological treatment, progression of Parkinson's disease normally results in a decline in general mobility and ability to ambulate safely.

Rigidity secondary to Parkinson's Disease often aggravates joint pain from osteoarthritis (Adams et al. 1997). The outcome of joint arthroplasty in these patients is effective in relieving pain, but the overall functional results have been found to be variable (Oni et al. 1985; Vince et al. 1989; Duffy et al. 1996; Koch et al. 1997; Weber et al. 2002; Shah et al. 2005; Kryzak et al. 2009; Kryzak et al. 2010). A report from the Scottish joint registry has found an annual prevalence of Parkinson's disease of 5% to 8% in patients undergoing total hip arthroplasty (Meek et al. 2006). Optimal management of the disease before, during and after surgery is a challenge due to the neurological disturbances in Parkinson's disease including tremor, rigidity, contractures and gait abnormalities.

We will firstly provide an overview of the difficulties faced when planning surgery in patients with Parkinson's disease before discussing specific pre-, intra- and post-operative measures that should be taken. Finally we will provide an overview of the evidence available for arthroplasty in Parkinson's disease specific to the three major joints replaced – hip, knee and shoulder.

2. Parkinson's disease and surgery

Patients with Parkinson's disease usually suffer from rigidity, contractures, tremor and gait abnormalities. People with Parkinson's disease who undergo surgery have longer hospital stays and increased mortality (Pepper et al. 1999). Preoperative fasting regimes can unnecessarily result in reduced or missed administration of dopaminergic medications and subsequent serious complications (Reed et al. 1992). Patients with mild Parkinson's disease are able to tolerate the fasting period but those patients with advanced Parkinson's disease, who are under high doses of levodopa are susceptible to the condition Neuroleptic Malignant Syndrome with associated fever, confusion, raised concentration of muscle enzymes and even death (Ueda et al. 1999). The disease itself predisposes these patients to increased risk of aspiration pneumonia and urinary tract infection compared to patients without the disease (Pepper et al. 1999).

Discharge from hospital after surgery is more difficult in those with Parkinson's disease. Patients are more likely to suffer from intra – operative and post-operative complication including falls and fractures. A longer duration of hospital stay than in patient without Parkinson's disease can be anticipated and appropriate planning is necessary (Mueller et al. 2009). Planning consists of medical and surgical optimisation and also appropriate consideration to prehabilitation, rehabilitation and convalescent requirements.

2.1 Pre – operative management
2.1.1 Pharmacologic management

Patients with Parkinson's disease require advance planning, appropriate medication and specialist neurological advice for optimisation of pharmacological management of the disease before, during and after surgery (Brennan et al. 2010). Ideally these patients are screened at the pre – assessment clinic, and advice should be sought from a neurologist or geriatrician. The neurologist can give advice about the patient treatment regimen for the period around the operation and to consider any additional measures required. Brennan and Genever have reported that oral medications should be continued until time of anaesthetic induction and that patients with Parkinson's disease are ideally placed at the start of the operating list. This facilitates greater predictability over the time of fasting and surgery.

Alternative Parkinson's drugs such as apomorphine and rotigontine can be used in the post-operative period, when post-operative ileus or delayed gastric emptying can be anticipated. Apomorphine is a potent dopamine agonist which is delivered subcutaneously, but can cause severe emesis and need the concomitant use of an anti-emetic such as domperidon. Rotigontine is delivered transdermally; it has ease of use and tolerability but may not provide adequate treatment in patients with severe Parkinson's disease (Brennan et al. 2010).

Parkinsonian medication should not be withheld prior to surgery. Although some can tolerate missed doses, there are reports of Neuroleptic Malignant Syndrome in cases where the regular dose has been omitted (Ueda et al. 1999). Mason et al have provided a detailed list of pre-anaesthetic assessments that should be carried out prior to surgery (Mason et al. 1996). This list details a number of features to look for by system and appropriate investigations (Table 1, page 511).

Respiratory complications are possible as a significant number of patients with Parkinson's Disease have an obstructive picture on pulmonary function testing (Neu et al. 1967). Orthostatic hypotension is a potential problem and agents that cause or contribute to peripheral vasodilatation can exacerbate this. Hypovolaemia secondary to surgical blood loss needs to be attended to as this can clearly contribute to lower blood pressure and risk of subsequent fall. Administration of medications such as tricyclic anti-depressants may also contribute to a fall in blood pressure and should be used with caution in this patient population (Nicholson et al. 2002).

2.1.2 Bone mineral density

Several studies have shown that patient with Parkinson's disease have decreased bone mineral density (BMD) and are prone to vitamin D deficiency when compared to the general

System	Assessment by history	Tests
Head and neck	Pharyngeal muscle dysfunction Dysphagia Sialorrhoea Blepharospasm	
Respiratory	Respiratory impairment from rigidity, bradykinesia or uncoordinated involuntary movement of the respiratory muscles	Chest radiograph Pulmonary function tests Arterial blood gases
Cardiovascular	Orthostatic hypotension Cardiac arrhythmias Hypertension Autonomic dysfunction	ECG
Gastrointestinal	Weight loss Poor nutrition Susceptibility to reflux	Serum albumin/transferrin Skin test allergy
Urological	Difficulty in micturition	
Endocrine	Abnormal glucose metabolism (selegiline)	Blood glucose concentration
Musculoskeletal	Muscle rigidity	
Central Nervous System	Muscle rigidity Akinesia Tremor Confusion Depression Hallucinations Speech impairment	

Table 1. Recommended assessment of the patient with Parkinson's disease(Mason et al. 1996)

population (Kao et al. 1994; Sato et al. 1997; Fink et al. 2005; Sato et al. 2005). Patients with Parkinson's disease tend to be less active than patients without the disease, and lack of sunlight absorption makes these patients more likely to be ostopenic. Rigidity and bradykinesia result in reduction in spontaneous movements, rendering the patient less mobile and active. Lack of mobilization stimulates bone calcium resorption, secondary to disuse and lack of weight bearing (Clouston et al. 1987; Gross et al. 1995; Inoue 2010). Patients with Parkinson's disease with low BMD are have twice as much the risk of fractures when compared with osteoporotic patients without the disease(Taylor et al. 2004).

Those with poor bone quality are at an increased are at increased risk of intraoperative fracture during joint arthroplasty particularly during femoral stem insertion in uncemented THA when hoop stresses are at their greatest (Hernigou et al. 2006). In an experimental *in vitro* study Thomsen et al found that patients with poor bone quality treated with uncemented THA are at higher risk of periprosthetic fracture and recommended that cemented stems should be used in this group of patients(Thomsen et al. 2008). Improving the patient bone density or preventing continuing bone loss is therefore important before joint arthroplasty is considered in patient with PD.

All patients with Parkinson's disease referred for orthopaedic assessment for possible joint arthroplasty should be screened for osteoporosis and treated appropriately. Bisphosphonates are known to reduce osteoclastic activity and immobilization induced bone loss has been successfully treated with these agents (Yates et al. 1984; Sato et al. 2007). In a randomized control trial in patients undergoing cemented TKA, Hilding et al. showed that daily treatment with 400mg of clodronate reduced tibial component migration by 25% when compared with placebo at 6 months following surgery(Hilding et al. 2000). Friedl et al. have identified reduced migration of cementless acetabular cups in THA over 2 years following a single dose of intravenous zoledronate in patients undergoing THA for avascular necrosis(Friedl et al. 2009). However, other authors have found the effect of bisphosphonates less promising with no beneficial effect of systemic bisphosphonates seen over 2 years after hybrid THA and cementless TKA(Wilkinson et al. 2005; Hansson et al. 2009).

Patients with PD are also reported to have abnormal bone metabolism(Sato et al. 2005) resulting from reduced parathyroid hormone. Recent studies using teriparatide, a recombinant human parathyroid hormone, for the treatment of reduced BMD are showing promising results (Aspenberg et al. 2010; Ma et al. 2011; Moricke et al. 2011) but so far none of the studies are related to patients with PD.

2.1.3 Physiotherapy

Physiotherapy has proven functional improvements in patients with PD and this needs to be considered in the planning for arthroplasty surgery (Formisano et al. 1992). Physiotherapy should not be left for the post-operative phase and emerging evidence suggests that it should play a greater role prior to surgery than we realize. Prehabilitation is fast growing to be a recognized as a potential key element in arthroplasty pathways and this has been particularly noted in patients undergoing total knee arthroplasty (Jaggers et al. 2007; Topp et al. 2009; Swank et al. 2011). Patients with PD should not be exempt from this more of preparation, and given the potential for poor mobility, loss of muscle mass and bone mineral density in this cohort, it may be even more prudent to direct these individuals for prehabilitation prior to surgery.

Nocera et al have found that knee extensor strength has a negative correlation with disease severity in PD and a positive correlation with dynamic stability (Nocera et al. 2010). Specific physical therapy programs for PD have been shown to be effective for mild to moderate disease severity(Ebersbach et al. 2010) . Allen et al in a randomized controlled trial setting have shown that a prescribed exercise program results in increased muscle strength and a reduced fear of falling in those with PD(Allen et al. 2010). While a painful degenerate joint can prohibit some prescribed exercises, gains made prior to surgery will be transcribed to potential gains made following surgery.

2.2 Intra – operative management

According to the literature, regional anaesthesia is preferred to general anaesthesia, especially in patients who require continues infusion of levodopa/carbidopa therapy during the procedure(Burton et al. 2004). Backus et al have reported a case of post-extubation laryngospasm in an un-anaesthetised patient(Backus et al. 1991). General anaesthesia has been shown to contribute to post-operative confusion, which adversely affects patient outcomes and prolongs hospital stay (Duffy et al. 1996; Koch et al. 1997; Weber et al. 2002) Propofol which is commonly used to induce general anaesthesia may temporarily supress the tremor associated with Parkinson's disease but it has been also shown to exacerbate dyskinesia (Anderson et al. 1994; Krauss et al. 1996). Wright et al have suggested that low dose ketamine may represent an alternative sedative for use pre-operatively as it reduces dyskinesia and controls Parkinsonian tremor(Wright et al. 2009).

Of the commonly used analgesics during surgery fentanyl and morphine can both result in increased muscular rigidity (Klausner et al. 1988; Berg et al. 1999). Alfentanil has been reported to have resulted in dystonic reactions(Mets 1991)

Succinylcholine can result in hyperkalaemia and should be avoided(Muzzi et al. 1989). Non-depolarizing muscle relaxants are considered safe(Nicholson et al. 2002).

2.2.1 Peri-articular infiltration

A number of randomized control studies (Andersen et al. 2007; Toftdahl et al. 2007; Andersen et al. 2010) show the effectiveness of intra operative local infiltration analgesia (LIA) in the post - operative period. LIA has been used both during TKA and THA with equal effectiveness in pain reduction and reduction in analgesic use in the post - operative period. In a randomized, double blinded, placebo controlled study, LIA was used in hip arthroplasty (Andersen et al. 2007). Patients treated with local infiltration analgesia experienced less pain up to two weeks postoperatively and resulted in less joint stiffness and better function one week after the procedure(Andersen et al. 2007).

Multimodal anaesthetic infiltration around the hip joint has been trialled and reports to date suggest that this is an efficacious way of controlling post-operative pain whilst reducing requirements for rescue analgesia. Busch et al have shown that peri-articular infiltration of a multi-modal analgesic regime has a positive effect on subjective pain following THA and results in a reduced requirement for rescue opiate use via PCA(Busch et al. 2010). Lee et al reported similar results noting that peri-articular infiltration conferred no increased risk for the patient in the post-operative setting. Their multi-modal injection consisted of morphine, ropivacaine and methylprednisolone. Parvataneni et al reported superior control of post-operative pain using peri-articular infiltration of bupivacaine, epinephrine, methylprednisolone, cefuroxime and morphine(Parvataneni et al. 2007). Use of periarticular infiltrations such as these, particularly in hip arthroplasty can minimise subsequent use of opiate based analgesics and reduce the risk of adverse events associated with opiate usage.

Recent studies show that periarticular infiltration at the end of TKA has several advantages over other approaches. In a randomized controlled study by Venditoli et al 42 patients who underwent TKA were randomized either to receive an intraoperative infiltration with ropivacaine followed by an infusion of ropivacaine through 16 gauge catheter on the first post-operative day or control group. Narcotic consumption was less in the first 40 hours post op with improved pain scores during rest and exercise for the first forty eight hours and fewer nausea symptoms during the first five post-operative days than the control group(Vendittoli et al. 2006). It is well known that morphine exerts its analgesic effect by binding to opioid receptors in the central nervous system and peripherally (Stein et al. 1989). In a double blinded, randomized clinical trial Tanaka et al. have shown that patient who were administered intra-articular morphine and bupivacaine had reduced pain scores, a much smaller requirement of systemic analgesia, longer duration between the operation and the first requirement of systemic analgesia and improvement in the range of motion of the knee joint at time of discharge(Tanaka et al. 2001). Andersen et al. have used a combination intraoperative infiltration of ropivacaine ketorolac and epinephrine combined with and intra-articular infusion of ropivacaine and ketorolac for the first 48 hours post operatively. They found out that peri and intra-articular analgesia with multi modal drugs provided superior pain relief and reduced opioid consumption compared with continuous epidural infusion with ropivacaine combined with intravenous ketorolac(Andersen et al. 2010). These protocols can be used in patients with Parkinson's disease to help reduce the use of opioids in the post-operative period and reducing the risk of multi drug interaction and side effects. Further studies are required, to assess the effectiveness of these protocols in patients with Parkinson's disease.

2.3 Post – operative management
2.3.1 Analgesic management
In joint arthroplasty, pain control after the procedure is one of the major elements in early mobilizations. Most patients are managed with opioid analgesics for the first 24 hours after surgery including the use of patient controlled analgesia (PCA). Opioid analgesics are well known to cause confusion especially in elderly patients.

This type of analgesics effect patients' mental state and can exacerbate Parkinsonian symptoms through the dopaminergic pathway (Chudler et al. 1995; Burton et al. 2004). Opioid analgesic has also been shown to increase the length of stay in hospital in a nationwide study done in Denmark(Husted et al. 2010).

Multimodal analgesia with non-steroidal anti-inflammatory drugs in patients with adequate renal function is reported to be as effective as opioid analgesia with fewer side effects (O'Hara et al. 1997; Post et al. 2010). When using multimodal analgesia, it is especially important to take early advice from the patient's neurologist for potential adverse interaction between the type of analgesic protocol used and the neurological medication regime.

2.3.2 Respiratory function
Post-operative nursing care and rehabilitation are an important factor in patients with Parkinson's disease because these patients are at high risk of for falls and fractures (Melton et al. 2006; Camicioli et al. 2010). Close attention to the respiratory status in this patient cohort following surgery is mandatory. As eluded to earlier, Parkinson's Disease is associated with an obstructive respiratory pattern. This is likely due to the incoordination of the upper airway seen in extra-pyramidal disorders(Vincken et al. 1984). Musculature around the larynx is likely to be affected by the neuromuscular abnormalities in Parkinson's disease. Patients are therefore prone to atelectasis, retained secretions and respiratory tract infections(Easdown et al. 1995). It has been noted that aspiration pneumonia is a not infrequent cause of death(Hughes et al. 1993). Pulmonary physiotherapy and early commencement of ambulation are essential components to help minimise the risk of these complications.

2.3.3 Physiotherapy
Patients with Parkinson's disease require more intensive monitoring than patients without the disease in order to prevent complications such as pressure sores. Earlier mobilization

and physiotherapy regimes improve motor function, respiratory function and may help in preventing muscle contractures (Gobbi et al. 2009; Dereli et al. 2010). The Royal Dutch Society for Physical Therapy (KNGF) has published evidenced based clinical practice guidelines in order to be able to deliver optimal care to patients with PD. These guidelines have been also adopted by the Association of Physiotherapist in Parkinson's disease Europe(Keus et al. 2007). The two treatment strategies recommended in these guidelines are cognitive movement strategies and cueing strategies. These guidelines also emphasize on training joint mobility and training strength which are essential in both the pre- and post-operative period. Hurwitz et al. showed that an exercise program focused on improving joint mobility, in combination with improving mobility and self-care also improved memory(Hurwitz 1989). In a randomized control trail, Schenkman et al. showed that an exercise program focused at improving joint mobility and coordinated moving incorporated in activities of daily living (ADL) improves functional axial rotation and reach(Schenkman et al. 1998). Exercise programs which are, focused on improving muscle strength, may also improve muscle strength in patients with PD (Toole et al. 2000; Hirsch et al. 2003).

Again, in the post-operative phase it is important to remain cognizant of the potential pharmacological interactions that may precipitate orthostatic hypotension and lead to a reduced mobility or increased risk of falling.

3. Parkinson's disease and arthroplasty

There is limited literature focusing on joint arthroplasty in patients with Parkinson's disease and so far there are only 17 studies. Seven studies dealt with fractures of the femoral neck treated with hemi-arthroplasty(Rothermel and Garcia 1972; Coughlin and Templeton 1980; Eventov, Moreno et al. 1983; Staeheli, Frassica et al. 1988; Turcotte, Godin et al. 1990; Clubb, Clubb et al. 2006; Kryzak, Sperling et al. 2010), 6 studies dealt with total knee arthroplasty in Parkinson's disease(Oni and Mackenney 1985; Vince, Insall et al. 1989; Fast, Mendelsohn et al. 1994; Duffy and Trousdale 1996; Erceg and Maricevic 2000; Shah, Hornyak et al. 2005), 2 studies dealt with total hip arthroplasty(Weber, Cabanela et al. 2002; Meek, Allan et al. 2006) and 2 dealt with total shoulder arthroplasty. In this section we will provide an overview of the evidence available for arthroplasty in PD specific to the three major joints replaced – hip, knee and shoulder.

3.1 Hip
3.1.1 Hemiarthroplasty for femoral neck fractures
The 7 studies (Rothermel et al. 1972; Coughlin et al. 1980; Eventov et al. 1983; Staeheli et al. 1988; Turcotte et al. 1990; Clubb et al. 2006; Kryzak et al. 2010), that discussed the outcome of hemi-arthroplasty in Parkinson's disease are not strictly applicable since the procedure is usually undertaken as an emergency or semi-elective procedure, but some inferences can be taken in terms of rates of dislocation and post-operative complications(Table.2. Page 516). However, it must be remembered that the biomechanics of a hemiarthroplasty are different to those in THA.

Turcotte, et al(Turcotte et al. 1990) reported that out of 41 patients undergoing 47 hemi-arthroplasty for a Garden III – IV fracture , five subsequently dislocated and four of these within the first month of surgery. Four patients had wound infections, one subsidence of the stem, one acetabular protrusion, one femoral shaft fracture, three decubitus ulcers on the operated limb and one patient died within the first 6 months. Four patients never walked

	Study type	Arthroplasty (type + numbers)	Mean age (yrs, range)	Length of follow up (yrs)	Implant type/surgical technique	Outcome
Weber et al	retrospective	THR(107)	72 (57 - 87)	7.1 (2 - 21)	94 acetabular cups and 103 femoral stems were cemented, 13 acetabular cups and 4 stems were uncemented	93% pain free, 6% dislocations, 3% aseptic loosening, 26% post oprative medical complication rate
Meek et al	retrospective	THR(2394)	N/A	N/A	N/A	0.46 annual dislocation rate
Kryzak et al	retrospective	Hemi hip		0.5 - 6 years	posterior approach, various types of endo prosthesis	6 month mortality 75%, 37% dislocation, 8.3% deep wound infection
Clubb et al	Literature review	Hemi hip	N/A	N/A	N/A	N/A
Eventov et al	retrospective	Hemi hip (62)	74 (61 - 90)	N/A	34 patients had a hemiarthroplasty using the posterolateral approach, 11 underwent plate and nail fixation , the rest were treated non operativly	31% mortality at 3 months, pneumonia most frequent cause of dead, complications highest in the operated group.
Rothermel et al	retrospective	Hemi hip (16)	63.5	N/A	7 treated with hemiarthroplasty, 3 McLaughlin nail, plate and screws, 1 miltiple pins 2 nail and plate and 2 on traction	12.5% flexion contractures,
Coughlin et al	retrospective	Hemi hip (13)	78	0.5 - 6 years	posterior approach, various types of endo prosthesis	6 month mortality 75%, 37% dislocation, 8.3% deep wound infection
Staeheli et al	retrospective	Hemi hip (50)	74.3 (47 - 92)	7.3 years	50% anterolateral approach, 40% posterior approach and 10 % trans trochanteric approach, various prosthesis used	2% dislocation, 20% mortality at 6 months, pneumonia was the most frequent cause of dead
Turcotte et al	retrospective	Hemi hip (47)	74 (51 - 89)	N/A	posterior approach	8.5% wound infection, 11% dislocated, , 2.1% subsidence, 2.1% protrusio acetabuli, 2.1% femoral shaft fracture, 6.4% decubitus ulcers, 15% mortality at 6 months

Table 2. Summary of the studies in patient with Parkinson's disease undergoing THR or Hemiarthroplasty.

again despite being ambulatory prior to surgery. Overall mortality in these patients was 15%(Turcotte et al. 1990) mainly due to increased medical complications.

Other studies had better outcomes with Staeheli et al(Staeheli et al. 1988) reporting only one dislocation out of a series of 49 patients undergoing hemi-arthroplasty for femoral neck fracture, while Eventov et al have reported a 3% dislocation rate (Eventov et al. 1983).

Some studies have reported mortality rates as high 47% within the first 6 months after hemi-arthroplasty of the hip(Coughlin et al. 1980). As in other studies the high mortality rate was mainly due to increased medical complications including myocardial infarction, urosepsis and pneumonia (Staeheli et al. 1988; Turcotte et al. 1990). Aggressive physiotherapy and early mobilization was advised for patients with Parkinson's disease undergoing hemi-arthroplasty(Coughlin et al. 1980; Eventov et al. 1983; Staeheli et al. 1988; Turcotte et al. 1990). Some of these studies have also advised that patients with Parkinson's disease should be treated with internal fixation of the fracture and that hemi-arthroplasty may be contraindicated (Coughlin et al. 1980; Turcotte et al. 1990).

3.1.2 Total hip arthroplasty

Total Hip Arthroplasty (THA) is usually performed in patients with osteoarthritis (OA) (Fig.1. Page 518 & Fig.2. Page 519) to relieve pain and improve joint function. In a review of total hip arthroplasty (THA) in patient with neurological conditions , Queally et al found only two studies in the literature which report the results of THA in patients with Parkinson's disease(Queally et al. 2009). These studies reported lower rates of dislocation than those noted in reported cohorts of hemiarthroplasty in the trauma setting. Meek et al have reported only two dislocations in 1467 patients with Parkinson's disease who underwent THA between 1996 and 2004 as reported in the Scottish National Arthroplasty Registry(Meek et al. 2006). They also found an annual incidence of Parkinson's disease 5% to 8% in patients undergoing THA (Meek et al. 2006).

Weber et al reported a high rate of post-operative complications (26%) in 98 patients with Parkinson's disease after THA at mean follow up at 7.1 years(Weber et al. 2002). An anterolateral approach was used in 56 patients, trans-trochanteric in 36, postero-lateral in 12, and direct lateral in three patients. No dislocations or wound infections were noted. They did note that THA provided a high level of long lasting pain relief and initial improvement in ambulation. Functional decline in the individuals was related to the neurological disease and was not joint specific. There were 6 dislocations in the revision THA group, which included 1 from the trans-trochanteric approach, 1 from the direct lateral and 4 from the anterolateral approach. The low rate of dislocation seen in these 2 studies is mostly related to both advancement in medical management of Parkinson's disease developed in recent years and the wider choice of biomaterials such as constrained liners and larger femoral heads which improve stability at the hip joint. These 2 studies are summarised in Table. 2 (page 516).

General decline in mobility in Parkinson's disease can lead to weakness in abductor muscle function. Application of biomechanical principles suggests that increasing the offset can optimize abductor function by lengthening the abductor lever arm. Contractures may develop in any individual after hip arthroplasty, limiting functional gains. This potential case is probably more likely in PD due to the lower mobility and associated problems with rigidity. Bhave et al have found that administration of botulinum toxin to the contracted muscle groups can help alleviate this problem. Injection to a variety of muscle group including the adductors, abductors and hip flexors resulted in lasting improvement in range of movement for 20 months or more(Bhave et al. 2009).

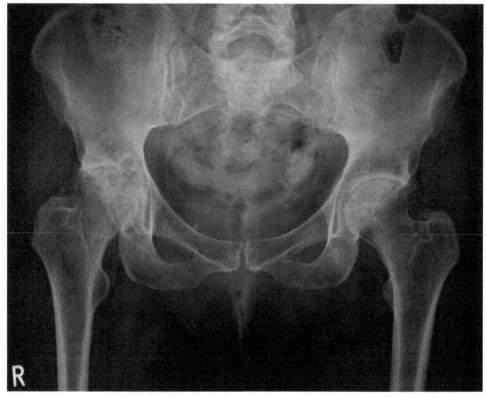

Fig. 1. Anteroposterior radiograph of the pelvis showing, right hip osteoarthritis with a triad of joint space narrowing, subchondral cysts and osteophyte formation.

3.2 Knee
3.2.1 Knee Arthroplasty
Total Knee Arthroplasty (TKA) has been condemned for patients with Parkinson's disease by Oni et al in 1985 when they reported 3 cases of TKA complicated by a persistent flexion contracture of the hamstrings induced by the operation itself(Oni et al. 1985). Quadriceps tendon rupture was also seen in two patients. All three patients died within six months of surgery.

Vince et al reported 13 TKA in 9 patients with Parkinson's disease at time of surgery(Vince et al. 1989). All knees showed fixed flexion before the arthroplasty. Ten joints had a posterior stabilised implant; one revision joint arthroplasty required a customized stem implant and the other two cases underwent a total condylar I and II. Nine of 12 primary knee replacement achieved excellent scores Hospital for Special Surgery knee rating system within the first year and the other 3 had good scores. Even though complications such as urinary tract infections, deep vein thrombosis and pulmonary embolism were common, all patients recovered. The authors' advice that with careful consideration of age and severity of disease TKA; may improve the function of patients with Parkinson's disease by alleviating the pain, correcting flexion deformity and restoring movement.

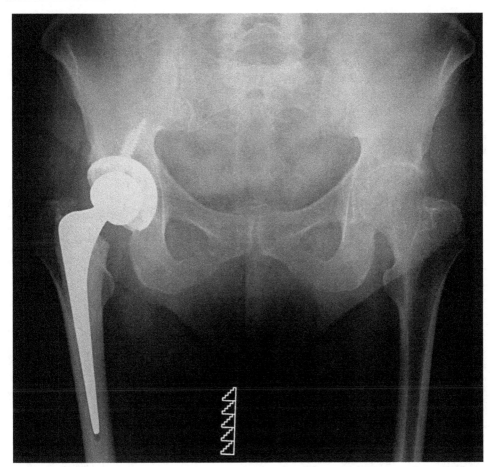

Fig. 2. Anteroposterior radiograph of the pelvis showing a right Hybrid (cemented stem/uncemented acetabular cup)THA and osteoarthritic left hip joint.

Duffy et al reported results from a retrospective review of 24 patients (33 knees) with Parkinson's disease who underwent TKA with patellar resurfacing(Duffy et al. 1996). All patients in this study continued levodopa/carbidopa up to the day of surgery and restarted it within 24 hours of surgery. Knee scores were assessed according to the Knee Society system at 2 months one year and mean follow up of 2.8 (2.2 - 6) years. Pain scores as determined by The Knee society scoring system, improved from a mean of 34 points before surgery to 89 points at the last follow up. On the other hand functional scores did not improve that much with 42 points pre – operatively to 68 points post operatively. Poor functional scores where reported due to progression of Parkinson's disease with increased imbalance, decreased muscle control, and increased rigidity(Duffy et al. 1996). In view of this the authors agree with Vince et al and recommend TKA in reliving the pain of arthritic knees in patient with Parkinson's disease(Vince et al. 1989; Duffy et al. 1996).

Two case reports have highlighted potential problems following TKR (Erceg et al. 2000; Shah et al. 2005). Erceg et al reported a case of recurrent dislocation with a posterior stabilized TKA in a patient with Parkinson's disease(Erceg et al. 2000). According to the authors, the recurrent posterior dislocation was mainly due to destruction of the cam of the polyethylene tibial insert caused by entrapped cement rather than progression of Parkinson's disease. Flexion contracture seems to be one of the most common complications after TKA in patients with Parkinson's disease (Oni et al. 1985; Duffy et al. 1996; Shah et al. 2005).

Shah et al describe a case which was effectively managed with a manipulation under anaesthesia and motor point blocks of the long head of the biceps femoris and semitendinosus with botulinum toxin type A(Shah et al. 2005). The authors recommend that motor block injection with Botulinum toxin type A may be a viable alternative to open hamstring release in treating flexion contractures in patients with Parkinson's disease(Shah et al. 2005). A summary of these papers is shown in Table. 3 (page 520).

	Study type	Arthroplasty (type + numbers)	Mean age (yrs, range)	Length of follow up (yrs)	Implant type/surgical technique	Outcome
Oni et al	case series	TKR(3)	76(72 - 83)	2	1 Stanmore , 2 Oxford meniscal TKA	Flexion contracture(3), quads rupture (2), death in 2 years(3)
Shah et al	case series	TKR(1)	61	6.5 months	N/A	Flexion contracture
Vince et al	retrospective	TKR(13)	70(64 - 75)	4.3(1-8)	Condylar type resurfacing arthroplasty, posterior stabilised TKA(10), Custom prosthetic (1), Total conylar I(1), total condoylar II(1), all cemented and all patella resurfaced	flexion contracture (5), patellar fracture 1, patellar subluxation(1), DVT(4), PE(2)
Erceg et al	case series	TKR(1)	65	1	PFC	Recurrent posterior tibial dislocation
Duffy et al	retrospective	TKR(33)	71	2.8(2.2 - 6)	cemented condylar TKA of a single design (press-fit condylar), Johnson & Johnson.	patellar subluxation (2), deep vein thrombosis (2), superficial infection (2), myositis ossificans (1), reoperation (4), patellar fracture (2), deep wound infection(2)

Table 3. Summary of the studies in patient with Parkinson's disease undergoing TKR.

Macauley et al have suggested a list of contraindications for total knee arthroplasty. These include any level of preoperative delirium, any contraindication to regional anaesthesia, re-operative fixed flexion deformity of greater than 25 degrees, a lack of a multidisciplinary team, and a Hoehn and Yahr rating greater than, or equal to, 3 (Table. 4. page 521)(Hoehn et al. 1967). They also propose that failure to respond to a diagnostic intra-articular infiltration of bupivacaine as a contraindication(Macaulay et al. 2010). Specific pre-operative planning should include appropriate implant selection. Cruciate retaining rather than cruciate substituting prostheses should be used. In severe disease constrained knees or hinged prostheses should be considered. The need for these considerations has been highlighted by the reports of dislocated prostheses (Macauley et al, 2010).

Femoral nerve blockade is contraindicated following knee arthroplasty – early quadriceps motor block could predispose to early development of a knee flexion deformity. Continuous Passive Motion (CPM) is not recommended as this can exacerbate the rigidity experienced.

3.3 Shoulder
3.3.1 Shoulder hemiarthroplasty for proximal humeral fractures
One report has assessed the outcomes of shoulder hemiarthroplasty for proximal humerus fractures (Kryzak et al. 2010). Their retrospective review of seven patients with a minimum of two years follow-up suggested that the surgical outcomes for patients with Parkinson's disease are poor. Mean achievable abduction was 97 degrees, external rotation 38 degrees and internal rotation to the level of the sacrum. Although there was one non-union and one mal-union no patient required revision surgery. On a scale of 1-5 the mean pain score remained as high as 2.5 and the authors concluded that the benefit of this surgical procedure in patients with Parkinson's disease is marginal. Consequently patients need to be counselled regarding the poor prognosis in surgery with anticipated persistent pain and restriction of movement.

Stage 1	Not disabling, mild, unilateral symptoms (e.g. tremor, posture, locomotion, and facial expression).
Stage 2	Bilateral involvement, without impairment of balance. Possibly already a light kyphotic posture, slowness and speech problems. Postural reflexes are still intact.
Stage 3	Significant slowing of body movements, moderate to severe symptoms, postural instability, walking is impaired, but still possible without help, physically independent in ADL
Stage 4	Severe symptoms, rigidity and bradykinesia, partly disabled, walking is impaired, but still possible without
Stage 5	Fully disabled, walking and standing impossible without help, continuous nursing care is necessary

Table 4. The Hoehn and Yahr scale for staging Parkinson's disease (Hoehn et al. 1967).

3.3.2 Total shoulder arthroplasty
There are two studies reviewing patients with Parkinson's disease that underwent a total shoulder arthroplasty (TSA)(Koch et al. 1997; Kryzak et al. 2009)(Table 5. Page 522).

The first study by Koch et al, reviewed 15 patients between 1979 and 1990 who underwent TSA in the Mayo clinic, Rochester(Koch et al. 1997). There were 16 TSA performed in 15 patients suffering from Parkinson's disease that were prospectively monitored as part of the total shoulder arthroplasty registry with average length of follow up of 5.3 years. Six of the patients in the study group were deceased at the most recent review and the average follow up was 2.1 years. The authors report that only 25% of the group achieved excellent results, 12.5% were rated satisfactory and 62.5% rated unsatisfactory. They also reported a significant reduction in external rotation after surgery. Three patients out of 15 required revision surgery, two for painful subluxation and one for glenoid loosening. The authors concluded that despite careful rehabilitation and medical management of Parkinson's disease, functional results are poor, particularly in patients older than 65 years of age.

Recently Kryzak et al have reported a series of 49 TSA performed in patients with Parkinson's disease for osteoarthritis of the shoulder(Kryzak et al. 2009). Mean age of patients at time of surgery was 69.7 years and 17 TSA were done in women while 32 were in men. Mean age of follow up was 8 years. Eight out of 49 shoulders were revised, three were revised in less than one year due to instability, four were revised due to loosening of the components and one due to periprosthetic fracture(Kryzak et al. 2009). The authors report a significant relief of pain with the average pain score decreasing from 4.6 pre-op to 1.8 post-op at last follow up. Overall they had 10 excellent (23%) results, 13 satisfactory (30%) results and 20 unsatisfactory (47%) results. The most common reason for unsatisfactory results were insufficient abduction, external rotation or a combination of both, instability requiring revision and continued pain.

	Study type	Arthroplasty (type + numbers)	Mean age (yrs, range)	Length of follow up (yrs)	Implant type/surgical technique	Outcome
Kryzak et al	retrospective	TSA (49)	69.7 (54 - 87)	8 years	31 Cofield (Smith and Nephew, Memphis, TN), 13Neer (Kirschner Medical, Fairlawn, NJ), 4 Tornier (Grenoble,France), and 1 Biomet humeral components (Warsaw, IN), 26 Cofield (Smith and Nephew), 18 Neer (KirschnerMedical), 4 Tornier (Grenoble, France), and 1 Biomet glenoidcomponents (Warsaw, IN)	16.3% of shoulders revised, 88% survival free of revision, 23% had excellent results, 30% satisfactory and 47% unsatisfactory
Koch et al	retrospective	TSA (16)	49 - 84 years	5.3 (1.2 - 15) years	standard deltopectoral approach was used, 12 cases used Neer (Kirschner Medical, Fairlawn, NJ), 4 cases treated with Cofield (Smith and Nephew, Memphis, TN)	40% of patient were dead at the most recent review, 25% rated as excellent, 12.5% rated as satisfactory and 62.5% rated as unsatisfactory results. 3 patients required revision 2 for subluxation and 1 for aseptic loosening

Table 5. Summary of the studies in patient with Parkinson's disease undergoing TKR.

4. Summary

Parkinson's disease affects a not inconsiderable proportion of the population and it is inevitable that the orthopaedic surgeon encounters these patients in practice. Arthroplasty of the hip, knee and shoulder are frequently used to alleviate pain from numerous arthropathies and hip and shoulder arthroplasty utilized in selected fracture patterns around the respective joints.

We have highlighted specific areas that require attention in the pre-, intra-, and post-operative management of patient with Parkinson's disease undergoing arthroplasty procedures. Although outcomes following elective arthroplasty procedures are promising, outcomes after shoulder hemiarthroplasty for trauma are less than encouraging.

Despite this, there is a distinct lack of evidence in the literature for many facets of care. We encourage physicians and surgeons alike to optimise the medical and surgical management of patients with Parkinson's disease to ensure best possible outcomes.

5. References

Adams, R. D., M. Victor and A. H. Ropper (1997). Principles of neurology. New York ; London, McGraw-Hill, Health Professions Division.

Allen, N. E., C. G. Canning, C. Sherrington, S. R. Lord, M. D. Latt, J. C. Close, S. D. O'Rourke, S. M. Murray and V. S. Fung (2010). "The effects of an exercise program on fall risk factors in people with Parkinson's disease: a randomized controlled trial." Mov Disord 25(9): 1217-1225.

Andersen, K. V., M. Bak, B. V. Christensen, J. Harazuk, N. A. Pedersen and K. Soballe (2010). "A randomized, controlled trial comparing local infiltration analgesia with epidural infusion for total knee arthroplasty." Acta Orthop 81(5): 606-610.

Andersen, K. V., M. Pfeiffer-Jensen, V. Haraldsted and K. Soballe (2007). "Reduced hospital stay and narcotic consumption, and improved mobilization with local and intraarticular infiltration after hip arthroplasty: a randomized clinical trial of an intraarticular technique versus epidural infusion in 80 patients." Acta Orthop 78(2): 180-186.

Andersen, L. J., T. Poulsen, B. Krogh and T. Nielsen (2007). "Postoperative analgesia in total hip arthroplasty: a randomized double-blinded, placebo-controlled study on peroperative and postoperative ropivacaine, ketorolac, and adrenaline wound infiltration." Acta Orthop 78(2): 187-192.

Anderson, B. J., P. V. Marks and M. E. Futter (1994). "Propofol--contrasting effects in movement disorders." Br J Neurosurg 8(3): 387-388.

Aspenberg, P. and T. Johansson (2010). "Teriparatide improves early callus formation in distal radial fractures." Acta Orthop 81(2): 234-236.

Backus, W. W., R. R. Ward, S. A. Vitkun, D. Fitzgerald and J. Askanazi (1991). "Postextubation laryngeal spasm in an unanesthetized patient with Parkinson's disease." J Clin Anesth 3(4): 314-316.

Berg, D., G. Becker and K. Reiners (1999). "Reduction of dyskinesia and induction of akinesia induced by morphine in two parkinsonian patients with severe sciatica." J Neural Transm 106(7-8): 725-728.

Bhave, A., M. G. Zywiel, S. D. Ulrich, M. S. McGrath, T. M. Seyler, D. R. Marker, R. E. Delanois and M. A. Mont (2009). "Botulinum toxin type A injections for the management of muscle tightness following total hip arthroplasty: a case series." J Orthop Surg Res 4: 34.

Brennan, K. A. and R. W. Genever (2010). "Managing Parkinson's disease during surgery." BMJ 341: c5718.

Burton, D. A., G. Nicholson and G. M. Hall (2004). "Anaesthesia in elderly patients with neurodegenerative disorders: special considerations." Drugs Aging 21(4): 229-242.

Busch, C. A., M. R. Whitehouse, B. J. Shore, S. J. MacDonald, R. W. McCalden and R. B. Bourne (2010). "The efficacy of periarticular multimodal drug infiltration in total hip arthroplasty." Clin Orthop Relat Res 468(8): 2152-2159.

Camicioli, R. and S. R. Majumdar (2010). "Relationship between mild cognitive impairment and falls in older people with and without Parkinson's disease: 1-Year Prospective Cohort Study." Gait Posture 32(1): 87-91.

Chudler, E. H. and W. K. Dong (1995). "The role of the basal ganglia in nociception and pain." Pain 60(1): 3-38.

Clouston, W. M. and H. M. Lloyd (1987). "Immobilization-induced hypercalcemia and regional osteoporosis." Clin Orthop Relat Res(216): 247-252.

Clubb, V. J., S. E. Clubb and S. Buckley (2006). "Parkinson's disease patients who fracture their neck of femur: a review of outcome data." Injury 37(10): 929-934.

Coughlin, L. and J. Templeton (1980). "Hip fractures in patients with Parkinson's disease." Clin Orthop Relat Res(148): 192-195.

Dereli, E. E. and A. Yaliman (2010). "Comparison of the effects of a physiotherapist-supervised exercise programme and a self-supervised exercise programme on quality of life in patients with Parkinson's disease." Clin Rehabil 24(4): 352-362.

Duffy, G. P. and R. T. Trousdale (1996). "Total knee arthroplasty in patients with parkinson's disease." J Arthroplasty 11(8): 899-904.

Easdown, L. J., M. J. Tessler and J. Minuk (1995). "Upper airway involvement in Parkinson's disease resulting in postoperative respiratory failure." Can J Anaesth 42(4): 344-347.

Ebersbach, G., A. Ebersbach, D. Edler, O. Kaufhold, M. Kusch, A. Kupsch and J. Wissel (2010). "Comparing exercise in Parkinson's disease--the Berlin LSVT(R)BIG study." Mov Disord 25(12): 1902-1908.

Erceg, M. and A. Maricevic (2000). "Recurrent posterior dislocation following primary posterior-stabilized total knee arthroplasty." Croat Med J 41(2): 207-209.

Eventov, I., M. Moreno, E. Geller, R. Tardiman and R. Salama (1983). "Hip fractures in patients with Parkinson's syndrome." J Trauma 23(2): 98-101.

Fink, H. A., M. A. Kuskowski, E. S. Orwoll, J. A. Cauley and K. E. Ensrud (2005). "Association between Parkinson's disease and low bone density and falls in older men: the osteoporotic fractures in men study." J Am Geriatr Soc 53(9): 1559-1564.

Formisano, R., L. Pratesi, F. T. Modarelli, V. Bonifati and G. Meco (1992). "Rehabilitation and Parkinson's disease." Scand J Rehabil Med 24(3): 157-160.

Friedl, G., R. Radl, C. Stihsen, P. Rehak, R. Aigner and R. Windhager (2009). "The effect of a single infusion of zoledronic acid on early implant migration in total hip arthroplasty. A randomized, double-blind, controlled trial." J Bone Joint Surg Am 91(2): 274-281.

Gobbi, L. T., M. D. Oliveira-Ferreira, M. J. Caetano, E. Lirani-Silva, F. A. Barbieri, F. Stella and S. Gobbi (2009). "Exercise programs improve mobility and balance in people with Parkinson's disease." Parkinsonism Relat Disord 15 Suppl 3: S49-52.

Gross, T. S. and C. T. Rubin (1995). "Uniformity of resorptive bone loss induced by disuse." J Orthop Res 13(5): 708-714.

Hansson, U., S. Toksvig-Larsen, L. Ryd and P. Aspenberg (2009). "Once-weekly oral medication with alendronate does not prevent migration of knee prostheses: A double-blind randomized RSA study." Acta Orthop 80(1): 41-45.

Hernigou, P., G. Mathieu, P. Filippini and A. Demoura (2006). "[Intra- and postoperative fractures of the femur in total knee arthroplasty: risk factors in 32 cases]." Rev Chir Orthop Reparatrice Appar Mot 92(2): 140-147.

Hilding, M., L. Ryd, S. Toksvig-Larsen and P. Aspenberg (2000). "Clodronate prevents prosthetic migration: a randomized radiostereometric study of 50 total knee patients." Acta Orthop Scand 71(6): 553-557.

Hirsch, M. A., T. Toole, C. G. Maitland and R. A. Rider (2003). "The effects of balance training and high-intensity resistance training on persons with idiopathic Parkinson's disease." Arch Phys Med Rehabil 84(8): 1109-1117.

Hoehn, M. M. and M. D. Yahr (1967). "Parkinsonism: onset, progression and mortality." Neurology 17(5): 427-442.

Hughes, A. J., S. E. Daniel, S. Blankson and A. J. Lees (1993). "A clinicopathologic study of 100 cases of Parkinson's disease." Arch Neurol 50(2): 140-148.

Hurwitz, A. (1989). "The benefit of a home exercise regimen for ambulatory Parkinson's disease patients." J Neurosci Nurs 21(3): 180-184.

Huse, D. M., K. Schulman, L. Orsini, J. Castelli-Haley, S. Kennedy and G. Lenhart (2005). "Burden of illness in Parkinson's disease." Mov Disord 20(11): 1449-1454.

Husted, H., H. C. Hansen, G. Holm, C. Bach-Dal, K. Rud, K. L. Andersen and H. Kehlet (2010). "What determines length of stay after total hip and knee arthroplasty? A nationwide study in Denmark." Arch Orthop Trauma Surg 130(2): 263-268.

Inoue, D. (2010). "[Musculoskeletal rehabilitation and bone. Mechanical stress on the skeletal system]." Clin Calcium 20(4): 503-511.

Jaggers, J. R., C. D. Simpson, K. L. Frost, P. M. Quesada, R. V. Topp, A. M. Swank and J. A. Nyland (2007). "Prehabilitation before knee arthroplasty increases postsurgical function: a case study." J Strength Cond Res 21(2): 632-634.

Kao, C. H., C. C. Chen, S. J. Wang, L. G. Chia and S. H. Yeh (1994). "Bone mineral density in patients with Parkinson's disease measured by dual photon absorptiometry." Nucl Med Commun 15(3): 173-177.

Keus, S. H., B. R. Bloem, E. J. Hendriks, A. B. Bredero-Cohen and M. Munneke (2007). "Evidence-based analysis of physical therapy in Parkinson's disease with recommendations for practice and research." Mov Disord 22(4): 451-460; quiz 600.

Klausner, J. M., J. Caspi, S. Lelcuk, A. Khazam, G. Marin, H. B. Hechtman and R. R. Rozin (1988). "Delayed muscular rigidity and respiratory depression following fentanyl anesthesia." Arch Surg 123(1): 66-67.

Koch, L. D., R. H. Cofield and J. E. Ahlskog (1997). "Total shoulder arthroplasty in patients with Parkinson's disease." J Shoulder Elbow Surg 6(1): 24-28.

Krauss, J. K., E. W. Akeyson, P. Giam and J. Jankovic (1996). "Propofol-induced dyskinesias in Parkinson's disease." Anesth Analg 83(2): 420-422.

Kryzak, T. J., J. W. Sperling, C. D. Schleck and R. H. Cofield (2009). "Total shoulder arthroplasty in patients with Parkinson's disease." J Shoulder Elbow Surg 18(1): 96-99.

Kryzak, T. J., J. W. Sperling, C. D. Schleck and R. H. Cofield (2010). "Hemiarthroplasty for proximal humerus fractures in patients with Parkinson's disease." Clin Orthop Relat Res 468(7): 1817-1821.

Ma, Y. L., F. Marin, J. Stepan, S. Ish-Shalom, R. Moricke, F. Hawkins, et al. (2011). "Comparative effects of teriparatide and strontium ranelate in the periosteum of iliac crest biopsies in postmenopausal women with osteoporosis." Bone.

Macaulay, W., J. A. Geller, A. R. Brown, L. J. Cote and H. A. Kiernan (2010). "Total knee arthroplasty and Parkinson disease: enhancing outcomes and avoiding complications." J Am Acad Orthop Surg 18(11): 687-694.

Mason, L. J., T. T. Cojocaru and D. J. Cole (1996). "Surgical intervention and anesthetic management of the patient with Parkinson's disease." Int Anesthesiol Clin 34(4): 133-150.

Meek, R. M., D. B. Allan, G. McPhillips, L. Kerr and C. R. Howie (2006). "Epidemiology of dislocation after total hip arthroplasty." Clin Orthop Relat Res 447: 9-18.

Melton, L. J., 3rd, C. L. Leibson, S. J. Achenbach, J. H. Bower, D. M. Maraganore, A. L. Oberg and W. A. Rocca (2006). "Fracture risk after the diagnosis of Parkinson's disease: Influence of concomitant dementia." Mov Disord 21(9): 1361-1367.

Mets, B. (1991). "Acute dystonia after alfentanil in untreated Parkinson's disease." Anesth Analg 72(4): 557-558.

Moricke, R., K. Rettig and T. D. Bethke (2011). "Use of Recombinant Human Parathyroid Hormone(1-84) in Patients with Postmenopausal Osteoporosis: A Prospective, Open-Label, Single-Arm, Multicentre, Observational Cohort Study of the Effects of Treatment on Quality of Life and Pain - the PROPOSE Study." Clin Drug Investig 31(2): 87-99.

Mueller, M. C., U. Juptner, U. Wuellner, S. Wirz, A. Turler, A. Hirner and J. Standop (2009). "Parkinson's disease influences the perioperative risk profile in surgery." Langenbecks Arch Surg 394(3): 511-515.

Muzzi, D. A., S. Black and R. F. Cucchiara (1989). "The lack of effect of succinylcholine on serum potassium in patients with Parkinson's disease." Anesthesiology 71(2): 322.

Neu, H. C., J. J. Connolly, Jr., F. W. Schwertley, H. A. Ladwig and A. W. Brody (1967). "Obstructive respiratory dysfunction in parkinsonian patients." Am Rev Respir Dis 95(1): 33-47.

Nicholson, G., A. C. Pereira and G. M. Hall (2002). "Parkinson's disease and anaesthesia." Br J Anaesth 89(6): 904-916.

Nocera, J. R., T. Buckley, D. Waddell, M. S. Okun and C. J. Hass (2010). "Knee extensor strength, dynamic stability, and functional ambulation: are they related in Parkinson's disease?" Arch Phys Med Rehabil 91(4): 589-595.

O'Hara, D. A., G. Fanciullo, L. Hubbard, T. Maneatis, P. Seuffert, L. Bynum and A. Shefrin (1997). "Evaluation of the safety and efficacy of ketorolac versus morphine by patient-controlled analgesia for postoperative pain." Pharmacotherapy 17(5): 891-899.

Oni, O. O. and R. P. Mackenney (1985). "Total knee replacement in patients with Parkinson's disease." J Bone Joint Surg Br 67(3): 424-425.

Parvataneni, H. K., V. P. Shah, H. Howard, N. Cole, A. S. Ranawat and C. S. Ranawat (2007). "Controlling pain after total hip and knee arthroplasty using a multimodal protocol with local periarticular injections: a prospective randomized study." J Arthroplasty 22(6 Suppl 2): 33-38.

Pepper, P. V. and M. K. Goldstein (1999). "Postoperative complications in Parkinson's disease." J Am Geriatr Soc 47(8): 967-972.

Post, Z. D., C. Restrepo, L. K. Kahl, T. van de Leur, J. J. Purtill and W. J. Hozack (2010). "A prospective evaluation of 2 different pain management protocols for total hip arthroplasty." J Arthroplasty 25(3): 410-415.

Queally, J. M., A. Abdulkarim and K. J. Mulhall (2009). "Total hip replacement in patients with neurological conditions." J Bone Joint Surg Br 91(10): 1267-1273.

Rajput, A. H., K. P. Offord, C. M. Beard and L. T. Kurland (1984). "Epidemiology of parkinsonism: incidence, classification, and mortality." Ann Neurol 16(3): 278-282.

Reed, A. P. and D. G. Han (1992). "Intraoperative exacerbation of Parkinson's disease." Anesth Analg 75(5): 850-853.

Rothermel, J. E. and A. Garcia (1972). "Treatment of hip fractures in patients with Parkinson's syndrome on levodopa therapy." J Bone Joint Surg Am 54(6): 1251-1254.

Sato, Y., Y. Honda and J. Iwamoto (2007). "Risedronate and ergocalciferol prevent hip fracture in elderly men with Parkinson disease." Neurology 68(12): 911-915.

Sato, Y., Y. Honda, J. Iwamoto, T. Kanoko and K. Satoh (2005). "Abnormal bone and calcium metabolism in immobilized Parkinson's disease patients." Mov Disord 20(12): 1598-1603.

Sato, Y., M. Kikuyama and K. Oizumi (1997). "High prevalence of vitamin D deficiency and reduced bone mass in Parkinson's disease." Neurology 49(5): 1273-1278.

Schenkman, M., T. M. Cutson, M. Kuchibhatla, J. Chandler, C. F. Pieper, L. Ray and K. C. Laub (1998). "Exercise to improve spinal flexibility and function for people with Parkinson's disease: a randomized, controlled trial." J Am Geriatr Soc 46(10): 1207-1216.

Shah, S. N., J. Hornyak and A. G. Urquhart (2005). "Flexion contracture after total knee arthroplasty in a patient with Parkinson's disease: successful treatment with botulinum toxin type A." J Arthroplasty 20(8): 1078-1080.

Staeheli, J. W., F. J. Frassica and F. H. Sim (1988). "Prosthetic replacement of the femoral head for fracture of the femoral neck in patients who have Parkinson disease." J Bone Joint Surg Am 70(4): 565-568.

Stein, C., M. J. Millan, T. S. Shippenberg, K. Peter and A. Herz (1989). "Peripheral opioid receptors mediating antinociception in inflammation. Evidence for involvement of mu, delta and kappa receptors." J Pharmacol Exp Ther 248(3): 1269-1275.

Swank, A. M., J. B. Kachelman, W. Bibeau, P. M. Quesada, J. Nyland, A. Malkani and R. V. Topp (2011). "Prehabilitation before total knee arthroplasty increases strength and function in older adults with severe osteoarthritis." J Strength Cond Res 25(2): 318-325.

Tanaka, N., H. Sakahashi, E. Sato, K. Hirose and S. Ishii (2001). "The efficacy of intra-articular analgesia after total knee arthroplasty in patients with rheumatoid arthritis and in patients with osteoarthritis." J Arthroplasty 16(3): 306-311.

Taylor, B. C., P. J. Schreiner, K. L. Stone, H. A. Fink, S. R. Cummings, M. C. Nevitt, P. J. Bowman and K. E. Ensrud (2004). "Long-term prediction of incident hip fracture risk in elderly white women: study of osteoporotic fractures." J Am Geriatr Soc 52(9): 1479-1486.

Thomsen, M. N., E. Jakubowitz, J. B. Seeger, C. Lee, J. P. Kretzer and M. Clarius (2008). "Fracture load for periprosthetic femoral fractures in cemented versus uncemented hip stems: an experimental in vitro study." Orthopedics 31(7): 653.

Toftdahl, K., L. Nikolajsen, V. Haraldsted, F. Madsen, E. K. Tonnesen and K. Soballe (2007). "Comparison of peri- and intraarticular analgesia with femoral nerve block after total knee arthroplasty: a randomized clinical trial." Acta Orthop 78(2): 172-179.

Toole, T., M. A. Hirsch, A. Forkink, D. A. Lehman and C. G. Maitland (2000). "The effects of a balance and strength training program on equilibrium in Parkinsonism: A preliminary study." NeuroRehabilitation 14(3): 165-174.

Topp, R., A. M. Swank, P. M. Quesada, J. Nyland and A. Malkani (2009). "The effect of prehabilitation exercise on strength and functioning after total knee arthroplasty." PM R 1(8): 729-735.

Turcotte, R., C. Godin, R. Duchesne and A. Jodoin (1990). "Hip fractures and Parkinson's disease. A clinical review of 94 fractures treated surgically." Clin Orthop Relat Res(256): 132-136.

Ueda, M., M. Hamamoto, H. Nagayama, K. Otsubo, C. Nito, T. Miyazaki, A. Terashi and Y. Katayama (1999). "Susceptibility to neuroleptic malignant syndrome in Parkinson's disease." Neurology 52(4): 777-781.

Vendittoli, P. A., P. Makinen, P. Drolet, M. Lavigne, M. Fallaha, M. C. Guertin and F. Varin (2006). "A multimodal analgesia protocol for total knee arthroplasty. A randomized, controlled study." J Bone Joint Surg Am 88(2): 282-289.

Vince, K. G., J. N. Insall and C. E. Bannerman (1989). "Total knee arthroplasty in the patient with Parkinson's disease." J Bone Joint Surg Br 71(1): 51-54.

Vincken, W. G., S. G. Gauthier, R. E. Dollfuss, R. E. Hanson, C. M. Darauay and M. G. Cosio (1984). "Involvement of upper-airway muscles in extrapyramidal disorders. A cause of airflow limitation." N Engl J Med 311(7): 438-442.

Weber, M., M. E. Cabanela, F. H. Sim, F. J. Frassica and W. S. Harmsen (2002). "Total hip replacement in patients with Parkinson's disease." Int Orthop 26(2): 66-68.

Wilkinson, J. M., A. C. Eagleton, I. Stockley, N. F. Peel, A. J. Hamer and R. Eastell (2005). "Effect of pamidronate on bone turnover and implant migration after total hip arthroplasty: a randomized trial." J Orthop Res 23(1): 1-8.

Wright, J. J., P. D. Goodnight and M. D. McEvoy (2009). "The utility of ketamine for the preoperative management of a patient with Parkinson's disease." Anesth Analg 108(3): 980-982.

Yates, A. J., T. H. Jones, K. I. Mundy, R. V. Hague, C. B. Brown, D. Guilland-Cumming and J. A. Kanis (1984). "Immobilisation hypercalcaemia in adults and treatment with clodronate." Br Med J (Clin Res Ed) 289(6452): 1111-1112.

Permissions

The contributors of this book come from diverse backgrounds, making this book a truly international effort. This book will bring forth new frontiers with its revolutionizing research information and detailed analysis of the nascent developments around the world.

We would like to thank Dr. Juliana Dushanova, for lending her expertise to make the book truly unique. She has played a crucial role in the development of this book. Without her invaluable contribution this book wouldn't have been possible. She has made vital efforts to compile up to date information on the varied aspects of this subject to make this book a valuable addition to the collection of many professionals and students.

This book was conceptualized with the vision of imparting up-to-date information and advanced data in this field. To ensure the same, a matchless editorial board was set up. Every individual on the board went through rigorous rounds of assessment to prove their worth. After which they invested a large part of their time researching and compiling the most relevant data for our readers. Conferences and sessions were held from time to time between the editorial board and the contributing authors to present the data in the most comprehensible form. The editorial team has worked tirelessly to provide valuable and valid information to help people across the globe.

Every chapter published in this book has been scrutinized by our experts. Their significance has been extensively debated. The topics covered herein carry significant findings which will fuel the growth of the discipline. They may even be implemented as practical applications or may be referred to as a beginning point for another development. Chapters in this book were first published by InTech; hereby published with permission under the Creative Commons Attribution License or equivalent.

The editorial board has been involved in producing this book since its inception. They have spent rigorous hours researching and exploring the diverse topics which have resulted in the successful publishing of this book. They have passed on their knowledge of decades through this book. To expedite this challenging task, the publisher supported the team at every step. A small team of assistant editors was also appointed to further simplify the editing procedure and attain best results for the readers.

Our editorial team has been hand-picked from every corner of the world. Their multi-ethnicity adds dynamic inputs to the discussions which result in innovative outcomes. These outcomes are then further discussed with the researchers and contributors who give their valuable feedback and opinion regarding the same. The feedback is then collaborated with the researches and they are edited in a comprehensive manner to aid the understanding of the subject.

Apart from the editorial board, the designing team has also invested a significant amount of their time in understanding the subject and creating the most relevant covers. They scrutinized every image to scout for the most suitable representation of the subject and create an appropriate cover for the book.

The publishing team has been involved in this book since its early stages. They were actively engaged in every process, be it collecting the data, connecting with the contributors or procuring relevant information. The team has been an ardent support to the editorial, designing and production team. Their endless efforts to recruit the best for this project, has resulted in the accomplishment of this book. They are a veteran in the field of academics and their pool of knowledge is as vast as their experience in printing. Their expertise and guidance has proved useful at every step. Their uncompromising quality standards have made this book an exceptional effort. Their encouragement from time to time has been an inspiration for everyone.

The publisher and the editorial board hope that this book will prove to be a valuable piece of knowledge for researchers, students, practitioners and scholars across the globe.

List of Contributors

Jessica Davies, Hoe Lee and Torbjorn Falkmer
School of Occupational Therapy and Social Work, Curtin Health Innovation Research Institute, Curtin University, Australia

Torbjorn Falkmer
School of Health Sciences, Jönköping University, Jönköping, Sweden
Department of Rehabilitation Medicine, IKE, Faculty of Health Sciences Linköping University, Sweden
School of Occupational Therapy, La Trobe University, Melbourne, VIC, Australia

I. Reuter and S. Mehnert
Dept. of Neurology, Justus-Liebig University, Giessen, Germany

M. Oechsner
Neurologisches Rehabilitationszentrum, HELIOS Klinik Zihlschlacht AG, Swiss

M. Engelhardt
Dept. of Orthopedic Surgery, Klinikum Osnabrück, Germany

Laura Pastor-Sanz, Mario Pansera, Jorge Cancela, Matteo Pastorino and María Teresa Arredondo Waldmeyer
Life Supporting Technologies, Universidad Politécnica de Madrid, Spain

L.T.B. Gobbi, F.A. Barbieri, R. Vitório, M.P. Pereira, C. Teixeira-Arroyo, A.P.T. Alves, R.A. Batistela, P.M. Formaggio, E. Lirani-Silva, L.C. Morais, P.H.S. Pelicioni, V. Raile, N.M. Rinaldi, P.C.R. Santos, C.B. Takaki, F. Stella and S. Gobbi
UNESP – Univ Estadual Paulista, Rio Claro, SP, Brazil

Gilles Orgeret
Regional Hospital, Poissy/Saint Germain en Laye, France

Lilian Beijer and Toni Rietveld
Sint Maartenskliniek Nijmegen, Section Research, Development & Education, The Netherlands

Toni Rietveld
Radboud University Nijmegen, Faculty of Arts, Department of Linguistics, The Netherlands

Jesús Seco Calvo and Inés Gago Fernández
University of León, Spain

Yoshiyuki Takahashi
Toyo University, Japan

Osamu Nitta
Tokyo Metropolitan University, Japan

Takashi Komeda
Shibaura Institute of Technology, Japan

Joao Costa, Francesc Valldeoriola and Josep Valls-Sole
Institute of Molecular Medicine, Lisbon Faculty of Medicine, Portugal

Joao Costa, Francesc Valldeoriola and Josep Valls-Sole
Neurology Department, Hospital Clínic, Centro de Investigación Biomédica en Red sobre Enfermedades Neurodegenerativas (CIBERNED) and Institut d'Investigacio Biomedica August Pi i Sunyer (IDIBAPS), Facultad de Medicina, Universitat de Barcelona, Spain

Naoki Tani and Youichi Saitoh
Department of Neurosurgery, Osaka University Graduate School of Medicine, Japan

Youichi Saitoh
Department of Neuromodulation and Neurosurgery, Osaka University, Japan

Sun Ha Paek
Movement Disorder Center, Department of Neurosurgery, Seoul National University Hospital, Seoul National University College of Medicine, South Korea

Adrian J. Cassar Gheiti, Joseph F. Baker and Kevin J. Mulhall
Orthopaedic Research and Innovation Foundation, Republic of Ireland

Printed in the USA
CPSIA information can be obtained
at www.ICGtesting.com
JSHW011454221024
72173JS00005B/1066